# Arrhythmias in Cardiomyopathies

*Editors*

MOHAMMAD SHENASA
MARK S. LINK
MARTIN S. MARON

# CARDIAC ELECTROPHYSIOLOGY CLINICS

www.cardiacEP.theclinics.com

*Consulting Editors*
RANJAN K. THAKUR
ANDREA NATALE

June 2015 • Volume 7 • Number 2

**ELSEVIER**

1600 John F. Kennedy Boulevard • Suite 1800 • Philadelphia, Pennsylvania, 19103-2899

http://www.theclinics.com

**CARDIAC ELECTROPHYSIOLOGY CLINICS Volume 7, Number 2**
**June 2015 ISSN 1877-9182, ISBN-13: 978-0-323-38878-8**

Editor: Adrianne Brigido
Developmental Editor: Barbara Cohen-Kligerman

*Cardiac Electrophysiology Clinics* (ISSN 1877-9182) is published quarterly by Elsevier Inc., 360 Park Avenue South, New York, NY 10010-1710. Months of issue are March, June, September, and December. Subscription prices are $200.00 per year for US individuals, $293.00 per year for US institutions, $105.00 per year for US students and residents, $225.00 per year for Canadian individuals, $331.00 per year for Canadian institutions, $285.00 per year for international individuals, $354.00 per year for international institutions and $150.00 per year for Canadian and international students/residents. To receive student/resident rate, orders must be accompanied by name of affiliated institution, date of term, and the signature of program/residency coordinator on institution letterhead. Orders will be billed at individual rate until proof of status is received. Foreign air speed delivery is included in all Clinics subscription prices. All prices are subject to change without notice. **POSTMASTER:** Send address changes to Cardiac Electrophysiology Clinics, Elsevier Health Sciences Division, Subscription Customer Service, 3251 Riverport Lane, Maryland Heights, MO 63043. **Customer Service: 1-800-654-2452 (US and Canada). From outside of the US and Canada, call 314-477-8871. Fax: 314-447-8029.** E-mail: JournalsCustomerService-usa@elsevier.com **(for print support);** JournalsOnlineSupport-usa@elsevier.com **(for online support).**

*Reprints.* For copies of 100 or more of articles in this publication, please contact the Commercial Reprints Department, Elsevier Inc., 360 Park Avenue South, New York, NY 10010-1710. Tel.: 212-633-3874; Fax: 212-633-3820; E-mail: reprints@elsevier.com.

*Cardiac Electrophysiology Clinics* is covered in *MEDLINE/PubMed (Index Medicus).*

# Contributors

## CONSULTING EDITORS

**RANJAN K. THAKUR, MD, MPH, MBA, FACC, FHRS**
Professor of Medicine and Director, Arrhythmia Service, Thoracic and Cardiovascular Institute, Sparrow Health System, Michigan State University, Lansing, Michigan

**ANDREA NATALE, MD, FACC, FHRS**
Executive Medical Director, Texas Cardiac Arrhythmia Institute, St. David's Medical Center, Austin, Texas; Consulting Professor, Division of Cardiology, Stanford University, Palo Alto, California; Adjunct Professor of Medicine, Heart and Vascular Center, Case Western Reserve University, Cleveland, Ohio; Director, Interventional Electrophysiology, Scripps Clinic, San Diego, California; Senior Clinical Director, EP Services, California Pacific Medical Center, San Francisco, California

## EDITORS

**MOHAMMAD SHENASA, MD**
Department of Cardiovascular Services, O'Connor Hospital, Heart and Rhythm Medical Group, San Jose, California

**MARTIN S. MARON, MD**
Division of Cardiology, Hypertrophic Cardiomyopathy Center, Tufts Medical Center, Boston, Massachusetts

**MARK S. LINK, MD**
Division of Cardiology, Hypertrophic Cardiomyopathy Center, Tufts Medical Center, Boston, Massachusetts

## AUTHORS

**DEEPAK ACHARYA, MD**
Assistant Professor of Medicine; Section of Advanced Heart Failure and Transplant Cardiology, Division of Cardiovascular Diseases, University of Alabama at Birmingham, Birmingham, Alabama

**SASIKANTH ADIGOPULA, MD**
Division of Cardiology, Department of Medicine, David Geffen School of Medicine, University of California, Los Angeles, Los Angeles, California

**SHONE O. ALMEIDA, MD**
Division of Cardiology, Department of Medicine, David Geffen School of Medicine, University of California, Los Angeles, Los Angeles, California

**REZA ARDEHALI, MD, PhD**
Division of Cardiology, Department of Medicine, David Geffen School of Medicine; Eli and Edyth Broad Stem Cell Research Center, University of California, Los Angeles, Los Angeles, California

**A. JOHN BAKSI, PhD, MRCP**
Cardiovascular Biomedical Research Unit, Royal Brompton Hospital & Harefield NHS Foundation Trust and Imperial College London; Cardiovascular Magnetic Resonance Unit, Royal Brompton Hospital, London, United Kingdom

**KATHLEEN HAYES BROWN, MD**
Clinical Cardiac Electrophysiology Service,
Division of Cardiology, Department of
Medicine, Rush University Medical Center,
Chicago, Illinois

**HUGH CALKINS, MD**
Division of Cardiology, Department of
Medicine, Johns Hopkins University School of
Medicine, Baltimore, Maryland

**ANDRE D'AVILA, MD, PhD**
Cardiac Arrhythmia Service, Hospital
Cardiologico, Florianopolis, Santa Catarina,
Brazil

**HARISH DOPPALAPUDI, MD**
Associate Professor of Medicine; Section of
Electrophysiology, Division of Cardiovascular
Diseases, University of Alabama at
Birmingham, Birmingham, Alabama

**NABIL EL-SHERIF, MD**
Professor of Medicine and Physiology, State
University of New York, Downstate Medical
Center; Chief, Cardiology Division, New York
Harbor VA Healthcare System, Brooklyn,
New York

**MICHAEL G. FRADLEY, MD**
Assistant Professor of Medicine; Director,
Cardio-Oncology Program, Division of
Cardiovascular Medicine, Morsani College of
Medicine, University of South Florida, Tampa,
Florida

**MICHAEL M. GIVERTZ, MD**
Medical Director, Heart Transplant and
Mechanical Circulatory Support, Brigham and
Women's Hospital; Associate Professor of
Medicine, Harvard Medical School, Boston,
Massachusetts

**WILLIAM J. GROH, MD, MPH**
Chief of Medicine, William Jennings Bryan
Dorn Veterans Affairs Medical Center;
Professor of Clinical Medicine, University
of South Carolina, Columbia, South Carolina

**CHRIS HEALY, MD**
Electrophysiology Fellow, Department of
Cardiac Electrophysiology, University of
Miami Miller School of Medicine, Miami,
Florida

**MICHAEL C. HONIGBERG, MD, MPP**
Clinical Fellow, Department of Medicine,
Brigham and Women's Hospital, Harvard
Medical School, Boston, Massachusetts

**ROY M. JOHN, MD, PhD**
Assistant Professor, Department of Medicine,
Brigham and Women's Hospital, Harvard
Medical School, Boston, Massachusetts

**G. SUNTHAR KANAGANAYAGAM, PhD,
MRCP**
Cardiovascular Biomedical Research Unit,
Royal Brompton Hospital & Harefield NHS
Foundation Trust and Imperial College London;
Cardiovascular Magnetic Resonance Unit,
Royal Brompton Hospital, London,
United Kingdom

**JEFFREY J. KIM, MD**
Associate Professor, Section of Pediatric
Cardiology, Department of Pediatrics, Baylor
College of Medicine, Texas Children's
Hospital, Houston, Texas

**KARTIK R. KUMAR, MBBS**
Department of Cardiology, Tufts Medical
Center, Boston, Massachusetts

**SAURABH KUMAR, BSc (Med), MBBS**
Department of Medicine, Brigham and
Women's Hospital, Harvard Medical School,
Boston, Massachusetts

**MARK S. LINK, MD**
Division of Cardiology, Hypertrophic
Cardiomyopathy Center, Tufts Medical Center,
Boston, Massachusetts

**CHRISTOPHER MADIAS, MD**
Clinical Cardiac Electrophysiology Service,
Division of Cardiology, Department of
Medicine, Rush University Medical Center,
Chicago, Illinois

**SWATI N. MANDLEYWALA, MBBS**
Department of Cardiology, Tufts Medical
Center, Boston, Massachusetts

**BARRY J. MARON, MD**
Director, Hypertrophic Cardiomyopathy
Center, Minneapolis Heart Institute
Foundation, Minneapolis, Minnesota;
Professor of Medicine, Mayo Clinic and
Tufts School of Medicine, Boston,
Massachusetts

**MARTIN S. MARON, MD**
Division of Cardiology, Hypertrophic
Cardiomyopathy Center, Tufts Medical Center,
Boston, Massachusetts

**CHRISTINA Y. MIYAKE, MD, MS**
Assistant Professor, Section of Pediatric
Cardiology, Department of Pediatrics, Baylor
College of Medicine, Texas Children's
Hospital, Houston, Texas

**DAVID MONTAIGNE, MD, PhD**
Lille University, Inserm U1011, European
Genomic Institute for Diabetes; Institut Pasteur
de Lille; Cardiovascular Explorations
Department, University Hospital of Lille, Lille,
France

**JAVID MOSLEHI, MD**
Assistant Professor of Medicine, Division of
Cardiovascular Medicine; Division of
Hematology-Oncology, Department of
Medicine, Vanderbilt-Ingram Cancer Center;
Director, Cardio-Oncology Program,
Vanderbilt University School of Medicine,
Nashville, Tennessee

**ANJU DUVA PENTIAH, MD**
Cardiovascular Explorations Department;
Division of Cardiomyopathy, Department of
Cardiology, University Hospital of Lille, Lille,
France

**SANJAY K. PRASAD, MD, FRCP, FESC**
Cardiovascular Biomedical Research Unit,
Royal Brompton Hospital & Harefield NHS
Foundation Trust and Imperial College London;
Cardiovascular Magnetic Resonance Unit,
Royal Brompton Hospital, London,
United Kingdom

**ARCHANA RAJDEV, MD**
Cardiac Electrophysiology Fellow, Krannert
Institute of Cardiology, Indiana University
School of Medicine, Indianapolis, Indiana

**JUAN D. RAMÍREZ, MD**
Electrophysiology Fellow, International
Arrhythmia Center, Cardioinfantil
Foundation-Cardiac Institute, Bogotá,
Colombia

**LUIS C. SÁENZ, MD**
Director, International Arrhythmia Center;
Section Head of Cardiac Pacing and
Electrophysiology, Department of

Cardiovascular Medicine, Cardioinfantil
Foundation-Cardiac Institute, Bogotá, Colombia

**WILLIAM H. SAUER, MD**
Associate Professor, Section of Cardiac
Electrophysiology, Division of Cardiology,
University of Colorado, Denver, Colorado

**ABHISHEK C. SAWANT, MD**
Division of Cardiology, Department of
Medicine, Johns Hopkins University School of
Medicine, Baltimore, Maryland

**HOSSEIN SHENASA, MD**
Department of Cardiovascular Services,
O'Connor Hospital; Heart and Rhythm Medical
Group, San Jose, California

**MOHAMMAD SHENASA, MD**
Department of Cardiovascular Services,
O'Connor Hospital, Heart and Rhythm Medical
Group, San Jose, California

**RHYS J. SKELTON, BS(Hons)**
Division of Cardiology, Department of
Medicine, David Geffen School of
Medicine, University of California, Los
Angeles, Los Angeles, California; Murdoch
Children's Research Institute, The Royal
Children's Hospital, Parkville, Victoria,
Australia

**MARIANA SOTO, MD**
Epidemiologist and Medical Researcher,
International Arrhythmia Center, Cardioinfantil
Foundation-Cardiac Institute, Bogotá,
Colombia

**WILLIAM G. STEVENSON, MD**
Professor, Department of Medicine, Brigham
and Women's Hospital, Harvard Medical
School, Boston, Massachusetts

**JOSÉ A. TALLAJ, MD**
Associate Professor of Medicine, Section of
Advanced Heart Failure and Transplant
Cardiology, Division of Cardiovascular
Diseases, University of Alabama at
Birmingham, Birmingham, Alabama

**RICHARD G. TROHMAN, MD, MBA**
Clinical Cardiac Electrophysiology Service,
Division of Cardiology, Department of
Medicine, Rush University Medical Center,
Chicago, Illinois

**JUAN F. VILES-GONZALEZ, MD**
Assistant Professor, Department of Cardiac
Electrophysiology, University of Miami Miller
School of Medicine, Miami, Florida

**MATTHEW M. ZIPSE, MD**
Electrophysiology Fellow, Section of Cardiac
Electrophysiology, Division of Cardiology,
University of Colorado, Denver, Colorado

# Contents

The implantable cardioverter–defibrillator (ICD) was not originally envisioned as a treatment to prevent sudden death (SD) in young people with genetic heart diseases. In the case of hypertrophic cardiomyopathy (HCM), initially it was not known whether the ICD would be effective in patients with a disease very different morphologically and functionally from coronary artery disease. Nevertheless, several observational clinical studies have shown that the ICD reliably terminates life-threatening ventricular tachyarrhythmias in HCM, and is largely responsible for reducing HCM mortality to 0.5% per year, by preventing SD and changing the natural course of the disease.

Hypertrophic cardiomyopathy (HCM) is an autosomal dominant disease caused by mutations in genes coding for cardiac sarcomeres. HCM is the most common inherited heart disease, with a prevalence of 0.2%. There are multiple genetic variants that cause pleomorphic clinical attributes and disease characterized by myocardial disarray and myocardial hypertrophy. Patients are at an increased risk of atrial and ventricular arrhythmias. Management of these arrhythmias is complex. Atrial fibrillation is associated with increased mortality and thromboembolism. Ventricular arrhythmias are life threatening and best treated with an implantable defibrillator.

Hypertrophic cardiomyopathy (HCM) is the most common cause of sudden death in young patients, but current risk stratification strategies do not identify all patients at risk. Contrast-enhanced cardiovascular magnetic resonance (CMR) with late gadolinium enhancement (LGE) can identify areas of abnormal myocardial substrate comprising fibrosis, the structural nidus for potentially life-threatening ventricular arrhythmias. More recently, follow-up studies have demonstrated a strong relationship between extent of LGE in patients with HCM and increased risk of adverse disease-related events, including sudden death.

Arrhythmogenic right ventricular dysplasia/cardiomyopathy (ARVD/C) is a rare cardiomyopathy associated with life-threatening arrhythmias and increased risk of sudden cardiac death. In addition to mutations in desmosomal genes, environmental factors such as exercise have been implicated in the pathogenesis of the disease. Recent studies have shown that exercise may be associated with adverse outcomes in ARVD/C patients. Based on current evidence, ARVD/C patients are recommended to limit exercise irrespective of their mutation status. In addition, some studies have suggested the presence of an entirely acquired form of the disease caused by exercise that has been dubbed exercise-induced ARVD/C.

Left ventricular hypertrophy (LVH) poses an independent risk of increased morbidity and mortality, including atrial arrhythmias, ventricular arrhythmias, and sudden cardiac death. The most common causes of LVH are hypertension and valvular heart disease. Electrocardiography and echocardiography are the first steps in the diagnosis and evaluation of therapy in patients with LVH. Cardiac MRI is the gold standard in diagnosis and assessment of response to therapy. Management of LVH should be based on etiology, evidence, and guideline adherence. Timely and optimal management of the underlying cause of LVH results in improvement (regression) of LVH and its related complications.

Patients with dilated cardiomyopathies (DCM) face a significant burden of arrhythmias, including conduction defects such as atrioventricular block and interventricular delay in the form of left bundle branch block, resulting in altered electromechanical coupling that can exacerbate heart failure. Atrial fibrillation is common and carries an adverse prognosis. Ventricular arrhythmias and sudden cardiac death generally occur late in the disease course. Sustained monomorphic ventricular tachycardia accounts for most of the sustained ventricular arrhythmias in DCM. This article summarizes common forms of arrhythmias encountered in patients with DCM, and reviews the relevant electrophysiologic basis of these arrhythmias and their management.

Myocardial involvement in patients with sarcoidosis can be difficult to diagnose, and requires a high index of suspicion and low threshold for screening. The presentation of cardiac sarcoidosis is variable, and can range from asymptomatic electrocardiographic changes to sudden cardiac death. This review provides an overview of the arrhythmic consequences of cardiac sarcoidosis, with emphasis on the electrophysiologist's role in recognition, diagnostic testing, and management of this rare disease.

Chagas disease, a chronic parasitosis caused by the protozoa *Trypanosoma cruzi*, is an increasing worldwide problem because of the number of cases in endemic areas and the migration of infected individuals to more developed regions. Chagas disease affects the heart through cardiac parasympathetic neuronal depopulation, immune-mediated myocardial injury, parasite persistence in cardiac tissue with secondary antigenic stimulation, and coronary microvascular abnormalities causing myocardial ischemia. A lack of knowledge exists for risk stratification, management, and prevention of ventricular arrhythmias in patients with chagasic cardiomyopathy. Catheter ablation can be effective for the management of recurrent ventricular tachycardia.

Acute viral myocarditis and acute pericarditis are self-limiting conditions that run a benign course and that may not involve symptoms that lead to medical assessment. However, ventricular arrhythmia is frequent in viral myocarditis. Myocarditis is thought to account for a large proportion of sudden cardiac deaths in young people without prior structural heart disease. Identification of acute myocarditis either with or without pericarditis is therefore important. However, therapeutic interventions are limited and nonspecific. Identifying those at greatest risk of a life-threatening arrhythmia is critical to reducing the mortality. This review summarizes current understanding of this challenging area in which many questions remain.

Fabry disease is an X-linked multisystem disorder caused by deficiency of the α-galactosidase A enzyme. Cardiovascular manifestations include hypertension, coronary disease, arrhythmias, valvular abnormalities, heart failure, and sudden death. Bradycardia and conduction system abnormalities are related initially to abnormal accumulation of glycolipids in the lysosomes of conduction tissues. Hypertrophy and eventual fibrosis provides a substrate for persistent conduction abnormalities and ventricular arrhythmias. Sudden cardiac death can be related to bradyarrhythmias or tachycardias. Enzyme replacement therapy can improve cardiac function and clinical outcomes. Pacemakers or defibrillators are important in the treatment of patients with Fabry disease who are at risk for arrhythmias.

Mitochondrial dysfunction has been shown to be involved in the pathophysiology of arrhythmia, not only in inherited cardiomyopathy due to specific mutations in the mitochondrial DNA but also in acquired cardiomyopathy such as ischemic or diabetic cardiomyopathy. This article briefly discusses the basics of mitochondrial physiology and details the mechanisms generating arrhythmias due to mitochondrial dysfunction. The clinical spectrum of inherited and acquired cardiomyopathies associated with mitochondrial dysfunction is discussed followed by general aspects of the management of mitochondrial cardiomyopathy and related arrhythmia.

In patients with muscular dystrophies, cardiac involvement leading to cardiomyopathy and arrhythmias occurs with variable prevalence, mirroring the phenotypic variability seen among and within the various hereditary myopathies. Knowledge of the incidence of arrhythmias and predictors of sudden death in the various hereditary myopathies can help guide screening and appropriate management of these patients, thereby improving survival. The noncardiac manifestations can lead to delayed recognition of symptoms, affect the decision to implant a prophylactic device, and once a decision is made to proceed with device implant, increase peri-procedural respiratory and anesthesia-related complications.

Peripartum cardiomyopathy (PPCM) is a complication of late pregnancy and the early postpartum period characterized by dilated cardiomyopathy and heart failure with reduced ejection fraction. Approximately half of women fail to recover left ventricular function. Standard management of heart failure is indicated, with some exceptions for women who are predelivery or breastfeeding. Atrial and ventricular arrhythmias are reported in PPCM, but the frequency of arrhythmias in this condition is not well characterized. Management of PPCM-associated arrhythmias may include antiarrhythmic drugs, catheter ablation, and wearable or implantable cardioverter-defibrillators. Further research is needed on the prevalence, natural history, and optimal management of arrhythmias in PPCM.

Left ventricular noncompaction (LVNC) is a newly recognized form of cardiomyopathy that has been associated with heart failure, arrhythmias, thromboembolic events, and sudden death. Both ventricular and supraventricular arrhythmias are now well described as prominent clinical components of LVNC. Throughout the spectrum of age, these arrhythmias have been associated with prognosis and outcome, and their clinical management is therefore an important aspect of patient care. The risk of sudden death seems to be associated with ventricular dilation, systolic dysfunction, and the presence of arrhythmias. Proposed management strategies shown to have efficacy include antiarrhythmic therapy, ablation techniques, and implantable cardioverter-defibrillator implantation.

Acute emotional or physical stress can trigger a catecholamine-mediated myocardial stunning known as takotstubo cardiomyopathy (TCM). Although TCM is generally reversible, it can be associated with significant morbidity, including secondarily to cardiac arrhythmia. Lethal arrhythmias such as heart block, ventricular tachycardia, and ventricular fibrillation have been described. Repolarization abnormalities associated with TCM can lead to characteristic T-wave abnormalities and QT prolongation that place patients at increased risk for ventricular arrhythmia, including torsades de pointes. This article focuses on the arrhythmic complications associated with TCM and explores the underlying etiology of these arrhythmias.

Many pharmaceutical agents interact with cardiac ion channels resulting in abnormal ventricular repolarization and prolongation of the QT interval. In rare circumstances, this has resulted in the development of the potentially life-threatening arrhythmia, torsades de pointes. It is recognized, however, that accurate measurement of the QT interval is challenging, and it is a poor predictor for the development of this arrhythmia. Nevertheless, QT interval monitoring is an essential part of pharmaceutical development, and significant increases in the QT interval may prevent a drug from gaining approval.

Stem cell regenerative therapies hold promise for treating diseases across the spectrum of medicine. While significant progress has been made in the preclinical stages, the clinical application of cardiac cell therapy is limited by technical challenges. Certain methods of cell delivery, such as intramyocardial injection, carry a higher rate of arrhythmias. Other potential contributors to the arrhythmogenicity of cell transplantation include reentrant pathways caused by heterogeneity in conduction velocities between graft and host as well as graft automaticity. In this article, the arrhythmogenic potential of cell delivery to the heart is discussed.

# CARDIAC ELECTROPHYSIOLOGY CLINICS

**THE CLINICS ARE AVAILABLE ONLINE!**
Access your subscription at:
www.theclinics.com

# Foreword
# Arrhythmias in Cardiomyopathies

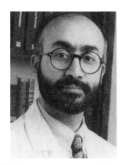
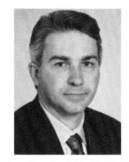

Ranjan K. Thakur, MD, MPH, MBA, FACC, FHRS      Andrea Natale, MD, FACC, FHRS

*Consulting Editors*

We are pleased to introduce this issue of the *Cardiac Electrophysiology Clinics* devoted to Arrhythmias in Cardiomyopathies.

The myocardium has a certain organizational structure and contractile and electrical functions. A disturbance in any of these, in isolation or in combination, can be described under the rubric of cardiomyopathy. Our initial appreciation of cardiomyopathy was in the setting of systolic left ventricular dysfunction; that appreciation has grown to include a vast number of entities that result in functional and/or electrical abnormalities. These are reflected in the table of contents of this volume: hypertrophic cardiomyopathy, arrhythmogenic right ventricular cardiomyopathy, peripartum cardiomyopathy, noncompaction syndrome, and so on.

Cardiomyopathies may be due to myocardial disorganization or metabolic abnormalities (such as in Fabry disease) and may occur after viral or parasitic infections or cellular/subcellular abnormalities (such as mitochondrial abnormalities). The field is still evolving as new research findings give us new insights. For example, recently the group from UCLA described arrhythmogenic inflammatory cardiomyopathy in patients with occult cardiac sarcoidosis.[1]

We congratulate Drs Shenasa, Link, and Maron on compiling this summary of the present understanding of cardiac arrhythmias in various forms of cardiomyopathy. They have enlisted leaders in the field to bring the readers up-to-date on their respective areas of focus. Electrophysiologists and cardiologists will find a lot of useful information "under one roof."

Ranjan K. Thakur, MD, MPH, MBA, FACC, FHRS
Sparrow Thoracic and Cardiovascular Institute
Michigan State University
1200 East Michigan Avenue, Suite 580
Lansing, MI 48912, USA

Andrea Natale, MD, FACC, FHRS
Texas Cardiac Arrhythmia Institute
Center for Atrial Fibrillation at
St. David's Medical Center
1015 East 32nd Street, Suite 516
Austin, TX 78705, USA

E-mail addresses:
thakur@msu.edu (R.K. Thakur)
andrea.natale@stdavids.com (A. Natale)

## REFERENCE

1. Bauer B, Tung R, Bradfield J, et al. Incidence of abnormal positron emission tomography in patients with idiopathic cardiomyopathy referred for ventricular arrhythmias: occult cardiac sarcoidosis and a new clinical entity of arrhythmogenic inflammatory cardiomyopathy. Heart Rhythm 2014;5(S):S29.

http://dx.doi.org/10.1016/j.ccep.2015.04.001
1877-9182/15/$ – see front matter © 2015 Published by Elsevier Inc.

cardiacEP.theclinics.com

# Preface

# Arrhythmias in Cardiomyopathies

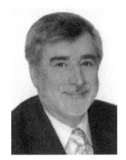 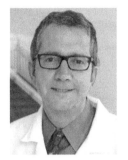 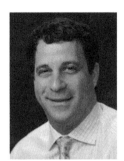

Mohammad Shenasa, MD     Mark S. Link, MD     Martin S. Maron, MD

*Editors*

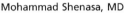

Cardiomyopathies constitute a large and diverse entity of myocardial, structural, and functional abnormalities. Hypertrophic cardiomyopathy is the most common abnormality with initially normal left ventricular cavity size and systolic function at one end of the spectrum and severe dilated nonischemic cardiomyopathy at the other end.

Almost all cardiomyopathies have a genetic basis that causes myocardial disarray that sets a substrate for arrhythmias of different mechanisms.

We are honored to have been invited as guest editors of this issue of *Cardiac Electrophysiology Clinics* dedicated to the "Arrhythmias in Cardiomyopathies." It is an important topic and as such there is currently no collective resource on the subject, although many reviews and articles are available on individual topics. We are privileged that a group of leading authors have accepted our invitation and provided their up-to-date evidence-based review on specific topics.

The articles begin with a historical perspective by Barry Maron, the godfather of hypertrophic cardiomyopathy. Next is "Atrial and Ventricular Arrhythmias in Hypertrophic Cardiomyopathy," followed by "The Role of Cardiovascular Magnetic Resonance in Sudden Death Risk Stratification in Hypertrophic Cardiomyopathy," "Relationship Between Arrhythmogenic Right Ventricular Dysplasia and Exercise," and "Left Ventricular Hypertrophy and Arrhythmogenesis." Subsequent articles focus on other cardiomyopathies, such as dilated cardiomyopathy, sarcoidosis; chagasic cardiomyopathy; viral myocarditis and pericarditis; Fabry cardiomyopathy; mitochondrial cardiomyopathy and related arrhythmias; arrhythmias in the muscular dystrophies; peripartum cardiomyopathy; left ventricular noncompaction; and

Card Electrophysiol Clin 7 (2015) xv–xvi
http://dx.doi.org/10.1016/j.ccep.2015.03.018
1877-9182/15/$ – see front matter © 2015 Published by Elsevier Inc.

Takotsubo cardiomyopathy. "QT Prolongation and Oncology Drug Development" is also included, with a final article on "Arrhythmia in Stem Cell Transplantation."

We are very pleased with the overall context of this issue and are confident that it will be useful to cardiology and electrophysiology fellows, cardiologists, and electrophysiologists as the most updated reference on this important topic, "Arrhythmias in Cardiomyopathies."

Mohammad Shenasa, MD
Department of Cardiovascular Services
O'Connor Hospital
Heart and Rhythm Medical Group
105 North Bascom Avenue, Suite 204
San Jose, CA 95128, USA

Mark S. Link, MD
Division of Cardiology
Hypertrophic Cardiomyopathy Center
Tufts Medical Center
800 Washington Street, Box 197
Boston, MA 02111, USA

Martin S. Maron, MD
Division of Cardiology
Hypertrophic Cardiomyopathy Center
Tufts Medical Center
800 Washington Street, Box 197
Boston, MA 02111, USA

E-mail addresses:
Mohammad.shenasa@gmail.com (M. Shenasa)
mlink@tuftsmedicalcenter.org (M.S. Link)
mmaron@tuftsmedicalcenter.org (M.S. Maron)

# Historical Perspectives on the Implantable Cardioverter–Defibrillator and Prevention of Sudden Death in Hypertrophic Cardiomyopathy

Barry J. Maron, MD

## KEYWORDS

• Implantable defibrillators • Sudden death • Hypertrophic cardiomyopathy

## KEY POINTS

- The implantable defibrillator has had a proven life-saving capability in coronary artery disease for 35 years.
- The defibrillator has been translated to hypertrophic cardiomyopathy (HCM) and has been effective in primary prevention of sudden death over the last 15 years in a range of patients.
- Risk stratification and selection of HCM patients for defibrillators has matured but is not yet complete.

## THE EARLY YEARS

Hypertrophic cardiomyopathy (HCM) is an important, if not the most common cause of unexpected and unanticipated nontraumatic sudden death (SD) in the young (including competitive athletes).[1–5] The often cited and remarkable paper of Donald Teare, coroner of London, reported 8 young people (15 to 45 years of age; mean 27) with SDs that he attributed to asymmetric left ventricular hypertrophy mimicking a cardiac tumor.[6] In addition to its focus on sudden and apparently arrhythmic death, Teare's detailed morphologic observations included the now acknowledged key features of HCM such as a disorganized arrangement of myocytes, extensive fibrosis, and familial occurrence, as well as the recognition that syncope and exercise can be risk factors.

Although SDs are now known to be relatively uncommon among the expansive disease spectrum of HCM (about 5% of patients), such events remain the most devastating potential disease complication, dominating the discourse on HCM both among patients and in the practicing cardiovascular community.[1–5] Indeed, for more than 3 decades following the initial recognition of HCM as a disease state, no effective treatment or intervention was available to prevent SD occurring predominantly in young people without symptoms or warning signs. Cardioactive drugs such as amiodarone, beta-blockers, verapamil, and antiarrhythmic medications (eg, procainamide or quinidine) had previously been administered to HCM patients as a means of preventing SD, but ultimately with no evidence of efficacy.[7]

## MIROWSKI, MOWER, AND THE IMPLANTABLE CARDIOVERTER–DEFIBRILLATOR

The impetus for creating an implantable defibrillator to abort impending sudden cardiac death was

Disclosure: Author receives grant from the Medtronic Corporation.
Hypertrophic Cardiomyopathy Center, Minneapolis Heart Institute Foundation, 920 East 28th Street, Suite 620, Minneapolis, MN 55407, USA
E-mail address: hcm.maron@mhif.org

fundamentally the vision of Michel Mirowski, and its development ultimately the work of Mirowski and Morton Mower at Sinai Hospital (Baltimore, Maryland) (**Fig. 1**).[8,9] Initially, they were working in a self-funded animal laboratory[8] and against multiple economic and other impediments including antagonism from the cardiology establishment.[10,11] After 10 years of investigation, the implantable cardioverter—defibrillator (ICD) was eventually placed into clinical trials. A major obstacle to overcome for Mirowski in the early development of the ICD came from Bernard Lown at Harvard Medical School, who regarded the defibrillator as a "gadget" and an "imperfect solution in search of a plausible and practical application," created only "because it was possible," and also taking the view that ventricular fibrillation does not recur.[10]

The initial ICD patient trial was conducted in 1980 at Johns Hopkins Hospital on 3 patients in the laboratory setting for whom ventricular fibrillation was reliably terminated and sinus rhythm immediately restored spontaneously by the defibrillator.[9] Notably, US Food and Drug Administration (FDA) approval required recruitment of patients who had

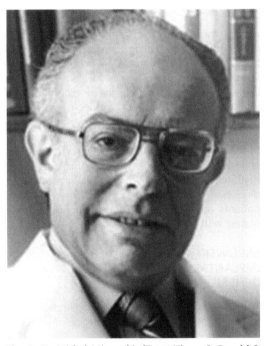

Fig. 1. Dr Michel Mirowski. (*From* Nisam S, Barold S. Historical evolution of the automatic implantable cardioverter defibrillator in the treatment of malignant ventricular tachyarrhythmias. In: Alt E, Klein H, Griffin JC, editors. The implantable cardioverter/defibrillator. Springer-Verlag Berlin Heidelberg: 1992. p. 3; with permission.)

survived 2 or more cardiac arrests, and 2 of the first 3 patients to receive ICDs were patients with HCM.

## LINKING THE IMPLANTABLE CARDIOVERTER–DEFIBRILLATOR TO HYPERTROPHIC CARDIOMYOPATHY

Clinical development and introduction of the ICD to the cardiology community began with the vast population of at-risk patients with atherosclerotic coronary artery disease following resuscitated cardiac arrest (ventricular fibrillation) or myocardial infarction (**Fig. 2**). With the development of transvenous lead systems in 1992, a number of large prospective and randomized secondary and primary prevention trials showed a survival benefit attributable to the ICD in patients with coronary artery disease (or nonischemic cardiomyopathy, eg, Antiarrhythmics versus Implantable Defibrillator Study [AVID], Multicenter Unsustained Tachycardia Trial [MUSTT], and Multicenter Automatic Defibrillator Implant Studies [MADIT I/II]).[12–16]

While this early evolutionary period for the ICD focused on prevention of SD due to ischemic heart disease, genetic heart diseases (including HCM) were largely ignored. Furthermore, at the onset, it was not at all certain that the standard ICD would be appropriate for a genetic disease such as HCM, being so different pathophysiologically from coronary artery disease (ie, with marked [if not extreme] increase in mass, left ventricular [LV] outflow obstruction and mitral regurgitation, diastolic dysfunction, and microvascular ischemia.[1–3]

The landmark clinical study that demonstrated for the first time the efficacy of the ICD specifically for patients with HCM was published in the New England Journal of Medicine in 2000 (see **Fig. 2**).[17] Translating the ICD to HCM represented a paradigm change in disease management by altering the natural course of the disease for many patients, including children implanted younger than 20 years of age with aggressive forms of HCM.[17–20]

Subsequently, a series of retrospective studies comprising hundreds of HCM patients judged to be at increased risk by the generally accepted stratification algorithm[1–3,21–25] proved the ICD to be highly effective in terminating potentially lethal ventricular tachyarrhythmias. A primary prevention appropriate intervention rate of 4% per year has been reported consistently (about 10% per year for secondary prevention),[18–20,26–28] with about 20% of devices intervening for ventricular tachycardia/ventricular fibrillation (VT/VF) about 4 years after implant (**Fig. 3**).[18] Indeed, in adult HCM patients, the ICD has been largely responsible for a reduction in HCM-related mortality to 0.5% per year, less than that expected for all-cause

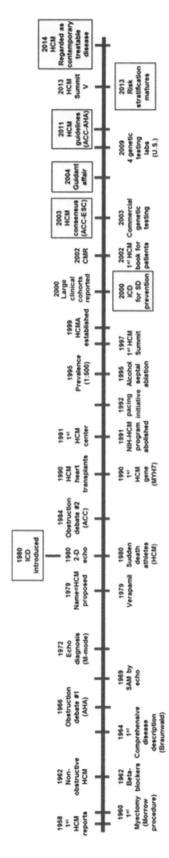

**Fig. 2.** Timeline of advances in HCM over 50 years, including introduction of the ICD. ACC, American College of Cardiology; AHA, American Heart Association; ESC, European Society of Cardiology; HCMA, Hypertrophic Cardiomyopathy Association; NIH, National Institutes of Health.

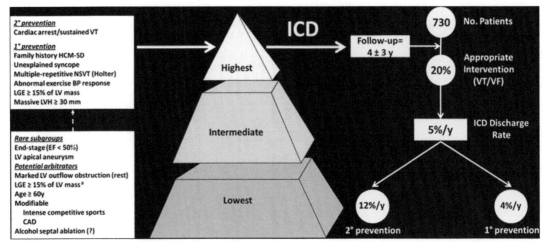

**Fig. 3.** Pyramid profile of risk stratification model currently used to identify patients at the highest risk who may be candidates for ICDs and sudden death prevention. Major and minor risk markers appear in boxes at the left. At right are the results of ICD therapy in 730 children, adolescents, and adults assembled from registry studies. BP, blood pressure; CAD, coronary artery disease; EF, ejection fraction; LGE, late gadolinium enhancement; LVH, left ventricular hypertrophy; NSVT, nonsustained ventricular tachycardia; VT/VF, ventricular tachycardia/ventricular fibrillation; y, years. [a] Extensive LGE can be a primary risk marker, but also an ICD decision arbitrator when assignment of high-risk status is ambiguous based on conventional risk markers. (*Adapted from* Maron BJ, Ommen SR, Semsarian C, et al. Hypertrophic cardiomyopathy: present and future, with translation into contemporary cardiovascular medicine. J Am Coll Cardiol 2014;64:83–99.)

mortality in the general US population.[29] Such changes in clinical practice have allowed HCM to achieve the status as a contemporary and treatable cardiac disease.[1]

Finally, a derivative of the ICD initiative in HCM has been prophylactic device therapy administered in other genetic heart diseases. This strategy has included effective ICD therapy for some patients with ion channelopathies[30–32] and arrhythmogenic right ventricular cardiomyopathy (ARVC).[33–35]

## MATURING OF RISK STRATIFICATION

The importance of identifying reliable risk markers for prediction of future SD events has accelerated and become a far more relevant issue after the ICD was introduced to the HCM patient population, and prevention of SD became a reality (see **Figs. 2** and **3**).[1–3] By virtue of numerous retrospective observational studies over 20 years, a risk stratification algorithm has been incrementally assembled, effective in identifying many high-risk patients who have benefited from prophylactic ICD therapy (see **Fig. 3**).[1–3,21–25]

The strategy of using one or more major risk markers, judged to be relevant within the individual patient's clinical profile, as the basis for consideration of a prophylactic ICD, has been the generally accepted management strategy for HCM patients in the United States.[1–3,17–25,36,37] Other

approaches have been advanced with limited success (particularly by European investigators), such as numerical summing of risk factors, highly mathematical/statistical modeling, and attempts to weight multiple risk factors in individual patients.[38,39] The most recent risk stratification marker to emerge takes advantage of quantitative contrast- cardiovascular magnetic resonance (CMR) to identify extensive late gadolinium enhancement as an arrhythmogenic substrate.[40]

## THE GUIDANT AFFAIR

In 2004, a 21-year-old college student with nonobstructive HCM and a high-risk profile died suddenly when his primary prevention defibrillator failed to defibrillate a lethal arrhythmia. Subsequently, it came to light that this patient's ICD model was prone to short-circuiting, and this possibility had been previously known only to the manufacturer (Guidant Corporation), while managing cardiologists, electrophysiologists, and patients had not been informed (see **Fig. 2**). Even while the defective defibrillators were being made public, Guidant continued to sell the same models to unaware consumers. Therefore, some patients with HCM (and other cardiac diseases) judged to be at risk for life-threatening arrhythmias were treated with devices that could not have been expected to reliably prevent SD.

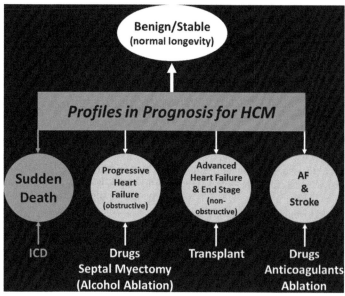

**Fig. 4.** Adverse pathways within the broad HCM clinical spectrum, including the risk for SD. Individual patients may be subject to disease progression with one or more of these complications, each of which is associated with potentially effective treatment options. Alternatively, most HCM patients probably experience a benign course without requiring major interventions. AF, atrial fibrillation.

The Guidant affair became highly visible publically,[41,42] ultimately creating greater transparency between industry, the fully informed patient, and practicing cardiology community, while paradoxically raising the visibility of the potential power of the ICD in preventing SD in HCM.

## SUMMARY

Historically, Mirowski did not envision the ICD as a treatment to prevent SD in young people with genetic heart diseases. In the case of HCM, initially it was not known whether the ICD would be effective in patients with a disease very different morphologically and functionally from coronary artery disease. Nevertheless, several observational clinical studies have convincingly shown that the ICD reliably senses and automatically terminates life-threatening ventricular tachyarrhythmias in HCM, and is responsible for reducing HCM mortality by preventing SD and changing the natural course of the disease. Indeed, the ICD has been a major determinant in the evolution of HCM to a contemporary and treatable disease (**Fig. 4**). However, research remains to refine risk stratification and reduce the number of ICDs implanted in patients who ultimately never require device intervention.

## REFERENCES

1. Maron BJ, Ommen SR, Semsarian C, et al. Hypertrophic cardiomyopathy: present and future, with translation into contemporary cardiovascular medicine. J Am Coll Cardiol 2014;64:83–99.
2. Maron BJ, Maron MS. Hypertrophic cardiomyopathy. Lancet 2013;381:242–55.
3. Maron BJ. Contemporary insights and strategies for risk stratification and prevention of sudden death in hypertrophic cardiomyopathy. Circulation 2010;121: 445–56.
4. Maron BJ, Braunwald E. Evolution of hypertrophic cardiomyopathy to a contemporary treatable disease. Circulation 2012;126:1640–4.
5. Maron BJ, Doerer JJ, Haas TS, et al. Sudden deaths in young competitive athletes: analysis of 1866 deaths in the United States, 1980–2006. Circulation 2009;119:1085–92.
6. Teare D. Asymmetrical hypertrophy of the heart in young adults. Br Heart J 1958;20:1–8.
7. Melacini P, Maron BJ, Bobbo F, et al. Evidence that pharmacological strategies lack efficacy for the prevention of sudden death in hypertrophic cardiomyopathy. Heart 2007;93:708–10.
8. Mirowski M, Mower MM, Langer A, et al. A chronically implanted system for automatic defibrillation in active conscious dogs. Experimental model for treatment of sudden death from ventricular fibrillation. Circulation 1978;58:90–4.
9. Mirowski M, Reid PR, Mower MM, et al. Termination of malignant ventricular arrhythmias with an implanted automatic defibrillator in human beings. N Engl J Med 1980;303:322–4.
10. Lown B, Axelrod P. Implanted standby defibrillators. Circulation 1972;46:637–9.

11. Mirowski M. The automatic implanted cardioverter-defibrillator: an overview. J Am Coll Cardiol 1985;6: 461–6.

12. Moss AJ, Hall WJ, Cannom DS, et al. Improved survival with an implanted defibrillator in patients with coronary disease at high risk for ventricular arrhythmia. Multicenter automatic defibrillator implantation trial investigators. N Engl J Med 1996; 335:1933–40.

13. Buxton AE, Lee KL, Fisher JD, et al. A randomized study of the prevention of sudden death in patients with coronary artery disease. Multicenter unsustained tachycardia trial investigators. N Engl J Med 1999;341:1882–90.

14. A comparison of antiarrhythmic drug therapy with implantable defibrillators in patients resuscitated from near-fatal ventricular arrhythmias. The antiarrhythmics versus implantable defibrillators (AVID) investigators. N Engl J Med 1997;337:1576–83.

15. Connolly SJ, Gent M, Roberts RS, et al. Canadian implantable defibrillator study (CIDS): a randomized trial of the implantable cardioverter defibrillator against amiodarone. Circulation 2000;101: 1297–302.

16. Kuck KH, Cappato R, Siebels J, et al. Randomized comparison of antiarrhythmic drug therapy with implantable defibrillators in patients resuscitated from cardiac arrest: the Cardiac Arrest Study Hamburg (CASH). Circulation 2000;102:748–54.

17. Maron BJ, Shen WK, Link MS, et al. Efficacy of implantable cardioverter–defibrillators for the prevention of sudden death in patients with hypertrophic cardiomyopathy. N Engl J Med 2000;342: 365–73.

18. Maron BJ, Spirito P, Shen WK, et al. Implantable cardioverter–defibrillators and prevention of sudden cardiac death in hypertrophic cardiomyopathy. JAMA 2007;298:405–12.

19. Maron BJ, Spirito P, Ackerman MJ, et al. Prevention of sudden cardiac death with implantable cardioverter–defibrillators in children and adolescents with hypertrophic cardiomyopathy. J Am Coll Cardiol 2013;61:1527–35.

20. Maron BJ, Spirito P. Implantable defibrillators and prevention of sudden death in hypertrophic cardiomyopathy. J Cardiovasc Electrophysiol 2008;19: 1118–26.

21. Maron BJ, McKenna WJ, Danielson GK, et al. American College of Cardiology/European Society of Cardiology Clinical expert consensus document on hypertrophic cardiomyopathy. A report of the American College of Cardiology task force on clinical expert consensus documents and the European Society of Cardiology Committee for Practice Guidelines Committee to develop an expert consensus document on hypertrophic cardiomyopathy. J Am Coll Cardiol 2003;42:1687–713.

22. Maron BJ, McKenna WJ, Danielson GK, et al. American College of Cardiology/European Society of Cardiology Clinical expert consensus document on hypertrophic cardiomyopathy. A report of the American College of Cardiology task force on clinical expert consensus documents and the European Society of Cardiology Committee for Practice Guidelines Committee to develop an expert consensus document on hypertrophic cardiomyopathy. Eur Heart J 2003;24:1965–91.

23. Gersh BJ, Maron BJ, Bonow RO, et al. 2011 ACCF/AHA guideline for the diagnosis and treatment of hypertrophic cardiomyopathy: executive summary: a report of the American College of Cardiology Foundation/American Heart Association task force on practice guidelines. Circulation 2011;124:2761–96.

24. Gersh BJ, Maron BJ, Bonow RO, et al. 2011 ACCF/AHA guideline for the diagnosis and Treatment of Hypertrophic Cardiomyopathy: a report of the American College of cardiology Foundation/American Heart Association Task Force on practice guidelines. Developed in collaboration with the American Association for Thoracic Surgery, American Society of Echocardiography, American Society of Nuclear Cardiology, Heart Failure Society Of America, Heart Rhythm Society, Society for Cardiovascular Angiography and Interventions, and Society of Thoracic Surgeons. J Am Coll Cardiol 2011;58:e212–60.

25. Gersh BJ, Maron BJ, Bonow RO, et al. 2011 ACCF/AHA guideline for the diagnosis and treatment of hypertrophic cardiomyopathy: a report of the American College of Cardiology Foundation/American Heart Association task force on practice guidelines. J Thorac Cardiovasc Surg 2011;142:e153–203.

26. Schinkel AF, Vriesendorp PA, Sijbrands EJ, et al. Outcome and complications after implantable cardioverter defibrillator therapy in hypertrophic cardiomyopathy: systematic review and meta-analysis. Circ Heart Fail 2012;5:552–9.

27. Christiaans I, van Engelen K, van Langen IM, et al. Risk stratification for sudden cardiac death in hypertrophic cardiomyopathy: systematic review of clinical risk markers. Europace 2010;12:313–21.

28. Vriesendorp PA, Schinkel AF, Van Cleemput J, et al. Implantable cardioverter–defibrillators in hypertrophic cardiomyopathy: patient outcomes, rate of appropriate and inappropriate interventions, and complications. Am Heart J 2013;166:496–502.

29. Maron BJ, Rowin EJ, Casey SA, et al. Hypertrophic cardiomyopathy in adulthood associated with low cardiovascular mortality with contemporary management strategies. J Am Coll Cardiol, in press.

30. Mönnig G, Köbe J, Löher A, et al. Implantable cardioverter-defibrillator therapy in patients with congenital long-QT syndrome: a long-term follow-up. Heart Rhythm 2005;2:497–504.

31. Zareba W, Moss AJ, Daubert JP, et al. Implantable cardioverter defibrillator in high-risk long QT syndrome patients. J Cardiovasc Electrophysiol 2003; 14:337–41.

32. Viskin S, Halkin A. Treating the long-QT syndrome in the era of implantable defibrillators. Circulation 2009;119:204–6.

33. Corrado D, Leoni L, Link MS, et al. Implantable cardioverter–defibrillator therapy for prevention of sudden death in patients with arrhythmogenic right ventricular cardiomyopathy/dysplasia. Circulation 2003;23(108):3084–91.

34. Wichter T, Paul M, Wollmann C, et al. Implantable cardioverter/defibrillator therapy in arrhythmogenic right ventricular cardiomyopathy: single-center experience of long-term follow-up and complications in 60 patients. Circulation 2004;109:1503–8.

35. Corrado D, Calkins H, Link MS, et al. Prophylactic implantable defibrillator in patients with arrhythmogenic right ventricular cardiomyopathy/dysplasia and no prior ventricular fibrillation or sustained ventricular tachycardia. Circulation 2010;122:1144–52.

36. Spirito P, Autore C, Rapezzi C, et al. Syncope and risk of sudden death in hypertrophic cardiomyopathy. Circulation 2009;119:1703–10.

37. Spirito P, Bellone P, Harris KM, et al. Magnitude of left ventricular hypertrophy and risk of sudden death in hypertrophic cardiomyopathy. N Engl J Med 2000; 342:1778–85.

38. Elliott PM, Anastasakis A, Borger MA, et al. 2014 ESC guidelines on diagnosis and management of hypertrophic cardiomyopathy: the task force for the diagnosis and management of hypertrophic cardiomyopathy of the European Society of Cardiology (ESC). Eur Heart J 2014;35:2733–79.

39. O'Mahony C, Jichi F, Pavlou M, et al. Hypertrophic cardiomyopathy outcomes investigators. A novel clinical risk prediction model for sudden cardiac death in hypertrophic cardiomyopathy (HCM risk-SCD). Eur Heart J 2014;35:2010–20.

40. Chan RH, Maron BJ, Olivotto I, et al. Prognostic value of quantitative contrast-enhanced cardiovascular magnetic resonance for the evaluation of sudden death risk in patients with hypertrophic cardiomyopathy. Circulation 2014;130:484–95.

41. Hauser RG, Maron BJ. Lessons from the failure and recall of an implantable cardioverter defibrillator. Circulation 2005;112:2040–2.

42. Steinbrook R. The controversy over Guidant's implantable defibrillators. N Engl J Med 2005;353: 221–4.

# Atrial and Ventricular Arrhythmias in Hypertrophic Cardiomyopathy

Kartik R. Kumar, MBBS, Swati N. Mandleywala, MBBS,
Mark S. Link, MD*

## KEYWORDS

- Arrhythmias • Atrial fibrillation • Ventricular fibrillation • Hypertrophic cardiomyopathy • Risk factors
- Electrophysiology

## KEY POINTS

- Atrial fibrillation (AF) is common finding in patients with hypertrophic cardiomyopathy (HCM) and contributes to poor outcomes as a result of the progression and exacerbation of heart failure in addition to the innate morbidity of AF.
- Ventricular tachycardia and fibrillation are life threatening, with the 5 most common risk factors being:
  - Left ventricular hypertrophy
  - Personal history of unexplained syncope
  - Family history of sudden cardiac death
  - Nonsustained ventricular tachycardia
  - Abnormal blood pressure response to exercise
- Management of AF in HCM is often difficult, and the risk of systemic thromboembolism is high.
- Ventricular arrhythmias are best managed with implantable cardioverter defibrillator implantation.

## INTRODUCTION

Hypertrophic cardiomyopathy (HCM) is an autosomal dominant disease caused by mutations in genes coding for cardiac sarcomeres. HCM is the most common inherited heart disease, with a prevalence of 0.2% or 1 in 500 persons.[1] There are multiple genetic variants that cause pleomorphic disease characterized by myocardial disarray and myocardial hypertrophy. Throughout the history of understanding this disease, we have come to learn that these patients are at an increased risk of atrial and ventricular arrhythmias and these contribute to the prognosis and mortality of the disease.[2]

## ATRIAL FIBRILLATION

Atrial fibrillation (AF) is the most common arrhythmia in patients with HCM. A landmark 2001 study[3] evaluated 480 patients with HCM with a mean follow-up of 9.1 years and found the prevalence of AF to be 22%. More recently, in 2009 a study in Japan [4] evaluated 261 patients with HCM and found that 74 (28%) patients had documented paroxysmal AF (PAF) or chronic AF at registration, and a 2014 systematic review[5] including several larger studies concluded an overall prevalence of 22.45%.

AF is an important prognostic indicator in patients with HCM, because these patients are typically at a higher New York Heart Association (NYHA) functional class and have a poorer outcome. This subgroup of patients with HCM are at an increased risk of cardiovascular morbidity and mortality in the form of thromboembolic events, heart failure, and sudden death.[6] A large cohort study including 293 patients with

The authors have nothing to disclose.
Department of Cardiology, Tufts Medical Center, 800 Washington Street, Boston, MA 02111, USA
* Corresponding author. Box #197, 800 Washington Street, Boston, MA 02111.
E-mail address: MLink@tuftsmedicalcenter.org

HCM with a median follow-up of 6 years found that 50 patients developed heart failure, of whom 32 (64%) had AF as a contributor. In addition, 18 of the 50 patients with heart failure who had died and on whom autopsy was performed, 5 had presence of thrombi in the left atrium (LA). All 5 of these hearts were in patients with HCM suffering from AF.[7] In 158 patients with HCM with AF and 496 patients with HCM without AF followed up for 4.2 ± 2.8 years, AF was associated with an increased risk for all-cause death ($P = .001$), cardiovascular death ($P<.001$), severe heart failure ($P<.001$), and ischemic stroke ($P<.001$) (**Table 1**).[8]

## Risk Factors

### Left atrial size

LA size is one of the most important determinants of AF occurrence in patients with HCM (**Table 2**). In 141 patients with HCM, 31 of whom had a history of PAF, maximum LA volume was the most sensitive and specific parameter for the occurrence of PAF in its study population.[10] A prospectively analyzed study looking at 612 patients with HCM from 1990 to 2007 found LA diameter (LAD) and brain natriuretic peptide to be independent predictors of occurrence of AF.[11] Cardiac magnetic resonance (CMR) in patients with HCM with AF has shown greater LA volume and higher mean extent of late gadolinium enhancement (LGE) when compared with patients with HCM without AF. LGE was inferior to LA dilation for predicting AF.[12–14]

A systematic review conducted in 2014[5] compiled 33 studies totaling 7381 patients with HCM and found that LA dimension and age were common predictors for AF. Meta-analysis of the included studies showed LAD of 38.03 mm (95% confidence interval [CI] 34.62%–41.44%) in

patients to be in sinus rhythm and an LAD of 45.37 mm (95% CI 41.64%–49.04%) in patients with AF. In addition, the study concluded the overall prevalence of thromboembolism in patients with HCM with AF to be 27.09% (95% CI 2.63%–3.54%).

### Left atrial function

In 427 consecutive patients with HCM, 41 of whom prospectively developed overt AF after study entry, LA ejection fraction and LA end diastolic volume were important markers of AF susceptibility. LA ejection fraction less than 38% and LA end diastolic volume of 118 mL or greater were associated with increased AF occurrence.[16]

### Myocardial fibrosis

In a small pathologic study published in 2001,[17] 10 HCM heart specimens were analyzed, 5 with AF and 5 without AF. The pathologists determined the extent of fibrosis and degree of intramyocardial small arterial stenosis to be greater and more extensive in the AF group. With more recent advances in imaging techniques, CMR imaging has been used to determine risk of AF. Delayed contrast enhancement on CMR may represent regions of myocardial fibrosis. Sixty-seven patients with HCM, 17 of whom had AF, were studied by CMR looking at left ventricular (LV) myocardial fibrosis as well as LV mass and volume. The study[18] concluded that AF was significantly more frequent in patients who had LV myocardial fibrosis compared with those without (42.1% versus 3.4%, respectively). The LA size was also larger in those patients with delayed contrast enhancement.

### Sleep-disordered breathing (sleep apnea)

Obstructive sleep apnea (OSA) is independently associated with cardiovascular disease and arrhythmias in non-HCM populations. Sleep apnea is also common in patients with HCM, being

---

**Table 1**
**Prevalence and outcomes of AF in patients with HCM**

| Study | Patients (n) | Prevalence (%) | Follow-up (y) | Outcomes |
|---|---|---|---|---|
| Olivotto et al,[3] 2001 | 480 | 22 | 9.1 ± 6.4 | 3% annual HCM-related mortality in patients with AF |
| Kubo et al,[4] 2009 | 261 | 74/261 patients = 28 | | |
| Melacini et al,[7] 2010 | 293 | | 6 | AF contributed to heart failure in 64% of patients |
| Tian et al,[8] 2013 | 654 | 17 | 4.2 ± 2.8 | AF is an independent risk factor for cardiovascular death and stroke-related death |
| Siontis et al,[9] 2014 | 3673 | 18 | 4.1 | Hazard ratio 1.48 (95% CI 1.27–1.71) for the effect of AF on overall mortality |

**Table 2**
**Risk factors for AF in patients with HCM**

| Study | Patients | Conclusion/Measure | LA Size, HCM + AF vs HCM No AF |
|---|---|---|---|
| Tani,[10] 2004 | 141 (22% had PAF) | Increased LAV = increased PAF | 41 ± 6 mm vs 37 ± 6 mm, P<.0006 |
| Han et al,[11] 2008 | 612–94 (15.4%) had AF - >43 (6.0%) sustained 51 (9.4%) PAF | Increased LAD/BNP | |
| Papavassiliu et al,[12] 2009 | 87 (42% had documented AF) | LGE/LAV | 68 ± 24 mL/m² vs 46 ± 18 mL/m², P<.0002 |
| Girasis et al,[15] 2013 | 30 (all with 1 documented PAF) | LA anteroposterior diameter, prolonged P-wave | 46.1 ± 5.9 vs 40.0 ± 4.7 mm,. P<.001 |
| Doi & Kitaoka[6] 2001 | 91 | LAD increased = increased AF | 43 ± 6 vs 36 ± 5 mm, P<.01 |
| Tian et al,[8] 2013 | 654 | LAD increased = AF increased | 45 ± 8 vs 39 ± 6 mm, P<.001 |
| Guttman,[5] 2014 Heart | 7381 | LAD is a predictor of AF | 45.37 mm (95% CI 41.64–49.04) vs 38.03 mm (95% CI 34.62%–41.44%) |

*Abbreviations:* BNP, brain natriuretic peptide; LAD, LA diameter; LAV, LA volume.

present in 32 of 80 patients with HCM studied by Pedrosa and colleagues.[19] The patients suffering from OSA in this study also had increased LADs compared with patients with HCM without OSA. AF was present in 31% of patients with HCM-OSA compared with 6% of patients with HCM without OSA. These findings were confirmed by another group, with OSA strongly associated with a higher prevalence of AF and also accompanied by a significantly increased LA volume.[20]

*P-wave*
Interatrial conduction alterations as shown by longer P-wave duration and P-wave morphology has also been postulated to be a marker for AF

(**Table 3**). A study found that patients with HCM have longer P-wave duration at 149 ± 22 milliseconds, whereas in healthy controls, it was 130 ± 16 milliseconds.[21]

*Genetic*
E334k cardiac myosin binding protein C mutations is a causative factor in HCM. In addition, it has recently been suggested to also cause ubiquitin-proteasome system impairment, which is a regulator of protein levels in cardiac channels. Modification of these cardiac channel levels can lead to electrophysiologic dysfunction and may partly contribute to the clinically observed arrhythmias in patients with HCM.[25]

**Table 3**
**Associations of P-wave abnormalities with AF**

| Study | Patients (n) | Conclusion |
|---|---|---|
| Cecchi et al,[22] 1997 | 110 | Patients with overt AF had greater PWD than those without AF: P-wave ≥140 ms was sensitive, specific, and PPV (56%, 83%, 66%) |
| Ozdemir et al,[23] 2004 | 27, cases vs 53 controls | $P_{max}$ >134.5 ms separated cases with AF and controls with sensitivity 92%, specificity 89%, and PPV 89%. PWD >52.5 ms, 96%, 91%, 84% |
| Kose et al,[24] 2003 | 22 cases 26 controls | PWD could identify patients with HCM. $P_{max}$ in cases = 134 ± 11 and $P_{max}$ control = 128 ± 13. PWD cases: 55 ± 6 and PWD control: 37 ± 8 ms |
| Girasis et al,[15] 2013 | 30 | PWD: 106.9 ± 24.6 vs 86.2 ± 14.3 |

*Abbreviations:* $P_{max}$, maximum P-wave duration; PPV, positive predictive value; PWD, P-wave duration.

Angiotensin-converting enzyme (ACE) insertion/insertion genotype may also be considered a significant risk factor for AF in patients with HCM. A total of 138 patients were genotyped by ACE whether insertion/deletion, deletion/deletion, and insertion/insertion (II). The highest documentation of AF was found in the II genotype of the ACE gene.[26] The endothelin-2 A985 allele was also found with higher frequency in patients who developed AF and may be considered a risk factor.[27] Another study[28] looking at familial HCM caused by Arg663His β-cardiac myosin heavy chain mutation also found 47% of affected individuals to eventually develop AF compared with ungenotyped FHC populations.

### Ischemic
Global hyperemic myocardial blood flow was significantly lower in patients with HCM and AF and with LAD and age was independently associated with AF.[29]

### Other possible risks
Insulin resistance is prevalent among nondiabetic patients with HCM, and its mechanism of causing AF seems to be through its association with LA size. A study[30] found that the strongest determinant of LA size was the homeostasis model assessment index, which can be used as an estimate of incremental vascular resistance. Epicardial adipose tissue (EAT) shows high metabolic activity and may alter activity of autonomic ganglia, leading to susceptibility to arrhythmias. Sixty-two patients with HCM underwent CMR to determine the extent of EAT. EAT area was significantly higher in the group of patients with HCM who were suffering from AF compared with those without AF.[31]

### Exercise intolerance and atrial fibrillation
A prospective study[32] of 86 patients using exercise echocardiography and arrhythmia monitoring was carried out. Thirty-nine of these patients developed arrhythmias (23 premature atrial contractions, 2 AF, 28 premature ventricular contractions [PVCs], 1 nonsustained ventricular tachycardia [NSVT]) during exercise testing. In follow-up of 2.6 ± 2.8 years, 3 deaths occurred along with 12 patients developing AF and 6 developing NSVT. The study concluded that increased exercise duration was associated with fewer events such as AF, sudden cardiac death (SCD), or NSVT. A recent retrospective study used expired gas analysis and exercise intolerance as defined by $Vo_2$ less than 20 mL/kg/min and evaluated an association between HCM and PAF. The study found 55 of the 265 recruited patients to have AF (28 PAF and 27 permanent). After age,

sex, and body mass index adjustment, exercise intolerance remained significantly associated with PAF.[33]

## WOLFF-PARKINSON-WHITE SYNDROME IN HYPERTROPHIC CARDIOMYOPATHY

Cases have been reported of HCM and Wolff-Parkinson-White (WPW) syndrome presenting concurrently, and this may represent a distinct form of HCM. However, whether these cases are primarily caused by HCM or other causes of cardiomyopathy is still under debate. Several case reports have documented the existence of WPW in cases of HCM, suggesting a particular genetic mutation that may account for both diseases.[34–37] A gene has been identified that maps to chromosome 7q35, and this may be the single autosomal dominant cause that accounts for the combination of HCM and WPW.[38]

### Treatment

#### Anticoagulation
Patients with HCM with AF are at high risk of thromboembolism, and thus, anticoagulation is important (Fig. 1). The $CHA_2DS_2$-VASC scoring system for risk of thromboembolism in patients with AF does not apply to patients with HCM. In Olivotto and colleagues' data,[3] patients with HCM and AF had 8-fold the risk of thromboembolic events compared with those patients with HCM without AF. Current American College of Cardiology (ACC)/American Heart Association (AHA)/European Society of Cardiology (ESC) guidelines[39] for the medical treatment of AF in HCM recommend oral vitamin K antagonist anticoagulation with goal international normalized ratio 2.0 to 3.0 for all patients with AF and HCM. Randomized trials of anticoagulant therapy in patients with HCM do not exist; yet, multiple retrospective studies have shown decreased rates of embolic events in patients on warfarin, and anticoagulation should be considered when AF persists for greater than 48 hours or when recurrence is probable.[3,39–41] It has even been suggested that warfarin should be initiated after the first AF paroxysm.[3] There are no HCM-specific data on the newer direct thrombin inhibitors (dabagitran) and the direct factor Xa inhibitors (rivaroxaban and apixaban). In large randomized clinical trials, these agents have been reported superior (dabagatran,[42] apixaban[43]) or noninferior (revaroxaban[44]) to warfarin in patients with AF, but these trials likely had few patients with HCM (also true for the warfarin trials). Yet, it is reasonable to believe that these novel anticoagulants would be useful in patients with HCM.

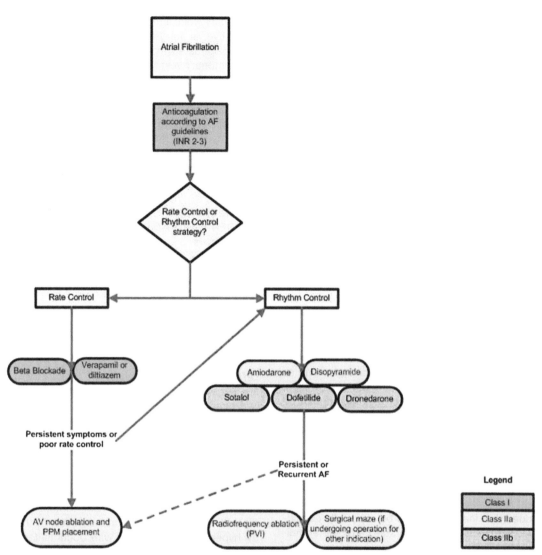

**Fig. 1.** Recommendations for the treatment of AF in patients with HCM. AF, atrial fibrillation; HCM, hypertrophic cardiomyopathy; INR, international normalized ratio; PPM, permanent pacemaker; PVI, pulmonary vein isolation. (*From* Gersh BJ, Maron BJ, Bonow RO, et al. 2011 ACCF/AHA guideline for the diagnosis and treatment of hypertrophic cardiomyopathy: a report of the American College of Cardiology Foundation/American Heart Association Task Force on Practice Guidelines. Developed in collaboration with the American Association for Thoracic Surgery, American Society of Echocardiography, American Society of Nuclear Cardiology, Heart Failure Society of America, Heart Rhythm Society, Society for Cardiovascular Angiography and Interventions, and Society of Thoracic Surgeons. J Am Coll Cardiol 2011;58:e244; with permission.)

### Rhythm control

Data for antiarrythmic agents in HCM are based on small and retrospective studies. Amiodarone is the most effective antiarrhythmic drug for the prevention of AF.[41,45] In 1 small retrospective study of 52 patients with HCM with PAF or chronic AF,[46] amiodarone use was associated with fewer episodes of AF and embolic events compared with class I drugs. In patients initially treated with standard therapy (including digoxin, β-blockers, calcium channel blockers, quinidine, and disopyramide), maintenance of sinus rhythm was achieved in 22 of 38 (58%) compared with 7 of 8 (87%) patients on amiodarone. Over time, 20 of the conventionally treated patients crossed over to amiodarone, and these patients have fewer cardioversions compared with when they were on conventional therapy. Another study[47] noted a return to sinus rhythm in most patients treated with amiodarone, whereas one other[3] found no difference.

Amiodarone therapy is not ideal in this population, given the early onset of the disease and need for long-term treatment.[48]

Disopyramide is used in patients with HCM because of its negative inotropic effects, yet disopyramide is also an antiarrhythmic agent, with some efficacy in AF. In the vast clinical experience of the use of disopyramide for LV outflow tract [LVOT] obstruction, the risk of SCD does not seem to be increased.[49] Yet, in this study, there was no difference in AF between those patients on disopyramide and those not on disopyramide. Sotalol is a class III agent that has efficacy in patients with structural heart disease. In a small study of 7 patients,[50] sotalol was effective in preventing supraventricular arrhythmias. The 2011 AHA guidelines on HCM[39] do list sotalol as an alternative agent in patients with HCM with AF. There are even fewer data on other antiarrhythmic agents. Data on dronedarone and dofetilide are largely anecdotal.

The 2010 ESC AF guidelines[51] promote amiodarone and disopyramide as antiarrhythmic agents for AF in HCM. The 2006 AHA AF guidelines[41] also list amiodarone and disopyramide as antiarrhythmic agents for AF in HCM. In addition, these guidelines state that sotalol should be avoided in substantial LV hypertrophy associated with hypertension. The 2011 AHA HCM guidelines give amiodarone and disopyramide a IIa rating (benefit > > risk; reasonable to use) as agents for rhythm control (see **Fig. 1**).[45] Sotalol, dofetilide, and dronedarone are given IIb status (benefit ≥ risk; use may be considered) but a proviso is added that their use should be especially considered in patients with implantable cardioverter defibrillators (ICDs). Flecainide and propafenone are not recommended.[45]

The 2014 AHA/ACC/Heart Rhythm Society guidelines have included catheter ablation as a treatment modality for rhythm control in patients with failed trials of antiarrhythmic or inability to tolerate medications.[52] However, many studies have found that repeat procedures are often necessary to achieve long-term control of AF. A large study[48] reported an overall 67% success rate. The study did note that 32 (52%) of the 61 patients required additional ablations. Patients requiring additional ablations were older, had larger LA volumes, and higher NYHA functional class. If AF is paroxysmal, success rates are higher (77%) compared with permanent AF (50%).[53] In 43 patients, 28% of whom were paroxysmal, there was a 91% success rate (mean of 1.6 procedures) at 1 year, yet, at the end of median follow-up of 42 months, only 49% of patients remained free of AF or atrial tachycardia.[54] In all patients, pulmonary vein antrum was isolated and found ineffective at long-term prevention of AF. The study suggested that other trigger areas outside the pulmonary vein antrum are most likely responsible for the late recurrences, and more extensive ablation is required for long-term effectiveness.

A diagnosis of AF may influence the decision of whether to undergo alcohol septal ablation or surgical myectomy in patients with symptomatic obstruction.[39] During a surgical myectomy, an LA maze procedure may also be performed, which offers real hope for a reduction of AF burden.

## VENTRICULAR TACHYARRHYTHMIAS/ SUDDEN CARDIAC DEATH
### Risk Factors

Five risk factors have been found to be associated with SCD: family history of sudden death, history of syncope, massive wall thickness, NSVT during Holter monitoring, and abnormal blood pressure response to exercise.[55–57] In addition, the same risk factors were found to be important even in a community-based cohort.[58]

### Left ventricular hypertrophy
In a large study, the magnitude of LV hypertrophy was directly related to the risk of SCD. The risk of sudden death increased progressively in relation to the maximal wall thickness.[59] Another study,[60] using two-dimensional (2D) echocardiography in 30 patients with HCM in whom ventricular tachycardia (VT) had been documented, the extent of LV hypertrophy was compared with a control group of 61 patients with HCM without documented VT. The study found significantly more LV hypertrophy in patients with documented VT (16 of 30, 53%) versus those without VT (13 of 61, 21%, P<.001).

A more recent study[61] including 157 patients with HCM undergoing 2D echocardiography evaluated the ventricular arrhythmia events over a median of 3.7 years. The study looked at maximal LV wall hypertrophy as well as regional hypertrophy such as basal anterior and equatorial inferior wall thickness. Maximal ventricular wall thickness and basal anterior thickness more than 15 mm was associated with a 4.5-fold increase in relative risk of ventricular arrhythmias. In addition, equatorial inferior thicknesses more than 19 mm had a 5.9-fold increase in relative risk. The 2 regional measures (basal and equatorial) were independently associated with arrhythmic risk.

### Syncope
Syncope is found in approximately 14% to 35% of patients suffering from HCM. Unexplained syncope is consistently found to be a predictor of

SCD.[62,63] A large cohort study looking at 1511 patients with HCM[62] found 205 patients to have unexplained or neurally mediated syncope. Over a mean follow-up of $5.6 \pm 5.2$ years, 74 of the 1511 patients died suddenly. Relative risk of sudden death was 1.78 (95% CI 0.00–3.51, $P = .08$) in patients with unexplained syncope and 0.91 (95% CI 0.00–3.83, $P = 1.0$) in those with neurally mediated syncope compared with patients with HCM without syncope. In addition, the study also found that the timing of unexplained syncope was also independently associated with SCD. Patients who had an episode of unexplained syncope within 6 months before initial evaluation had a 5-fold increase in risk compared with patients without syncope (hazard ratio [HR] 4.89%, 95% CI 2.19–10.94). A similar study[64] examining 174 consecutive patients with HCM and with a follow-up of 74 $\pm$ 22 months reported 8 cardiovascular deaths. All 8 patients had a reported history of syncope.

### Family history of sudden death
Family history of sudden death was found as a significant risk factor for sudden death in patients with HCM. Alone, family history has a 1.9 (95% CI 0.8–4.5; $P = .15$) risk ratio. However, when taken with history of syncope, the combined risk ratio is 5.3 (95% CI 1.9–14.9; $P = .002$).[65]

### Nonsustained ventricular tachycardia
In 1380 patients, 24 had NSVT during exercise and 3 had VF.[66] Eight patients of the 27 NSVT or ventricular fibrillation (VF) on exercise group died or had a cardiac event requiring ICD discharge or implant compared with 150 patients without exercise NSVT/VF ($P = .008$). Patients with NSVT or VF had a 3.73-fold increase in risk of sudden death or an ICD discharge (HR 95% CI: 1.61–8.63, $P = .002$). In another study with Holter monitoring,[67] the estimated rate for sudden death was 1.8% per year in patients with NSVT compared with 0.8% in those without NSVT. NSVT has conflicting reports as to its contribution to SCD. In a study in an unselected patient population with HCM,[68] NSVT was not associated with adverse prognosis.

### Abnormal blood pressure response to exercise
Abnormal blood pressure response to exercise was proposed as a marker for increased disease-related mortality in a study by Olivotto and colleagues.[69] An abnormal response to exercise was considered when there was a hypotensive response or a failure to increase blood pressure. Of the 126 patients, 19 had failure of blood pressure to increase and 9 had a hypotensive response. On follow-up of $4.7 \pm 3.7$ years, 9 patients had HCM-related deaths. Four of these 9 had an abnormal

blood pressure response to exercise, and survival analysis found that patients aged 50 years or younger had an increased risk for cardiovascular mortality. However, the positive predictive accuracy was low and the negative predictive accuracy was high, allowing it to possibly be used as a screening test to identify low-risk patients.

### Fibrosis
Myocardial fibrosis is a common finding in patients with HCM that can be determined by LGE. Multiple studies have found associations between the percentage of myocardial fibrosis/scarring as seen by LGE and ventricular tachyarrhythmias.[14,70–73] In the largest study of 1293 patients undergoing CMR, fibrosis as found by LGE correlated linearly with risk of ventricular arrhythmias.[73] LGE of 15% or greater of LV mass showed a 2-fold increase in SCD event risk. In addition, certain locations of scarring may be at an increased likelihood of ventricular arrhythmias. Patients with basal septal scarring on CMR were shown to have higher VT frequency than those patients without (27% vs 5%, $P = .03$),[74] and another study[75] found the number of scarred segments is also a significant factor in the increased arrhythmogenicity of basal septal hypertrophy. In addition, a study looking at signal intensities of LGE found that intermediate signal intensity was a better predictor of ventricular tachyarrhythmias, including NSVT, ventricular couplets, and PVCs, compared with high-intensity LGE (**Table 4**).[13]

### Electrocardiographic parameters
**Heart rate** A recent study of 106 patients with HCM[79] evaluated cardiovascular event end points and Holter monitoring for arrhythmias as a prognostic factor, over a mean of 10.1 years follow-up. The study found no evidence of differences in heart rate on Holter monitoring between patients with or without cardiovascular events. However, the study did note that average heart rates were lower in patients with cardiovascular events (64.7 $\pm$ 11.2 beats/min) versus patients without cardiovascular events (73.7 $\pm$ 10.2 beats/min) ($P = .001$). Average heart rate may be another factor in long-term prognosis in patients with HCM, and further studies are needed to confirm these findings.

**Fragmented QRS** Surface electrocardiographic (ECG) findings have been evaluated to assess risk for future arrhythmic events. Using appropriate ICD therapies as a surrogate, fragmented QRS (fQRS) as seen on surface ECG at ICD implant was found to predict arrhythmic events in patients with HCM along with history of VT/VF. fQRS in the lateral location increased the risk of appropriate ICD therapy ($P<.0001$).[80]

**Table 4**
**Other noninvasive markers of myocardial fibrosis**

| Study | Test/Marker | Patients (n) | Conclusion |
|-------|-------------|--------------|------------|
| Zachariah et al,[76] 2012, | Matrix metalloproteinases (MMP3) | 45 | Circulating MMP3 can be reflective of myocardial fibrosis. MMP3 significantly higher in patients with history of VAs, 12.9 μg vs 5.8 μg |
| Almaas et al, [77] 2013 | Strain echocardiography | 32 | Reduced longitudinal septal strain may be a better correlate with interstitial and total fibrosis compared with LGE |
| Almaas et al,[77] 2013 | Strain echocardiography | 63 | Patients with VA had lower septal longitudinal strain compared with those patients without VA. Reduced longitudinal strain correlated with interstitial fibrosis but not replacement fibrosis |
| Shiozaki et al,[78] 2013 | Myocardial fibrosis mass detected by cardiac computed tomography | 26 | ≥18 g of myocardial fibrosis had a sensitivity for appropriate ICD therapy for 73% and specificity of 71% |
| Chan et al,[73] 2014 | CMR with LGE | 1293 | LGE of ≥15% of LV mass showed a 2-fold increase in SCD event risk |

*Abbreviation:* VA, ventricular arrhythmia.

**QT intervals/dispersions** QT variables have also been evaluated as a part of noninvasive risk stratification. A study found that patients with ECG abnormalities and echo-determined LV hypertrophy (LVH) had maximum QTc interval and QT dispersion significantly longer than patients without ECG abnormalities and echo-determined LVH. Follow-up also showed that 4 SCDs and 1 VF event were observed in this group compared with fewer events in the group without QT dispersion.[81] A large study of 479 patients[82] found the mean QTc to be 440 ± 28 milliseconds and 13% of patients also exceeded 480 milliseconds. The study found that QT prolongation (QTc > 480 milliseconds) to be present in 1 of 8 patients with HCM and should be an important parameter to assess, because it can partly reflect the degree of cardiac hypertrophy and LVOT obstruction in addition to its proarrhythmic potential.

**T-wave alternans** In one study,[83] 53 patients, 27 of whom had T-wave alternans (TWA), which was associated with an increased maximal number of successive ventricular ectopic beats and NSVT as well as histopathologic disarray score. The patients in the previous studies were taken off antiarrhythmics, β-blockers, and calcium channel blockers for at least 5 times their respective half-lives. Another similar study conducted many years later[84] found that TWA cannot be used as a noninvasive test for predicting SCD in HCM; however, this study measured TWA while the patients were maintained on antiarrhythmic medications. A recent third study[85] performing TWA exercise testing and follow-up found TWA to be associated with maximal and regional LV wall thickness, which in itself may increase the arrhythmic vulnerability of patients with HCM.

## PREVENTION OF SUDDEN CARDIAC DEATH
### Medical Management

Medical management of patients with HCM for the prevention of SCD has never been proved.

Amiodarone, β-blockers, calcium antagonists, and type I-A antiarrhythmic agents have been advocated in the hope that they would prevent SCD.[86] Although early reports suggested amiodarone as potentially protective,[47,68,86,87] it is clear that amiodarone does not provide absolute protection from sudden death in patients with HCM.[59,88,89] In addition, amiodarone is associated with significant cumulative toxicity, making it unsuitable for use in young patients.[86]

## Implantable Cardioverter Defibrillators

ICDs in patients with HCM are effective in preventing SCD.[56,86,88–92] The increased heart mass and thickened substrate in HCM have made some question whether ICDs could reliably terminate ventricular arrhythmia; yet, ICDs have been shown to terminate VT and VF.[89,93] High-risk patients with ICDs have annual appropriate discharge rates of 4% to 7%/y, with appropriate

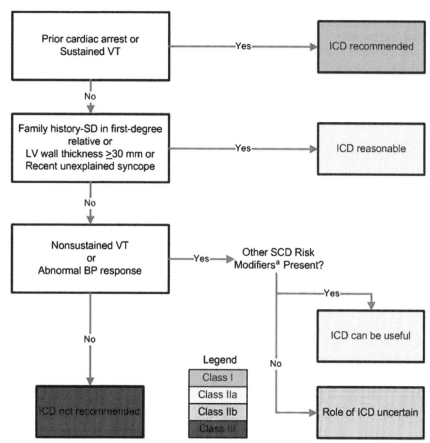

**Fig. 2.** Guidelines for implantation of ICDs in patients with HCM. Patients who survive a cardiac arrest should receive an ICD. For primary prophylaxis, the 3 major risk factors are massively thick myocardium, family history of SCD, and personal history of syncope. [a]For those with NSVT or hypotensive response to exercise, additional risk modifiers (LVOT obstruction, LGE on CMR imaging, LV apical aneurysm, genetic mutations [especially multiple]) may offer guidance in the decision for implantation of an ICD. Regardless of the level of recommendation put forth in these guidelines, the decision for placement of an ICD must involve prudent application of individual clinical judgment, thorough discussions of the strength of evidence, the benefits, and the risks (including but not limited to inappropriate discharges, lead and procedural complications) to allow active participation of the fully informed patient in ultimate decision making. BP, blood pressure; CMR, cardiac magnetic resonance; HCM, hypertrophic cardiomyopathy; ICD, implantable cardioverter defibrillator; LGE, late gadolinium enhancement; LV, left ventricular; LVOT, left ventricular outflow tract obstruction; NSVT, nonsustained ventricular tachycardia; SCD, sudden cardiac death; SD, sudden death. (*From* Gersh BJ, Maron BJ, Bonow RO, et al. 2011 ACCF/AHA guideline for the diagnosis and treatment of hypertrophic cardiomyopathy: a report of the American College of Cardiology Foundation/American Heart Association Task Force on Practice Guidelines. Developed in collaboration with the American Association for Thoracic Surgery, American Society of Echocardiography, American Society of Nuclear Cardiology, Heart Failure Society of America, Heart Rhythm Society, Society for Cardiovascular Angiography and Interventions, and Society of Thoracic Surgeons. J Am Coll Cardiol 2011;58:e240; with permission.)

treatment occurring more frequently when placed for secondary prevention (7%–11%/y) compared with primary prevention (3%–5%/y).[56,89,90,94] In the 2011 AHA HCM guidelines,[39] it is recommended that patients who survive a cardiac arrest should receive an ICD (**Fig. 2**). For primary prophylaxis, the 3 major risk factors are massively thick myocardium, family history of SCD, and personal history of syncope. For those with NSVT or hypotensive response to exercise, additional risk modifiers (LVOT obstruction, LGE on CMR imaging, LV apical aneurysm, genetic mutations [especially multiple]) may offer guidance in the decision for implantation of an ICD. Inappropriate discharges are also common in patients with HCM, with up to 25% receiving inappropriate shocks.[56,89,90,95] Younger age and AF have been associated with inappropriate ICD shocks.[56,90,94] Inappropriate discharge caused by sinus tachycardia, AF, or lead malfunction are the most common ICD complications in HCM, followed by infection, hemorrhage/thrombosis, lead fracture, dislodgement, and oversensing, which are found at rates similar to the general population of patients with pacemakers and ICDs.[95]

## SUMMARY

Atrial and ventricular arrhythmias are common in HCM and contribute to the morbidity and mortality in this condition. Treatment of AF importantly includes anticoagulation. AF rhythm control is difficult and limited by the few antiarrhythmic agents that may be used. Ablation is less successful than in non-HCM patients. The only effective treatment of prevention of SCD is the ICD. Yet, the ICD is not without its own risks in this often young population.

## REFERENCES

1. Maron BJ, Gardin JM, Flack JM, et al. Prevalence of hypertrophic cardiomyopathy in a general population of young adults. Echocardiographic analysis of 4111 subjects in the CARDIA Study. Coronary Artery Risk Development in (Young) Adults. Circulation 1995;92:785–9.
2. Bockstall KE, Link MS. A primer on arrhythmias in patients with hypertrophic cardiomyopathy. Curr Cardiol Rep 2012;14:552–62.
3. Olivotto I, Cecchi F, Casey SA, et al. Impact of atrial fibrillation on the clinical course of hypertrophic cardiomyopathy. Circulation 2001;104:2517–24.
4. Kubo T, Kitaoka H, Okawa M, et al. Clinical impact of atrial fibrillation in patients with hypertrophic cardiomyopathy. Results from Kochi RYOMA Study. Circ J 2009;73:1599–605.
5. Guttmann OP, Rahman MS, O'Mahony C, et al. Atrial fibrillation and thromboembolism in patients with hypertrophic cardiomyopathy: systematic review. Heart 2014;100:465–72.
6. Doi Y, Kitaoka H. Hypertrophic cardiomyopathy in the elderly: significance of atrial fibrillation. J Cardiol 2001;37(Suppl 1):133–8.
7. Melacini P, Basso C, Angelini A, et al. Clinicopathological profiles of progressive heart failure in hypertrophic cardiomyopathy. Eur Heart J 2010;31:2111–23.
8. Tian T, Wang Y, Sun K, et al. Clinical profile and prognostic significance of atrial fibrillation in hypertrophic cardiomyopathy. Cardiology 2013;126:258–64.
9. Siontis KC, Geske JB, Ong K, et al. Atrial fibrillation in hypertrophic cardiomyopathy: prevalence, clinical correlations, and mortality in a large high-risk population. J Am Heart Assoc 2014;3:e001002.
10. Tani T, Tanabe K, Ono M, et al. Left atrial volume and the risk of paroxysmal atrial fibrillation in patients with hypertrophic cardiomyopathy. J Am Soc Echocardiogr 2004;17:644–8.
11. Han ZH, Li Y, Jiang TY, et al. The incidence and predictors of atrial fibrillation in hypertrophic cardiomyopathy. Zhonghua Nei Ke Za Zhi 2008;47:475–7 [in Chinese].
12. Papavassiliu T, Germans T, Fluchter S, et al. CMR findings in patients with hypertrophic cardiomyopathy and atrial fibrillation. J Cardiovasc Magn Reson 2009;11:34.
13. Appelbaum E, Maron BJ, Adabag S, et al. Intermediate-signal-intensity late gadolinium enhancement predicts ventricular tachyarrhythmias in patients with hypertrophic cardiomyopathy. Circ Cardiovasc Imaging 2012;5:78–85.
14. Oka K, Tsujino T, Nakao S, et al. Symptomatic ventricular tachyarrhythmia is associated with delayed gadolinium enhancement in cardiac magnetic resonance imaging and with elevated plasma brain natriuretic peptide level in hypertrophic cardiomyopathy. J Cardiol 2008;52:146–53.
15. Girasis C, Vassilikos V, Efthimiadis GK, et al. Patients with hypertrophic cardiomyopathy at risk for paroxysmal atrial fibrillation: advanced echocardiographic evaluation of the left atrium combined with non-invasive P-wave analysis. Eur Heart J Cardiovasc Imaging 2013;14:425–34.
16. Maron BJ, Haas TS, Maron MS, et al. Left atrial remodeling in hypertrophic cardiomyopathy and susceptibility markers for atrial fibrillation identified by cardiovascular magnetic resonance. Am J Cardiol 2014;113:1394–400.
17. Yamaji K, Fujimoto S, Yutani C, et al. Does the progression of myocardial fibrosis lead to atrial fibrillation in patients with hypertrophic cardiomyopathy? Cardiovasc Pathol 2001;10:297–303.

18. Pujadas S, Vidal-Perez R, Hidalgo A, et al. Correlation between myocardial fibrosis and the occurrence of atrial fibrillation in hypertrophic cardiomyopathy: a cardiac magnetic resonance imaging study. Eur J Radiol 2010;75:e88–91.

19. Pedrosa RP, Drager LF, Genta PR, et al. Obstructive sleep apnea is common and independently associated with atrial fibrillation in patients with hypertrophic cardiomyopathy. Chest 2010;137:1078–84.

20. Konecny T, Brady PA, Orban M, et al. Interactions between sleep disordered breathing and atrial fibrillation in patients with hypertrophic cardiomyopathy. Am J Cardiol 2010;105:1597–602.

21. Holmqvist F, Platonov PG, Carlson J, et al. Variable interatrial conduction illustrated in a hypertrophic cardiomyopathy population. Ann Noninvasive Electrocardiol 2007;12:227–36.

22. Cecchi F, Montereggi A, Olivotto I, et al. Risk for atrial fibrillation in patients with hypertrophic cardiomyopathy assessed by signal averaged P wave duration. Heart 1997;78:44–9.

23. Ozdemir O, Soylu M, Demir AD, et al. P-wave durations as a predictor for atrial fibrillation development in patients with hypertrophic cardiomyopathy. Int J Cardiol 2004;94:163–6.

24. Kose S, Aytemir K, Sade E, et al. Detection of patients with hypertrophic cardiomyopathy at risk for paroxysmal atrial fibrillation during sinus rhythm by P-wave dispersion. Clin Cardiol 2003;26:431–4.

25. Bahrudin U, Morikawa K, Takeuchi A, et al. Impairment of ubiquitin-proteasome system by E334K cMyBPC modifies channel proteins, leading to electrophysiological dysfunction. J Mol Biol 2011;413:857–78.

26. Ogimoto A, Hamada M, Nakura J, et al. Relation between angiotensin-converting enzyme II genotype and atrial fibrillation in Japanese patients with hypertrophic cardiomyopathy. J Hum Genet 2002;47:184–9.

27. Nagai T, Ogimoto A, Okayama H, et al. A985G polymorphism of the endothelin-2 gene and atrial fibrillation in patients with hypertrophic cardiomyopathy. Circ J 2007;71:1932–6.

28. Gruver EJ, Fatkin D, Dodds GA, et al. Familial hypertrophic cardiomyopathy and atrial fibrillation caused by Arg663His beta-cardiac myosin heavy chain mutation. Am J Cardiol 1999;83:13H–8H.

29. Sciagra R, Sotgia B, Olivotto I, et al. Relationship between atrial fibrillation and blunted hyperemic myocardial blood flow in patients with hypertrophic cardiomyopathy. J Nucl Cardiol 2009;16:92–6.

30. Shigematsu Y, Hamada M, Nagai T, et al. Risk for atrial fibrillation in patients with hypertrophic cardiomyopathy: association with insulin resistance. J Cardiol 2011;58:18–25.

31. Muhib S, Fujino T, Sato N, et al. Epicardial adipose tissue is associated with prevalent atrial fibrillation in patients with hypertrophic cardiomyopathy. Int Heart J 2013;54:297–303.

32. Bunch TJ, Chandrasekaran K, Ehrsam JE, et al. Prognostic significance of exercise induced arrhythmias and echocardiographic variables in hypertrophic cardiomyopathy. Am J Cardiol 2007;99:835–8.

33. Azarbal F, Singh M, Finocchiaro G, et al. Exercise capacity and paroxysmal atrial fibrillation in patients with hypertrophic cardiomyopathy. Heart 2014;100:624–30.

34. Ghosh S, Avari JN, Rhee EK, et al. Hypertrophic cardiomyopathy with preexcitation: insights from noninvasive electrocardiographic imaging (ECGI) and catheter mapping. J Cardiovasc Electrophysiol 2008;19:1215–7.

35. Popov VG, Sedov VP. Familial forms of hypertrophic cardiomyopathy. Ter Arkh 1986;58:68–70.

36. Angel J, Armendariz JJ, del Castillo HG, et al. Idiopathic hypertrophic subaortic stenosis and Wolff-Parkinson-White syndrome. Changes of obstruction in left ventricular outflow depending on the type of ventricular activation. Chest 1975;68:248–50.

37. Perosio AM, Suarez LD, Bunster AM, et al. Pre-excitation syndrome and hypertrophic cardiomyopathy. J Electrocardiol 1983;16:29–40.

38. MacRae CA, Ghaisas N, Kass S, et al. Familial hypertrophic cardiomyopathy with Wolff-Parkinson-White syndrome maps to a locus on chromosome 7q3. J Clin Invest 1995;96:1216–20.

39. Gersh BJ, Maron BJ, Bonow RO, et al. 2011 ACCF/AHA guideline for the diagnosis and treatment of hypertrophic cardiomyopathy: a report of the American College of Cardiology Foundation/American Heart Association Task Force on Practice Guidelines. Developed in collaboration with the American Association for Thoracic Surgery, American Society of Echocardiography, American Society of Nuclear Cardiology, Heart Failure Society of America, Heart Rhythm Society, Society for Cardiovascular Angiography and Interventions, and Society of Thoracic Surgeons. J Am Coll Cardiol 2011;58:e212–60.

40. Maron BJ. Hypertrophic cardiomyopathy; a systemic review. JAMA 2002;287:1308–20.

41. Fuster V, Ryden LE, Cannom DS, et al. ACC/AHA/ESC 2006 guidelines for the management of patients with atrial fibrillation: a report of the American College of Cardiology/American Heart Association Task Force on Practice Guidelines and the European Society of Cardiology Committee for Practice Guidelines (writing committee to revise the 2001 guidelines for the management of patients with atrial fibrillation): developed in collaboration with the European Heart Rhythm Association and the Heart Rhythm Society. Circulation 2006;114:e257–354.

42. Connolly SJ, Ezekowitz MD, Yusuf S, et al. Dabigatran versus warfarin in patients with atrial fibrillation. N Engl J Med 2009;361:1139–51.

43. Granger CB, Alexander JH, McMurray JJ, et al. Apixaban versus warfarin in patients with atrial fibrillation. N Engl J Med 2011;365:981–92.

44. Patel MR, Mahaffey KW, Garg J, et al. Rivaroxaban versus warfarin in nonvalvular atrial fibrillation. N Engl J Med 2011;365:883–91.

45. Gersh BJ, Maron BJ, Bonow RO, et al. 2011 ACCF/AHA guideline for the diagnosis and treatment of hypertrophic cardiomyopathy: a report of the American College of Cardiology Foundation/American Heart Association Task Force on Practice Guidelines. Circulation 2011;124:e783–831.

46. Robinson K, Frenneaux MP, Stockins B, et al. Atrial fibrillation in hypertrophic cardiomyopathy: a longitudinal study. J Am Coll Cardiol 1990;15:1279–85.

47. McKenna WJ, Harris L, Rowland E, et al. Amiodarone for long-term management of patients with hypertrophic cardiomyopathy. Am J Cardiol 1984;54:802–10.

48. Di Donna P, Olivotto I, Delcre SD, et al. Efficacy of catheter ablation for atrial fibrillation in hypertrophic cardiomyopathy: impact of age, atrial remodelling, and disease progression. Europace 2010;12:347–55.

49. Sherrid MV, Barac I, McKenna WJ, et al. Multicenter study of the efficacy and safety of disopyramide in obstructive hypertrophic cardiomyopathy. J Am Coll Cardiol 2005;45:1251–8.

50. Tendera M, Wycisk A, Schneeweiss A, et al. Effect of sotalol on arrhythmias and exercise tolerance in patients with hypertrophic cardiomyopathy. Cardiology 1993;82:335–42.

51. Camm AJ, Kirchhof P, Lip GY, et al. Guidelines for the management of atrial fibrillation: the task force for the management of atrial fibrillation of the European Society of Cardiology (ESC). Eur Heart J 2010;31:2369–429.

52. January CT, Wann LS, Alpert JS, et al. 2014 AHA/ACC/HRS guideline for the management of patients with atrial fibrillation: executive summary: a report of the American College of Cardiology/American Heart Association Task Force on Practice Guidelines and the Heart Rhythm Society. J Am Coll Cardiol 2014;64:2246–80.

53. Gaita F, Di Donna P, Olivotto I, et al. Usefulness and safety of transcatheter ablation of atrial fibrillation in patients with hypertrophic cardiomyopathy. Am J Cardiol 2007;99:1575–81.

54. Santangeli P, Di Biase L, Themistoclakis S, et al. Catheter ablation of atrial fibrillation in hypertrophic cardiomyopathy: long-term outcomes and mechanisms of arrhythmia recurrence. Circ Arrhythm Electrophysiol 2013;6:1089–94.

55. Dimitrow PP, Chojnowska L, Rudzinski T, et al. Sudden death in hypertrophic cardiomyopathy: old risk factors re-assessed in a new model of maximalized follow-up. Eur Heart J 2010;31:3084–93.

56. Maron BJ, Spirito P, Ackerman MJ, et al. Prevention of sudden cardiac death with implantable cardioverter-defibrillators in children and adolescents with hypertrophic cardiomyopathy. J Am Coll Cardiol 2013;61:1527–35.

57. Gersh BJ, Maron BJ, Bonow RO, et al. 2011 ACCF/AHA guideline for the diagnosis and treatment of hypertrophic cardiomyopathy: executive summary: a report of the American College of Cardiology Foundation/American Heart Association Task Force on Practice Guidelines. Circulation 2011;124:2761–96.

58. Anastasakis A, Theopistou A, Rigopoulos A, et al. Sudden cardiac death: investigation of the classical risk factors in a community-based hypertrophic cardiomyopathy cohort. Hellenic J Cardiol 2013;54:281–8.

59. Spirito P, Bellone P, Harris KM, et al. Magnitude of left ventricular hypertrophy and risk of sudden death in hypertrophic cardiomyopathy. N Engl J Med 2000;342:1778–85.

60. Spirito P, Watson RM, Maron BJ. Relation between extent of left ventricular hypertrophy and occurrence of ventricular tachycardia in hypertrophic cardiomyopathy. Am J Cardiol 1987;60:1137–42.

61. Puntmann VO, Yap YG, McKenna W, et al. Significance of maximal and regional left ventricular wall thickness in association with arrhythmic events in patients with hypertrophic cardiomyopathy. Circ J 2010;74:531–7.

62. Spirito P, Autore C, Rapezzi C, et al. Syncope and risk of sudden death in hypertrophic cardiomyopathy. Circulation 2009;119:1703–10.

63. Fananapazir L, Chang AC, Epstein SE, et al. Prognostic determinants in hypertrophic cardiomyopathy. Prospective evaluation of a therapeutic strategy based on clinical, Holter, hemodynamic, and electrophysiological findings. Circulation 1992;86:730–40.

64. Kyriakidis M, Triposkiadis F, Anastasakis A, et al. Hypertrophic cardiomyopathy in Greece: clinical course and outcome. Chest 1998;114:1091–6.

65. Elliott PM, Poloniecki J, Dickie S, et al. Sudden death in hypertrophic cardiomyopathy: identification of high risk patients. J Am Coll Cardiol 2000;36:2212–8.

66. Gimeno JR, Tome-Esteban M, Lofiego C, et al. Exercise-induced ventricular arrhythmias and risk of sudden cardiac death in patients with hypertrophic cardiomyopathy. Eur Heart J 2009;30:2599–605.

67. Adabag AS, Casey SA, Kuskowski MA, et al. Spectrum and prognostic significance of arrhythmias on ambulatory Holter electrocardiogram in hypertrophic cardiomyopathy. J Am Coll Cardiol 2005;45:697–704.

68. Cecchi F, Olivotto I, Montereggi A, et al. Prognostic value of non-sustained ventricular tachycardia and the potential role of amiodarone treatment in hypertrophic cardiomyopathy: assessment in an unselected non-referral based patient population. Heart 1998;79:331–6.

69. Olivotto I, Maron BJ, Montereggi A, et al. Prognostic value of systemic blood pressure response during exercise in a community-based patient population with hypertrophic cardiomyopathy. J Am Coll Cardiol 1999;33:2044–51.

70. Kwon DH, Setser RM, Popovic ZB, et al. Association of myocardial fibrosis, electrocardiography and ventricular tachyarrhythmia in hypertrophic cardiomyopathy: a delayed contrast enhanced MRI study. Int J Cardiovasc Imaging 2008;24:617–25.

71. Adabag AS, Maron BJ, Appelbaum E, et al. Occurrence and frequency of arrhythmias in hypertrophic cardiomyopathy in relation to delayed enhancement on cardiovascular magnetic resonance. J Am Coll Cardiol 2008;51:1369–74.

72. Leonardi S, Raineri C, De Ferrari GM, et al. Usefulness of cardiac magnetic resonance in assessing the risk of ventricular arrhythmias and sudden death in patients with hypertrophic cardiomyopathy. Eur Heart J 2009;30:2003–10.

73. Chan RH, Maron BJ, Olivotto I, et al. Prognostic value of quantitative contrast-enhanced cardiovascular magnetic resonance for the evaluation of sudden death risk in patients with hypertrophic cardiomyopathy. Circulation 2014;130:484–95.

74. Kwon DH, Smedira NG, Rodriguez ER, et al. Cardiac magnetic resonance detection of myocardial scarring in hypertrophic cardiomyopathy: correlation with histopathology and prevalence of ventricular tachycardia. J Am Coll Cardiol 2009;54:242–9.

75. Amano Y, Kitamura M, Tachi M, et al. Delayed enhancement magnetic resonance imaging in hypertrophic cardiomyopathy with basal septal hypertrophy and preserved ejection fraction: relationship with ventricular tachyarrhythmia. J Comput Assist Tomogr 2014;38:67–71.

76. Zachariah JP, Colan SD, Lang P, et al. Circulating matrix metalloproteinases in adolescents with hypertrophic cardiomyopathy and ventricular arrhythmia. Circ Heart Fail 2012;5:462–6.

77. Almaas VM, Haugaa KH, Strom EH, et al. Increased amount of interstitial fibrosis predicts ventricular arrhythmias, and is associated with reduced myocardial septal function in patients with obstructive hypertrophic cardiomyopathy. Europace 2013;15:1319–27.

78. Shiozaki AA, Senra T, Arteaga E, et al. Myocardial fibrosis detected by cardiac CT predicts ventricular fibrillation/ventricular tachycardia events in patients with hypertrophic cardiomyopathy. J Cardiovasc Comput Tomogr 2013;7:173–81.

79. Kawasaki T, Sakai C, Harimoto K, et al. Holter monitoring and long-term prognosis in hypertrophic cardiomyopathy. Cardiology 2012;122:44–54.

80. Femenia F, Arce M, Van Grieken J, et al. Fragmented QRS as a predictor of arrhythmic events in patients with hypertrophic obstructive cardiomyopathy. J Interv Card Electrophysiol 2013;38:159–65.

81. Uchiyama K, Hayashi K, Fujino N, et al. Impact of QT variables on clinical outcome of genotyped hypertrophic cardiomyopathy. Ann Noninvasive Electrocardiol 2009;14:65–71.

82. Johnson JN, Grifoni C, Bos JM, et al. Prevalence and clinical correlates of QT prolongation in patients with hypertrophic cardiomyopathy. Eur Heart J 2011;32:1114–20.

83. Kuroda N, Ohnishi Y, Yoshida A, et al. Clinical significance of T-wave alternans in hypertrophic cardiomyopathy. Circ J 2002;66:457–62.

84. Fuchs T, Torjman A. The usefulness of microvolt T-wave alternans in the risk stratification of patients with hypertrophic cardiomyopathy. Isr Med Assoc J 2009;11:606–10.

85. Puntmann VO, Yap YG, McKenna W, et al. T-wave alternans and left ventricular wall thickness in predicting arrhythmic risk in patients with hypertrophic cardiomyopathy. Circ J 2010;74:1197–204.

86. Maron BJ, Estes NA 3rd, Maron MS, et al. Primary prevention of sudden death as a novel treatment strategy in hypertrophic cardiomyopathy. Circulation 2003;107:2872–5.

87. McKenna WJ, Oakley CM, Krikler DM, et al. Improved survival with amiodarone in patients with hypertrophic cardiomyopathy and ventricular tachycardia. Br Heart J 1985;53:412–6.

88. Melacini P, Maron BJ, Bobbo F, et al. Evidence that pharmacological strategies lack efficacy for the prevention of sudden death in hypertrophic cardiomyopathy. Heart 2007;93:708–10.

89. Maron BJ, Shen WK, Link MS, et al. Efficacy of implantable cardioverter-defibrillators for the prevention of sudden death in patients with hypertrophic cardiomyopathy. N Engl J Med 2000;342:365–73.

90. Maron BJ, Spirito P, Shen WK, et al. Implantable cardioverter-defibrillators and prevention of sudden cardiac death in hypertrophic cardiomyopathy. JAMA 2007;298:405–12.

91. Epstein AE, DiMarco JP, Ellenbogen KA, et al. ACC/AHA/HRS 2008 guidelines for device-based therapy for cardiac rhythm abnormalities: a report of the American College of Cardiology/American Heart Association Task Force on Practice Guidelines (writing committee to revise the ACC/AHA/NASPE 2002 guideline update for implantation of cardiac pacemakers and antiarrhythmia devices) developed in collaboration with the American Association for Thoracic Surgery and Society of Thoracic Surgeons. J Am Coll Cardiol 2008;51:e1–62.

92. Zipes DP, Camm AJ, Borggrefe M, et al. ACC/AHA/ESC 2006 guidelines for management of patients with ventricular arrhythmias and the prevention of sudden cardiac death: a report of the American College of Cardiology/American Heart Association Task Force and the European Society of Cardiology

Committee for Practice Guidelines (writing committee to develop guidelines for management of patients with ventricular arrhythmias and the prevention of sudden cardiac death): developed in collaboration with the European Heart Rhythm Association and the Heart Rhythm Society. Circulation 2006;114:e385–484.

93. Alsheikh-Ali AA, Link MS, Semsarian C, et al. Ventricular tachycardia/fibrillation early after defibrillator implantation in patients with hypertrophic cardiomyopathy is explained by a high-risk subgroup of patients. Heart Rhythm 2013;10:214–8.

94. Woo A, Monakier D, Harris L, et al. Determinants of implantable defibrillator discharges in high-risk patients with hypertrophic cardiomyopathy. Heart 2007;93:1044–5.

95. Lin G, Nishimura RA, Gersh BJ, et al. Device complications and inappropriate implantable cardioverter defibrillator shocks in patients with hypertrophic cardiomyopathy. Heart 2009;95:709–14.

# The Role of Cardiovascular Magnetic Resonance in Sudden Death Risk Stratification in Hypertrophic Cardiomyopathy

Martin S. Maron, MD

## KEYWORDS

- Hypertrophic cardiomyopathy • Cardiovascular magnetic resonance • Sudden death
- Myocardial fibrosis • Late gadolinium enhancement

## KEY POINTS

- Hypertrophic cardiomyopathy (HCM) is the leading cause of sudden death in young patients; although current risk factor strategy is very effective, not all high-risk patients are identified.
- Contrast-enhanced cardiovascular magnetic resonance (CMR) with late gadolinium enhancement (LGE) can identify areas of myocardial fibrosis where potentially life-threatening ventricular arrhythmias originate.
- HCM patients with LGE have a 7-fold greater risk for nonsustained ventricular tachycardia compared with patients without LGE.
- Extensive LGE ($\geq$15% of left ventricular [LV] mass) is an emerging risk marker for sudden death events, even in HCM patients without conventional risk factors.
- The absence of LGE in patients with HCM is associated with low risk and is a measure of reassurance for patients.
- Other high-risk HCM subgroups can be reliably identified with CMR, including patients who develop LV apical aneurysm and those with massive LV hypertrophy.

## INTRODUCTION

Hypertrophic cardiomyopathy (HCM) is the most common genetic heart disease and the leading cause of sudden death in young people, including competitive athletes.[1,2] Recently, cardiovascular magnetic resonance (CMR), with its high spatial resolution and tomographic imaging capability, has emerged as an important complementary imaging technique to echocardiography with the opportunity to provide unique clinical information.[3–6] For example, CMR can precisely characterize the location, distribution, and extent of left ventricular (LV) hypertrophy, and can be superior to echocardiography for HCM diagnosis by identifying areas of segmental hypertrophy not reliably visualized by echocardiography (or underestimated in terms of extent), which can improve diagnostic strategies.[7–9]

However, over the last decade it is the unique capability of contrast-enhanced CMR with late gadolinium enhancement (LGE) to identify myocardial fibrosis, the structural nidus for the generation of potentially life-threatening ventricular arrhythmias,[10] which has generated the greatest enthusiasm for the notion that LGE may enhance risk stratification in HCM.[6] These

The author has nothing to disclose.
Division of Cardiology, Hypertrophic Cardiomyopathy Center, Tufts Medical Center, #70, 800 Washington Street, Boston, MA 02111, USA
E-mail address: mmaron@tuftsmedicalcenter.org

observations underscore an important role for CMR in the contemporary assessment of patients with HCM, providing important information that affects diagnosis and risk stratification.

## CURRENT RISK STRATIFICATION STRATEGY IN HYPERTROPHIC CARDIOMYOPATHY

Sudden death remains the most devastating consequence of HCM and the most frequent cause of sudden death in competitive athletes in the United States.[1,2] Sudden death in HCM occurs most commonly in young patients and significantly less in patients of advanced ages ($\geq$60 years), and is often the initial clinical manifestation of HCM.[1] However, intense vigorous exertional activity, such as with most organized competitive sports, is also associated with an increased risk of sudden death in patients with HCM.[2,11] The mechanism of sudden death is primary ventricular tachycardia/ fibrillation (VT/VF) originating from an unstable electrophysiologic substrate, which includes an abnormal arrangement of hypertrophied myocytes, with an expanded extracellular space composed of interstitial fibrosis and replacement scar resulting from bursts of silent microvascular ischemia (caused by structurally abnormal intramural coronary arteries).[1,10]

Over the last 5 decades, several noninvasive risk markers have emerged to comprise a primary prevention risk stratification model, in an effort to identify HCM patients at highest risk for potentially life-threatening VT/VF.[2,12] These risk factors include: (1) family history of premature HCM-related sudden death, in close or multiple relatives; (2) unexplained syncope judged nonneurocardiogenic, particularly if recent and in young patients; (3) nonsustained VT on serial ambulatory electrocardiogram (ECG), particularly when bursts are multiple, repetitive, or prolonged; (4) hypotensive or attenuated blood pressure response to exercise; and (5) extreme LV hypertrophy (wall thickness $\geq$30 mm).[2,12] Secondary prevention with an implantable cardioverter-defibrillator (ICD) is indicated in patients with a history of prior cardiac arrest or spontaneous, sustained VT.[1,12]

Risk for sudden death is increased in proportion to the absolute number of risk factors.[12] However, one risk factor alone may be sufficient to increase the risk enough in an HCM patient for that individual to be considered for life-saving therapy with primary prevention ICD, particularly in a patient with 1 of the 3 strongest risk markers: massive LV hypertrophy, family history of sudden death, or recent unexplained syncope.[13] For those patients considered at high risk (ie, patients with 1 or more of the previously stated primary risk factors) the ICD has proved efficacious at preventing sudden death (Fig. 1).[1,2,13] In a recent multicenter study with more than 500 HCM patients, the ICD delivered an appropriate shock for VT/VF in 20% of patients, who were implanted for primary or secondary prevention, over a follow-up period of less than 4 years.[13] Appropriate device interventions occurred at 11% per year for secondary prevention and 4% per year for those patients implanted for primary prevention. The current risk stratification strategy and the ICD seem to have substantially affected the natural history of HCM, with HCM-related mortality rates decreasing to very low and less than those of the pre-ICD treatment era.[1]

## LIMITATIONS OF RISK STRATIFICATION IN HYPERTROPHIC CARDIOMYOPATHY

Although the noninvasive clinical risk markers have proved to be highly effective in identifying many HCM patients at increased risk for sudden death who will benefit from primary prevention ICDs, the HCM risk algorithm is incomplete.[14] For example, sudden death risk in patients without conventional risk markers is 0.5% per year, meaning that a minority of high-risk patients remains unrecognized with the current risk stratification algorithm.[14] In addition, nearly half of clinically identified HCM patients have 1 or more risk factors so a substantial proportion of the HCM patient population could be considered at risk, leading to overtreatment with ICDs in some patients.[12] Furthermore, high-risk stratus remains ambiguous (ie, "gray zone") in a subgroup of patients (particularly those with 1 risk factor), making decision making about ICDs complex. These observations underscore the need for additional strategies to improve risk prediction for sudden death.

## CONTRAST-ENHANCED CARDIOVASCULAR MAGNETIC RESONANCE

Following the intravenous injection of gadolinium, contrast-enhanced CMR images can detect areas of high signal intensity LGE in the LV myocardium (Fig. 2). Several observations support the principle that LGE represents the arrhythmogenic substrate of myocardial fibrosis in HCM. For example, in ventricular septal tissue removed from HCM patients at the time of surgical myectomy, there is a strong association between the extent of fibrosis assessed by histologic examination and LGE (as determined from preoperative contrast-enhanced CMR studies).[15] In addition, CMR findings of LGE correlate to areas of myocardial fibrosis by histologic evaluation in HCM patients undergoing transplant.[16]

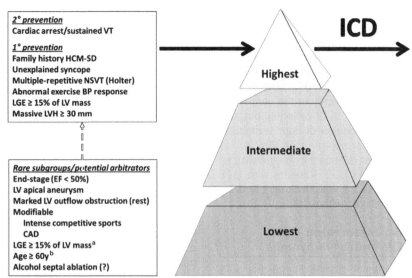

**Fig. 1.** Pyramid profile of risk stratification model currently used to identify patients at the highest risk who may be candidates for ICDs and prevention of sudden death. Major and minor risk markers appear in boxes at the left. [a] Extensive LGE is a novel primary risk marker that can also be used as an arbitrator when conventional risk assessment is ambiguous. [b] Sudden death events uncommon after age 60 years, even with conventional risk factors. CAD, coronary artery disease; EF, ejection fraction; HCM, hypertrophic cardiomyopathy; ICD, implantable cardioverter-defibrillator; LGE, late gadolinium enhancement; LV, left ventricular; LVH, left ventricular hypertrophy; NSVT, nonsustained ventricular tachycardia; SD, sudden death; VT/VF, ventricular tachycardia/ventricular fibrillation; y, years. (*Adapted from* Maron BJ, Ommen SR, Semsarian C, et al. Hypertrophic cardiomyopathy: present and future, with translation into contemporary cardiovascular medicine. J Am Coll Cardiol 2014;64:89; with permission.)

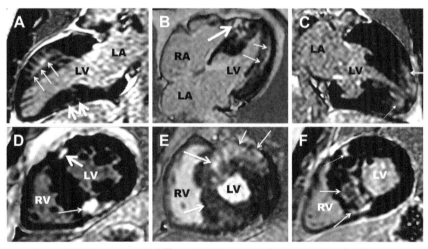

**Fig. 2.** Contrast-enhanced CMR images in 6 different HCM patients demonstrating the diverse pattern and extent of late gadolinium enhancement (LGE) in this disease. (*A*) extensive transmural LGE in the anterior wall (*small arrows*) with smaller focal area in the inferior wall (*large arrows*). (*B*) mid-myocardial LGE in the lateral wall (*small arrows*) and diffuse LGE in the ventricular septum that extends into the RV wall (*large arrow*) in a 26-year-old man with end-stage phase HCM with an ejection fraction of 40%. (*C*) LGE confined to the LV apex (*arrows*). (*D*) LGE localized to the insertion area of the RV wall into the anterior (*large arrow*) and posterior ventricular septum (*small arrow*). (*E*) transmural LGE involving most of the ventricular septum (*large arrow*) and lateral wall (*small arrows*). (*F*) Basal short-axis image with transmural LGE located predominantly in the ventricular septum (*arrows*). LA, left atrium; LV, left ventricle; RA, right atrium; RV, right ventricle. (*From* Maron MS. Clinical utility of cardiovascular magnetic resonance in hypertrophic cardiomyopathy. J Cardiovasc Magn Reson 2012;14:13.)

Areas of LGE can be quantified and expressed as a percentage of the total LV mass. Approximately 50% of HCM patients demonstrate LGE which, when present, occupies on average 10% of the overall LV myocardial volume.[6,17] LGE can be observed in any location or distribution in HCM, although most frequently in the ventricular septum and free wall (>30% of patients), but less often the apex and the areas of right ventricular insertion into ventricular septum (see **Fig. 2**).[17] A significant but modest relationship is present between hypertrophy and LGE. Patients with LGE have greater maximal LV wall thickness and LV mass index than patients without LGE.[17]

### Late Gadolinium Enhancement and Nonsustained Ventricular Tachycardia

Several cross-sectional studies in patients with HCM have demonstrated a strong association between the presence of LGE and ventricular tachyarrhythmias on ambulatory 24-hour Holter ECG. HCM patients with LGE have up to a 7-fold increased risk for ambulatory nonsustained ventricular tachyarrhythmias compared with those without LGE (**Fig. 3**).[10] These observations suggest that LGE represents the unstable arrhythmogenic substrate responsible for ventricular tachyarrhythmias in HCM. As NSVT is an independent risk factor for sudden death in this disease, the relationship between ambulatory ventricular tachyarrhythmia and LGE raised the possibility that contrast-enhanced CMR could represent a novel risk marker to identify HCM patients at increased risk of sudden death and candidates for ICD preventive therapy.[6]

### Sudden Death

Several prospective outcome studies have demonstrated an association between the

presence of LGE and a combined end-point of adverse HCM-related events.[17-22] However, these studies have conflicting results regarding the relation between LGE and sudden death and the appropriate therapy for VT/VF.[22] When data from these studies were combined, LGE was more common in patients who experienced sudden death or an appropriate ICD discharge than those who did not, resulting in a significant but weak relationship between the presence of LGE and the risk for sudden death.[22]

Another point in establishing clinical relevance for contrast-enhanced CMR is the relationship of presence versus extent of LGE with respect to outcome. Most follow-up contrast-enhanced CMR studies have reported only an association between the presence of LGE and sudden death.[17,20-22] However, the reported prevalence of LGE is greater than 50%.[6,17-22] Therefore, even if some relationship could be derived between the presence of LGE and sudden death, LGE alone would not qualify as a practical risk marker because simply too many HCM patients would be identified for primary prevention ICDs.[10] Therefore, for contrast-enhanced CMR to be a clinically useful tool for management decisions, it will likely be necessary to ultimately demonstrate that risk of adverse outcome is related to the extent of LGE.[1,6,18]

More recently, a large, multicenter, international prospective study of nearly 1300 HCM patients was completed, in which extent of LGE emerged as a strong predictor of future sudden death risk.[18] Indeed, a continuous relationship was present between the amount of LGE and sudden death risk, with substantial LGE ($\geq$15% of LV mass) associated with a 2-fold greater risk of sudden death compared with patients without LGE, even in patients without conventional sudden death risk factors (**Fig. 4**).[18] On the other hand,

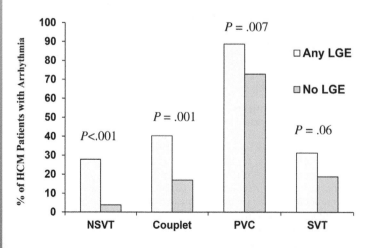

Fig. 3. Prevalence of arrhythmia on 24-hour Holter ECG with respect to presence of LGE in patients with HCM. HCM, hypertrophic cardiomyopathy. PVC, premature ventricular contraction; SVT, supraventricular tachycardia. (Adapted from Adabag AS, Maron BJ, Appelbaum E, et al. Occurrence and frequency of arrhythmias in hypertrophic cardiomyopathy in relation to delayed enhancement on cardiovascular magnetic resonance. J Am Coll Cardiol 2008;51:1371; with permission.)

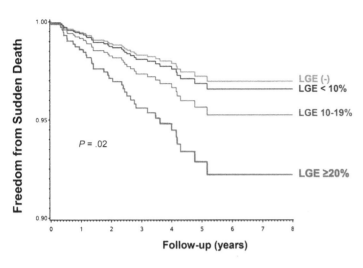

**Fig. 4.** Relation between extent of late gadolinium enhancement (LGE) and sudden death events in 1293 patients with HCM. Hazard plot based on multivariable Cox regression analysis ($P = .02$). Continuous relationship between amount of LGE and risk of SD. This relationship was independent of several other relevant clinical variables that could influence SD. (*From* Chan RH, Maron BJ, Olivotto I, et al. Prognostic value of quantitative contrast-enhanced cardiovascular magnetic resonance for the evaluation of sudden death risk in patients with hypertrophic cardiomyopathy. Circulation 2014;130:490; with permission.)

patients without LGE had a relatively benign course and low risk for adverse events, providing a measure of reassurance (see **Fig. 4**).[18] In addition, when the results of contrast-enhanced CMR were used in conjunction with the traditional sudden death risk factors, the extent of LGE strengthened the current sudden death risk model by providing information that improved the ability to identify high-risk patients (**Fig. 5**).

These findings suggest that the results of contrast-enhanced CMR can be used to improve on the current risk stratification strategy in HCM in 2 important areas. First, extensive LGE can identify a novel subgroup of relatively young, asymptomatic HCM patients without conventional sudden death risk factors (and who therefore would be considered without clinical evidence of high-risk status), but who nevertheless are at increased risk for sudden death (see **Fig. 4**).[1,18] These patients may benefit from consideration of ICDs to prevent a catastrophic event. Second, results of contrast-enhanced CMR may also help resolve complex decisions regarding ICDs for patients in whom sudden death risk remains ambiguous after standard risk stratification. For example, in many HCM patients the importance of a single risk marker may be poorly or incompletely defined (the "gray zone" of HCM risk stratification) such as young HCM patients with only 1 burst of NSVT on ambulatory Holter monitoring or older HCM patients with unexplained syncope.[1,18] In these clinical scenarios, extensive LGE can potentially act as an arbitrator by swaying toward a recommendation for ICD and away from device therapy in those with no (or little) LGE (see **Fig. 5**).

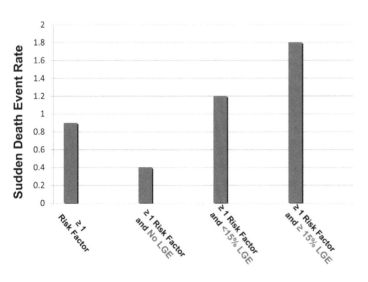

**Fig. 5.** Relation between extent of late gadolinium enhancement (LGE) and sudden death events in 1293 patients with HCM with 1 or more conventional sudden death risk factors. LGE improves or strengthens the SD risk model. The model performance metrics (area under the curve, integrated discrimination improvement, net reclassification index) also demonstrate improvement of the conventional SD risk model after adding LGE. (*Data from* Chan RH, Maron BJ, Olivotto I, et al. Prognostic value of quantitative contrast-enhanced cardiovascular magnetic resonance for the evaluation of sudden death risk in patients with hypertrophic cardiomyopathy. Circulation 2014;130:484–95.)

## End-Stage Hypertrophic Cardiomyopathy

A small subgroup of HCM patients develop systolic dysfunction (ejection fraction <50%), as a result of a process of accelerated myocardial fibrosis leading to adverse LV remodeling.[23] The end-stage phase of HCM is associated with an increased risk for sudden death and progressive symptoms of heart failure.[1,2,23] Extensive LGE (≥20% of the total LV mass) has also emerged as a marker to prospectively identify HCM patients with preserved systolic function who are at increased risk for future progression and development to the end-stage phase of HCM.[18] The capability to identify patients who will progress to the end-stage before adverse LV remodeling associated with systolic dysfunction is evident, is clinically relevant by permitting potentially important changes in management strategies, including tailored drug administration and early consideration for heart transplantation and prophylactic defibrillators.[1,2,23]

## ADDITIONAL HIGH-RISK SUBGROUPS
### Left Ventricular Apical Aneurysm

The ability with CMR to provide imaging of the distal LV chamber at high spatial resolution, not encumbered by thoracic and pulmonary parenchyma, has resulted in the increased recognition and visibility in clinical cardiovascular practice of a unique subgroup of HCM patients with LV apical aneurysm.[24] The junction of scarred aneurysm rim and LV myocardium provides another nidus for the generation of ventricular tachyarrhythmias (in addition to an already myopathic ventricle),[25] and a focus of blood stasis in the aneurysm and thrombus formation.[24] Recognition of these patients is critical, as they are a high-risk subgroup remaining at increased risk of sudden death and thromboembolic events, prompting consideration for certain management interventions including primary prevention ICD therapy, anticoagulation with coumadin to prevent stroke, and VT ablation.[1,2,24,25] CMR can identify apical aneurysm (particularly when small in size) when not detected by echocardiography, in addition to the presence and extent of fibrosis contained within the aneurysm rim and in adjacent areas of myocardium.[24]

### Massive Left Ventricular Hypertrophy

Noninvasive imaging of LV wall thickness has been proved to have a role in risk stratification, with massive LV hypertrophy of 30 mm or larger that is demonstrated by 2-dimensional echocardiography anywhere in the LV chamber identifies those HCM patients at highest risk and potentially deserving of ICD therapy for primary prevention of sudden death.[1,2] Indeed, the presence of massive hypertrophy alone, in the absence of any additional risk markers, may be enough to recommend ICD therapy for primary prevention of sudden death.[2] Therefore, accurate assessment of maximal wall thickness is an essential part of the initial evaluation of all HCM patients. In this regard, measures of LV wall thickness in some patients may also be underestimated by echocardiography relative to CMR. This point may have important management implications, particularly in those HCM patients in whom massive LV hypertrophy (wall thickness ≥30 mm, and an independent risk factor for sudden death) is detected by CMR but in whom a lesser extent of wall thickening was seen with echocardiography.[9]

### Left Ventricular Mass

Because of the variable distribution of LV hypertrophy in regions of the LV chamber remote from maximal wall thickness, CMR-derived LV mass provides the most accurate assessment of the overall extent of LV hypertrophy.[26] As a result, LV mass may represent a marker for adverse risk and would therefore seem to hold promise for aiding in risk stratification. However, long-term prospective CMR studies are needed before establishing the precise relationship between LV mass and outcome in this disease.

## SUMMARY

CMR with LGE has emerged as an important imaging technique to improve diagnosis and risk assessment in patients with HCM. Extensive areas of fibrosis are associated with increased risk for sudden death events, even in HCM patients without conventional risk factors, and may identify patients for potentially life-saving therapy with primary prevention ICD. In addition, for those patients in the "gray zone" of risk stratification, extensive LGE may arbitrate complex ICD decision making. The absence of LGE is associated with lower risk and is a source of reassurance to patients. In addition, CMR may identify other high-risk subgroups within the diverse HCM disease spectrum, including patients with LV apical aneurysm and massive LV hypertrophy.

## REFERENCES

1. Maron BJ, Ommen SR, Semsarian C, et al. Hypertrophic cardiomyopathy: present and future, with translation into contemporary cardiovascular medicine. J Am Coll Cardiol 2014;64:83–99.

2. Gersh BJ, Maron BJ, Bonow RO, et al. 2011 ACCF/AHA guidelines for the diagnosis and treatment of hypertrophic cardiomyopathy. J Am Coll Cardiol 2011;58:e212–60. Circulation. 2011;124:2761–96.

3. Maron MS, Maron BJ, Harrigan C, et al. Hypertrophic cardiomyopathy phenotype revisited after 50 years with cardiovascular magnetic resonance. J Am Coll Cardiol 2009;54:220–8.

4. Pennell DJ. Cardiovascular magnetic resonance. Circulation 2010;121:692–705.

5. Reichek N, Gupta D. Hypertrophic cardiomyopathy: cardiac magnetic resonance imaging changes the paradigm. J Am Coll Cardiol 2008;52:567–8.

6. Maron MS. Clinical utility of cardiovascular magnetic resonance in hypertrophic cardiomyopathy. J Cardiovasc Magn Reson 2012;14:13.

7. Rickers C, Wilke NM, Jerosch-Herold M, et al. Utility of cardiac magnetic resonance imaging in the diagnosis of hypertrophic cardiomyopathy. Circulation 2005;112:855–61.

8. Moon JC, Fisher NG, McKenna WJ, et al. Detection of apical hypertrophic cardiomyopathy by cardiovascular magnetic resonance in patients with non-diagnostic echocardiography. Heart 2004;90:645–9.

9. Maron MS, Lesser JR, Maron BJ. Management implications of massive left ventricular hypertrophy in hypertrophic cardiomyopathy significantly underestimated by echocardiography but identified by cardiovascular magnetic resonance. Am J Cardiol 2010;105:1842–3.

10. Adabag AS, Maron BJ, Appelbaum E, et al. Occurrence and frequency of arrhythmias in hypertrophic cardiomyopathy in relation to delayed enhancement on cardiovascular magnetic resonance. J Am Coll Cardiol 2008;51:1369–74.

11. Maron BJ, Ackerman MJ, Nishimura RA, et al. Task Force 4: hypertrophic cardiomyopathy and other cardiomyopathies, mitral valve prolapse, myocarditis and Marfan syndrome. J Am Coll Cardiol 2005;45:1340–5.

12. Elliott PM, Poloniecki J, Dickie S, et al. Sudden death in hypertrophic cardiomyopathy: identification of high risk patients. J Am Coll Cardiol 2000;36:2212–8.

13. Maron BJ, Spirito P, Shen WK, et al. Implantable cardioverter-defibrillators and prevention of sudden cardiac death in hypertrophic cardiomyopathy. JAMA 2007;298:405–12.

14. Spirito P, Autore C, Formisano F, et al. Risk of sudden death and outcome in patients with hypertrophic cardiomyopathy with benign clinical presentation and without risk factors. Am J Cardiol 2014;113:1550–5.

15. Moravsky G, Ofek E, Rakowski H, et al. Myocardial fibrosis in hypertrophic cardiomyopathy: accurate reflection of histopathological findings by CMR. JACC Cardiovasc Imaging 2013;6:587–96.

16. Moon JC, Reed E, Sheppard MN, et al. The histologic basis of late gadolinium enhancement cardiovascular magnetic resonance in hypertrophic cardiomyopathy. J Am Coll Cardiol 2004;43:2260–4.

17. Maron MS, Appelbaum E, Harrigan CJ, et al. Clinical profile and significance of delayed enhancement in hypertrophic cardiomyopathy. Circ Heart Fail 2008; 1:184–91.

18. Chan RH, Maron BJ, Olivotto I, et al. Prognostic value of quantitative contrast-enhanced cardiovascular magnetic resonance for the evaluation of sudden death risk in patients with hypertrophic cardiomyopathy. Circulation 2014;130:484–95.

19. O'Hanlon R, Grasso A, Roughton M, et al. Prognostic significance of myocardial fibrosis in hypertrophic cardiomyopathy. J Am Coll Cardiol 2010; 56:867–74.

20. Bruder O, Wagner A, Jensen CJ, et al. Myocardial scar visualized by cardiovascular magnetic resonance imaging predicts major adverse events in patients with hypertrophic cardiomyopathy. J Am Coll Cardiol 2010;56:875–87.

21. Rubinshtein R, Glockner JF, Ommen SR, et al. Characteristics and clinical significance of late gadolinium enhancement by contrast-enhanced magnetic resonance imaging in patients with hypertrophic cardiomyopathy. Circ Heart Fail 2010;3:51–8.

22. Green JJ, Berger JS, Kramer CM, et al. Prognostic value of late gadolinium enhancement in clinical outcomes for hypertrophic cardiomyopathy. JACC Cardiovasc Imaging 2012;5:370–7.

23. Harris KM, Spirito P, Maron MS, et al. Prevalence, clinical profile, and significance of left ventricular remodeling in the end-stage phase of hypertrophic cardiomyopathy. Circulation 2006;114:216–25.

24. Maron MS, Finley JJ, Bos JM, et al. Prevalence, clinical significance, and natural history of left ventricular apical aneurysms in hypertrophic cardiomyopathy. Circulation 2008;118:1541–9.

25. Lim KK, Maron BJ, Knight BP. Successful catheter ablation of hemodyamically unstable monomorphic ventricular tachycardia in a patient with hypertrophic cardiomyopathy and apical aneurysm. J Cardiovasc Electrophysiol 2009;20:445–7.

26. Olivotto I, Maron MS, Autore C, et al. Assessment and significance of left ventricular mass by cardiovascular magnetic resonance in hypertrophic cardiomyopathy. J Am Coll Cardiol 2008;52:559–66.

# Relationship Between Arrhythmogenic Right Ventricular Dysplasia and Exercise

Abhishek C. Sawant, MD, Hugh Calkins, MD*

## KEYWORDS

- Arrhythmogenic right ventricular dysplasia/cardiomyopathy • Exercise • Sudden cardiac death
- Exercise-induced cardiomyopathy

## KEY POINTS

- In patients with a risk of ARVD/C, exercise participation has been shown to be associated with an increased risk of developing disease and adverse outcomes.
- The pathogenesis of arrhythmogenic right ventricular dysplasia/cardiomyopathy (ARVD/C) ranges across a spectrum from exercise-induced cardiomyopathy to a pure familial disease.
- The physician should recommend that index patients and family members inheriting a pathogenic ARVD/C mutation limit exercise participation.
- At present, according to the American Heart Association guidelines, individuals with inherited cardiomyopathies such as ARVD/C are recommended to limit exercise participation to only a few recreational sports.
- Future studies are warranted focusing on a "safe exercise dose" to determine if ARVD/C patients can participate in and continue to gain the health benefits of exercise, and maintain overall cardiovascular health.
- Further research is also needed to study the mechanisms by which exercise causes right ventricular cardiomyopathy and to identify genes that may be involved in pathways influenced by exercise.

## INTRODUCTION

Arrhythmogenic right ventricular dysplasia/cardiomyopathy (ARVD/C) is a rare cardiomyopathy associated with right ventricular (RV) dysfunction, ventricular arrhythmias, and increased risk of sudden cardiac death (SCD).[1–4] Since the first major description of this disorder in 1982,[1] much has been learned about this condition. Although initial data suggested that ARVD/C predominantly involves the right ventricle, subsequently a left-dominant form has been observed.[5] The pathologic hallmark of the disease is myocyte loss and fibrofatty replacement of the myocardium. In the past decade, pathogenic ARVD/C-associated mutations have been identified in 5 desmosomal

Disclosures: Dr H. Calkins receives research support from the Dr. Francis P. Chiaramonte Private Foundation, St. Jude Medical, and Medtronic. Dr A.C. Sawant reports no conflict of interest.

Sources of Funding: The Johns Hopkins ARVD/C Program is supported by the Leyla Erkan Family Fund for ARVD Research, the Dr Satish, Rupal, and Robin Shah ARVD Fund at Johns Hopkins, the Bogle Foundation, the Healing Hearts Foundation, the Campanella Family, the Patrick J. Harrison Family, the Peter French Memorial Foundation, and the Wilmerding Endowments.

Division of Cardiology, Department of Medicine, Johns Hopkins University School of Medicine, 1800 Orleans Street, Baltimore, MD 21287, USA

* Corresponding author. Division of Cardiology, Department of Medicine, The Johns Hopkins Hospital, 1800 Orleans Street/Zayed Tower 7125R, Baltimore, MD 21287.

E-mail address: hcalkins@jhmi.edu

cardiacEP.theclinics.com

genes (*PKP2*, *DSG2*, *DSP*, *DSC2*, and *JUP*), which are identified in approximately 60% of index cases.[6–12] The inheritance is typically autosomal dominant, although nondominant forms have been reported. Recent studies have also identified mutations in genes coding for nonjunctional proteins[13,14] and adherens junction proteins,[15,16] which have been implicated in the pathogenesis of the disease.

This article has 3 overarching goals. First, a focused review of ARVD/C is presented. Next, data supporting the relationship between ARVD/C and exercise are examined in detail, and recommendations are provided regarding exercise participation for patients who at risk or have already developed ARVD/C. Finally, the authors review the evidence supporting the recent concept that some high level ultra-endurance athletes may develop an ARVD/C-like condition referred to as exercise-induced arrhythmogenic cardiomyopathy, which, in contrast to ARVD/C, is not an inherited disease and is exclusively caused by intense exercise.

## OVERVIEW OF ARRHYTHMOGENIC RIGHT VENTRICULAR DYSPLASIA/CARDIOMYOPATHY
### Natural History

ARVD/C is a rare disease with an estimated prevalence in the general population of 1 in 5000.[17] However, in specific geographic regions such as the Venito region in Italy the prevalence is much higher,[18] and is a major cause of SCD in the young (age <35 years).[3,19] The disease is slightly more common in males, and patients usually present in the second to fifth decade of life,[20] although older age at presentation has been observed. The natural history of ARVD/C includes 4 clinical-pathologic stages, which may have significant overlap. The earliest "concealed" stage is usually asymptomatic and associated with ultrastructural or microscopic changes in the myocardium. However, SCD may be the first presenting symptom in this stage.[21] Diagnosis of ARVD/C may be challenging during this stage, although recent advances in risk stratification have improved the identification of high-risk patients.[22,23] The next stage is the overt stage characterized by ventricular arrhythmias of left bundle branch morphology, which is suggestive of RV origin of the arrhythmias, and leads to symptoms including palpitations (27%), syncope (26%), lightheadedness (25%), and sudden death (23%).[4] Overt RV structural and functional abnormalities may become evident on noninvasive imaging.[24] ARVD/C may commonly be misdiagnosed as sarcoidosis during this phase, owing to overlap of electrocardiographic and structural features, and may require additional electrophysiologic testing and imaging for further discrimination.[25] The third stage is characterized by progressive RV dysfunction, often with subtle left ventricular involvement. The final stage involves the myocardial degenerative process and is associated with global dilatation and biventricular involvement, leading to overt heart failure in a small percentage (6%–13%) of patients.[4,26]

### Etiology

ARVD/C is largely an inherited disease with an autosomal dominant pattern of inheritance with variable penetrance and expressivity. The initial association of ARVD/C with mutations in genes coding for desmosomal proteins was recognized after identification of plakoglobin (*JUP*) and desmoplakin (*DSP*) as the genes responsible for causing Naxos disease and Carvajal syndrome, respectively.[27,28] Based on these seminal observations it was suspected that mutations in other desmosomal genes may be the genetic cause of typical ARVD/C. In 2004, Gerull and colleagues[6] reported that plakophilin-2 (*PKP2*) mutations were present in a significant proportion of ARVD/C patients. Subsequently, in the last decade, mutations in other desmosomal proteins such as desmoglein-2 (*DSG2*),[11,12] desmoplakin (*DSP*),[7] and desmocollin-2 (*DSC2*)[8] have been reported. As shown in **Fig. 1**, desmosomes are composed of 3 major groups of proteins: (1) the desmosomal cadherins (desmogleins and desmocollin), which are transmembrane proteins providing the actual mechanical coupling between individual cells; (2) the "plakin family protein" desmoplakin, which anchors the desmosomal structure to the intermediate filaments, and (3) the "armadillo proteins" including plakoglobin and plakophilin, which link desmoplakin and the cadherin tails. The most common genes implicated in ARVD/C are plakophilin-2 and desmoglein-2, accounting for roughly 45% and 9% of patients, respectively. Data from the North American ARVD/C registry showed that 86% of patients had a single heterozygous gene mutation, 7% showed compound heterozygosity, 7% showed digenic heterozygosity, and 1% had homozygous mutation.[9,20] These data are important, as clinicians need to be aware that some individuals with ARVD/C may have more than 1 mutation in a gene or mutations in genes for multiple desmosomal proteins. Patients with multiple mutations seem to have early disease onset and a worse arrhythmic course.[29]

In the past decade, there has been increasing evidence to suggest that ARVD/C is a disease of the intercalated disc.[15] Mutations in the *CTNNA3* gene coding for α T-catenin protein in the area

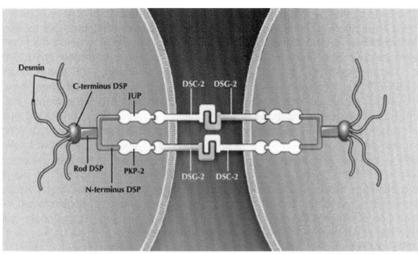

**Fig. 1.** The cardiac desmosomes. The desmoglein-2 (DSG)-2 and desmocollin-2 (DSC)-2 transmembrane proteins provide structural integrity and mechanical coupling between cardiac myocytes. Their intracellular portions bind to the armadillo family proteins plakophilin-2 (PKP-2) and plakoglobin (JUP), which bind to the N-terminal domain of the plakin family protein desmoplakin (DSP). The C-terminal portion anchors the desmosomes to the desmin intermediate filaments. (*From* Sen-Chowdhry S, Syrris P, McKenna WJ. Role of genetic analysis in the management of patients with arrhythmogenic right ventricular dysplasia/cardiomyopathy. J Am Coll Cardiol 2007;50:1814; with permission.)

composita (composed of both desmosomal and adherens junctional proteins), which specifically interacts with *PKP2* desmosomal protein, has been shown to be associated with ARVD/C.[16] A reduced expression of connexin-43, is a key gap-junction protein observed during ultrastructural examination of myocytes in ARVD/C patients, further supports the role of intercalated disc proteins in ARVD/C.[30,31] The presence of mutations in genes encoding for extra desmosomal proteins such as transmembrane protein 43 (*TMEM43*),[32] transforming growth factor β3 (*TGFβ3*),[33] and ryanodine receptor (*RYR2*),[34] have also been shown to be associated with ARVD/C. There is also a growing body of evidence showing that mutations in genes coding for nonjunctional proteins such as desmin (*DES*),[35] lamin A/C (*LMNA*),[13] titin (*TTN*),[36] and phospholamban (*PLN*)[14] may also be involved in the pathogenesis of ARVD/C.

## Pathogenesis

Although several hypotheses have been proposed, the pathogenic mechanisms involved in ARVD/C remain unclear. A simple structural model proposes that recurrent myocardial strain may lead to mechanical uncoupling of the desmosomal proteins, which may already be weakened by mutations.[28] This process leads to an inflammatory condition associated with fibrofatty scar formation, which predisposes to ventricular arrhythmias. This model suggests that the dominant RV involvement is due to the relatively thinner wall and

disproportionately greater strain exerted on the right ventricle compared with the left ventricle during exercise. The theory also supports the observation of increased risk of sudden death among young athletes resulting from increased strain on the myocardium secondary to prolonged strenuous exertion.[37] However, the variable penetrance and expressivity seen in ARVD/C patients cannot be fully explained by this theory. Studies have shown that compound and digenic heterozygosity is associated with a severe phenotype suggestive of a "second hit" hypothesis.[38] Thus, presence of modifier genes or environmental factors such as exercise may contribute to the phenotypic heterogeneity.

## Diagnosis

The diagnosis of ARVD/C is based on a set of Task Force Criteria (TFC) first developed in 1994 and revised in 2010,[39] relying on demonstration of defects in RV morphology and systolic function, depolarization/repolarization abnormalities on electrocardiograms (ECG), pathologic tissue characteristics, ventricular arrhythmias, and family history and genetics. The diagnosis of ARVD/C is based on the presence of 2 major, 1 major and 2 minor, or 4 minor criteria. T-wave inversion (TWI) is the most common repolarization abnormality in ARVD/C seen commonly in precordial leads, which can also extend to V4-V6 and inferior leads. However, in the presence of a right bundle branch block (RBBB), which is commonly seen in

ARVD/C, TWI criteria cannot be applied for diagnosing ARVD/C. The authors have shown that an R/S ratio of less than 1 in lead V1 can be used as a reliable parameter for diagnosing ARVD/C, with sensitivity of 88% and specificity of 86% in the presence of RBBB.[40] Depolarization abnormalities seen in ARVD/C include an epsilon wave, which is a small-amplitude postexcitation electrical potential occurring in the ST segment after the QRS complex, and the presence of terminal activation delay, defined as duration greater than 55 milliseconds from S-wave nadir to the end of all depolarizations. However, there is a significant interobserver variability in identification of these depolarization abnormalities, owing to the significant difficulty in determining the beginning and end of QRS deflections. In addition, signal-averaged ECG (SAECG) can be used to identify depolarization abnormalities. A SAEGC is considered abnormal in the presence of 1 or more of these abnormalities: (1) filtered QRS duration (fQRS) greater than 114 milliseconds; (2) terminal low amplitude (<40 μV) signal duration 38 milliseconds or longer; and (3) root mean square voltage of the terminal 40 milliseconds of the filtered QRS complex (RMS40) less than 20 μV. The presence of sustained or nonsustained ventricular tachycardia (VT) of left bundle branch block (LBBB) morphology suggestive of RV origin can be used to diagnose ARVD/C. Ambulatory Holter monitoring for the presence of more than 500 frequent ectopic beats and exercise stress testing for occurrence of sustained/nonsustained VT during exercise are inexpensive tests that can be used for diagnosing ARVD/C. Assessment of RV structure and function using transthoracic echocardiography and cardiac magnetic resonance (CMR) imaging is paramount for the diagnosis of ARVD/C. The presence of both global/segmental RV wall motion abnormalities (hypokinesis/akinesis) along with RV cavity dilatation or reduced RV systolic function are required for diagnosing ARVD/C. It is important that although CMR has emerged as the imaging modality of choice for ARVD/C, significant experience is needed for accurately diagnosing ARVD/C using CMR, and the diagnosis should not be solely based on abnormalities found on CMR alone. Lastly, endomyocardial biopsies, though rarely performed, can aid in differentiating ARVD/C from conditions such as sarcoidosis, which often mimic ARVD/C.

## Management

The cornerstone of management for ARVD/C involves prevention of SCD. Patients sustaining a life-threatening ventricular arrhythmia are always recommended to have an implantable cardioverter-defibrillator (ICD) for secondary prevention. For primary prevention, probands and family members who meet 2010 TFC are recommended to undergo ICD implantation. The Johns Hopkins ARVD/C Registry has shown in a large cohort of 1001 ARVD/C patients that among probands, implantation of an ICD is associated with reduced SCD and improved long-term outcomes.[26] Several studies have shown that up to 80% of ARVD/C probands receive appropriate ICD therapies.[41] Predictors on appropriate ICD therapies include inducibility at electrophysiologic study, occurrence of nonsustained ventricular arrhythmias, cardiogenic syncope, and increased ventricular ectopy.[42] ICD placement for primary prevention among family members, however, remains controversial. In a combined North American and Dutch cohort of family members, researchers found that meeting TFC independent of family history and presence of genetic mutation had higher prognostic value for developing ventricular arrhythmias and should be used for arrhythmic risk stratification before undergoing ICD implantation.[43] Among ARVD/C patients undergoing ICD implantation at a young age, the risks of long-term device complications and poorer psychological adjustment also need to be considered.[44]

The pharmacologic treatment is usually directed toward reducing the arrhythmia burden using class III antiarrhythmic agents such as sotalol and amiodarone.[45] β-Blockers and angiotensin-converting enzyme inhibitors are frequently used given their benefit in other cardiomyopathies, although there is paucity of data to support their use in ARVD/C. Among ARVD/C patients who have sustained a ventricular arrhythmia, radiofrequency ablation has been used as an important treatment option for reducing arrhythmic burden by reducing the frequencies of arrhythmic events. At the Johns Hopkins ARVD/C program, the authors prefer a combined endocardial and epicardial approach as a first-line ablation strategy, and have shown it to be a safe and effective option for reducing both VT recurrence and burden.[46] However, because ARVD/C is a progressive disease, ablation should not be considered as curative and an alternative for ICD implantation. A minority of ARVD/C patients eventually require cardiac transplantation, mostly for development of stage D heart failure and less commonly for incessant ventricular arrhythmias.[47] Patients undergoing cardiac transplantation often present at an early age and usually have a prolonged clinical course.

## RELATIONSHIP BETWEEN ARRHYTHMOGENIC RIGHT VENTRICULAR DYSPLASIA/ CARDIOMYOPATHY AND EXERCISE
### Studies Linking Exercise and Arrhythmogenic Right Ventricular Dysplasia/Cardiomyopathy

The association of exercise stems from the observation that SCD in ARVD/C patients often occurred during exertion.[48] Thiene and colleagues[3] found that among 60 consecutive cases presenting with SCD, ARVD/C was identified as the diagnosis on postmortem examination in 12 patients. On evaluation of the circumstances of death, most of these ARVD/C patients (10 of 12) were found to have died during exertion. These investigators also reported that young athletes in the Veneto region of Italy had a 5-fold risk of dying of ARVD/C in comparison with nonathletes.[37] Kirchhof and colleagues[49] showed that endurance training of the transgenic plakoglobin-deficient mouse was associated with RV enlargement, RV conduction slowing, and significantly increased ventricular arrhythmias originating from the RV free wall or septum in comparison with wild-type hearts. Subsequently, Fabritz and colleagues[50] showed that load-reducing therapy prevented RV enlargement, conduction slowing, and inducibility of ventricular arrhythmias, thus preventing development of the ARVD/C phenotype in these mice. Surprisingly, in both studies the investigators failed to find evidence of fibrosis, fibrofatty replacement, or cardiomyocyte hypertrophy in the right ventricle among trained plakoglobin-deficient mice on comparison with wild-type littermates. The results of these and other studies support the hypothesis that repeated strenuous exercise is an important factor that could increase the chance of development of ARVD/C, especially in patients with a desmosomal mutation.

### Role of Exercise in Desmosomal Arrhythmogenic Right Ventricular Dysplasia/ Cardiomyopathy

The first study evaluating the role of exercise in ARVD/C patients inheriting a pathogenic desmosomal mutation was performed by James and colleagues.[51] The authors studied 87 probands and family members from the Johns Hopkins ARVD/C Registry who underwent direct sequencing of the desmosomal genes *PKP2*, *DSG2*, *DSC2*, *DSP*, and *JUP* and were identified to carry a single copy of a pathogenic mutation in 1 of these genes. All patients participated in an exercise interview detailing their exercise history for leisure/recreation, work, and transportation. Study participants provided information about the duration of exercise (hours per year) and intensity (light, moderate, and vigorous) of exercise participation from age

10 years until clinical presentation. Participants were classified as an endurance athlete if they performed 50 h/y or more of vigorous-intensity sports with a high dynamic demand (>70% maximum $O_2$), as defined by the 36th Bethesda Conference Classification of Sports (Task Force 8).[52] The study had several key findings regarding exercise and clinical outcomes. First, the investigators found that ARVD/C patients who were endurance athletes became symptomatic at an earlier age than nonathletes. Second, endurance exercise and higher duration of exercise participation were both associated with an increasing likelihood of developing manifest ARVD/C (**Fig. 2**A). Third, endurance exercise was associated with worse survival from a ventricular arrhythmia and heart failure (see **Fig. 2**B). Lastly, those individuals who continued to participate in the top quartile for hours of annual exercise after presentation had worse survival from first ventricular arrhythmia compared with individuals who reduced their exercise after presentation. The study thus confirmed the role of exercise as a disease modifier in ARVD/C patients with a desmosomal mutation.

The authors subsequently evaluated the role of exercise among 10 families (9 probands and 28 family members) inheriting a pathogenic plakophilin-2 (*PKP2*) mutation.[53] Again, structured interviews were performed focusing on the duration (hours per year), intensity (metabolic equivalent [MET]-hours per year), and participation in endurance exercise. Family members who were endurance athletes and participated in higher duration and intensity of exercise were found to be more likely to develop disease. This association remained significant even after adjusting for family membership. In addition, family members who were endurance athletes were more likely to develop structural abnormalities and had significantly lower RV ejection fraction in comparison with nonathletes. Of interest, the authors also found that family members who participated in sports with a high dynamic component were more likely to develop ARVD/C.[53]

### Role of Exercise in Nondesmosomal arrhythmogenic Right Ventricular Dysplasia/ Cardiomyopathy

A subsequent study was performed by researchers at Johns Hopkins to evaluate the role of exercise in ARVD/C patients without a pathogenic desmosomal mutation.[54] The authors examined the role of duration and intensity of exercise participation among 43 probands without a desmosomal mutation (nondesmosomal) and compared it with that of 39 probands with

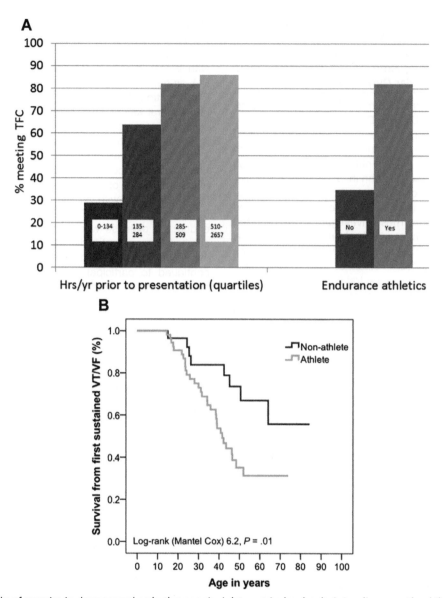

**Fig. 2.** Role of exercise in desmosomal arrhythmogenic right ventricular dysplasia/cardiomyopathy. (*A*) Participation in endurance exercise and higher durations of exercise were both associated with increased likelihood of meeting 2010 Task Force Criteria (TFC) for ARVD/C. (*B*) Kaplan-Meier survival curves show worse survival from ventricular arrhythmias (VT/VF) among endurance athletes in comparison with nonathletes. (*From* James CA, Bhonsale A, Tichnell C, et al. Exercise increases age-related penetrance and arrhythmic risk in arrhythmogenic right ventricular dysplasia/cardiomyopathy-associated desmosomal mutation carriers. J Am Coll Cardiol 2013;62:1294; with permission.)

desmosomal mutations, all of whom met the 2010 TFC. Among nondesmosomal patients, those participating in the highest quartile of MET-h/y exercise presented at a significantly earlier age, and had worse structural abnormalities on CMR and significantly poorer survival from a ventricular arrhythmia during follow-up. Next, the authors compared exercise participation stratified by mutation status and family history. Although nondesmosomal ARVD/C patients had performed annual

exercise of similar duration as desmosomal carriers; their exercise was significantly more intense, with significantly higher participation in endurance sports and expending greater MET-h/y of exercise in comparison with desmosomal patients. Lastly, ARVD/C nondesmosomal patients with no family history performed the highest MET-h/y exercise when compared with nondesmosomal patients with a family history and desmosomal mutation carriers (**Fig. 3**). Because the nondesmosomal

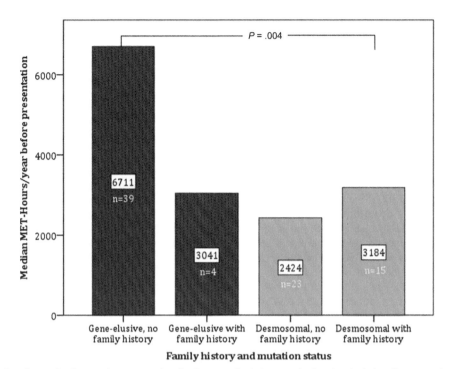

**Fig. 3.** Role of exercise in nondesmosomal arrhythmogenic right ventricular dysplasia/cardiomyopathy. Nondesmosomal nonfamilial patients participated in higher-intensity exercise (MET-hours/year) than nondesmosomal patients with family history and desmosomal carriers. (*From* Sawant AC, Bhonsale A, Te Riele AS, et al. Exercise has a disproportionate role in the pathogenesis of arrhythmogenic right ventricular dysplasia/cardiomyopathy in patients without desmosomal mutations. J Am Heart Assoc 2014;3(6):e001471.)

patients without family history performed the highest-intensity exercise, the authors concluded that exercise may be the key environmental factor driving disease pathogenesis in that subgroup. When annual pre-presentation MET-hours and endurance exercise participation during youth (age ≤25 years) were compared, higher-intensity exercise during youth was found to be associated with earlier age of presentation in both desmosomal and nondesmosomal ARVD/C patients. Prior studies have shown that although the components of the intercalated disc (gap junctions, adherens junctions, and desmosomes) typically assemble within 1 year after birth, their localization and maturation often continues until adolescence.[55] Thus, additional environmental factors such as exercise from the postnatal period until adolescence may influence the maturation and localization of these components, especially in the presence of mutations.[56]

In a recent study, Saberniak and colleagues[57] focused on the role of exercise and cardiac function among ARVD/C patients and family members with and without desmosomal mutations. Exercise participation was measured by MET-minutes per week, and those patients participating in vigorous (≥6 METs) physical activity for ≥4 h/wk (≥1440

MET-min/wk) were classified as athletes. The investigators found that both RV and left ventricular function assessed using echocardiography and CMR was significantly reduced in athletes when compared with nonathletes. Next, the amount of physical activity correlated with the RV ejection fraction (%) measured using CMR and left ventricular ejection fraction (%) measured by echocardiography. Lastly, patients who sustained a ventricular arrhythmia were significantly more likely to be athletes and had higher MET-minutes per week of physical activity. The investigators thus concluded that exercise participation influences biventricular function and arrhythmic outcomes in ARVD/C patients and asymptomatic family members with and without desmosomal mutations. These studies add to the growing body of evidence supporting the role of duration, intensity, and timing of exercise in the pathogenesis of ARVD/C patients with and without desmosomal mutations.[58]

## Exercise Recommendations

The most widely used guidelines, from the 36th Bethesda Conference Eligibility Recommendations for Competitive Athletes with Cardiovascular

Abnormalities, recommend avoidance of all competitive activities for patients with probable or definite diagnosis of ARVD/C except for class I-A sports with a low cardiovascular demand.[59] The European Society of Cardiology recommendations are similar where athletes diagnosed with ARVD/C are excluded from most competitive sports, except those without arrhythmias or absence of exercise-related symptoms who can be allowed to participate in low-intensity sports only.[60] The American Heart Association (AHA) has a grading system for recommendations regarding participation in recreational sports, ranking them on a scale of 0 to 5.[61] In general, ARVD/C patients are prohibited from participating in all competitive sports and recreational sports requiring 4 or more METs. Based on the growing body of literature outlined herein and their own clinical experience, the authors have become strong believers that patients with ARVD/C or those at risk for developing ARVD/C should limit exercise. As exercise participation affects structure and outcomes, those patients diagnosed with ARVD/C by meeting 4 or more TFC points should limit exercise irrespective of their mutation status. Because lifestyle changes are not easy to make, especially in individuals used to exercising regularly, limiting exercise will be a negotiation and will require frequent reinforcement. Another important group to consider is the family members of patients with diagnosed ARVD/C. Specifically, family members who are identified to carry a pathogenic mutation should be recommended to limit exercise participation. However, the authors recommend approaching these family members on a case-by-case basis. Those family members without evidence of disease and who are allowed to participate in endurance sports should be monitored closely with frequent follow-up. In addition, participation in endurance sports should not be allowed for extended periods of time and should be discontinued immediately if there is any evidence of disease progression. For family members of probands without an identified mutation, one should be less inclined to limit exercise because the a priori risk seems to be lower. In this situation, the authors advise serial screening, with more frequent screening in the highest-level athletes.

## EXERCISE-INDUCED CARDIOMYOPATHY

In the last decade there has been increasing interest in determining whether exercise in itself can induce cardiomyopathy that leads to life-threatening arrhythmias. Heidbuchel and colleagues[62] have published literature propagating the hypothesis of exercise-induced ARVC,

whereby exercise alone has been shown to cause an ARVD/C-like phenotype. These investigators proposed that recurrent bouts of strenuous exercise typically performed by competitive athletes may not allow for sufficient recovery, leading to maladaptive changes including inflammation and fibrosis in the right ventricle, eventually resulting in exercise-induced ARVC (**Fig. 4**). Several mechanisms have been hypothesized by which the right ventricle may be disproportionately affected by endurance exercise. Because the pulmonary circulation has lesser compliance than the systemic circulation, there is a significant increase in pulmonary pressures caused by increased cardiac output during exercise. This phenomenon may be even more pronounced in athletes, owing to the relatively higher cardiac outputs achieved during peak exercise. La Gerche and colleagues[63] compared end-systolic wall stress using CMR imaging and echocardiography among 39 endurance athletes and 14 age-matched and sex-matched nonathletes. Compared with at rest, the RV wall stress at peak exercise in athletes rose by 170%, compared with a 23% increase in left ventricular wall stress. In addition, it was shown that this disproportionate wall stress may predispose the right ventricle to greater dilatation and eventual dysfunction in comparison with the left ventricle. These findings have also been confirmed in large epidemiologic cohorts such as the Multi-Ethnic Study of Atherosclerosis (MESA) where higher-intensity exercise was associated with increased RV mass and volumes in comparison with the left ventricle.[64]

As shown in **Fig. 4**, recurrent strenuous exercise causing myocardial injury may eventually lead to pathologic remodeling and fibrosis, which may act as a substrate for life-threatening arrhythmias.[65,66] The cardiac remodeling and fibrosis, although initially reversible, may eventually become permanent, likely because of repeated damage and persistent myocardial injury.[62] In another small cohort of endurance athletes, Heidbüchel[67] found a high prevalence of ventricular arrhythmias originating from the right ventricle whereby 37 of 46 (80%) athletes developed VT with an LBBB morphology. Among the 46 athletes, 27 (59%) met definite ($\geq$4 points) and 14 (30%) met probable ($\geq$2 points) diagnosis of ARVD/C based on the 1994 TFC. One athlete had a significant family history whereby his brother was diagnosed with ARVD. Given the paucity of family history, and evidence of RV origin of arrhythmias and RV structural abnormalities in most of these athletes, Heidbüchel's group proposed a causal relationship between exercise and RV dysfunction, which they dubbed

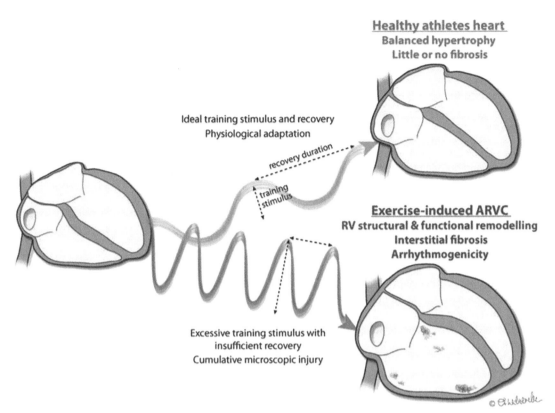

Fig. 4. Comparison between healthy athlete's heart and exercise-induced arrhythmogenic right ventricular cardiomyopathy (ARVC). Repeated bouts of excessive endurance exercise without time for recovery may cause disproportionate wall stress on the right ventricle, eventually leading to inflammation and fibrosis instead of the balanced hypertrophy seen in the healthy athlete's heart. (*From* Heidbuchel H, Prior DL, La Gerche A. Ventricular arrhythmias associated with long-term endurance sports: what is the evidence? Br J Sports Med 2012;46(Suppl 1):i45).

exercise-induced ARVC, and also proposed that exercise-induced ARVC has a less severe phenotype than familial ARVD/C, with a more benign course.[68] Although the authors found that exercise does plays a key role in both desmosomal and nondesmosomal ARVD/C, as described earlier, they did not find any phenotypic differences among athletes with or without

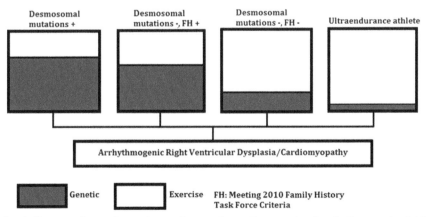

Fig. 5. Relative influence of exercise and genetics on the pathogenesis of arrhythmogenic right ventricular dysplasia/cardiomyopathy. (*From* Sawant AC, Bhonsale A, Te Riele AS, et al. Exercise has a disproportionate role in the pathogenesis of arrhythmogenic right ventricular dysplasia/cardiomyopathy in patients without desmosomal mutations. J Am Heart Assoc 2014;3(6):e001471.)

desmosomal mutations. The pathogenesis of ARVD/C may actually be represented by a spectrum with varying underlying genetic risk modulated by environmental factors such as exercise, which eventually leads to an ARVD/C phenotype (**Fig. 5**).

## SUMMARY

Exercise participation has been shown in both animal models and humans to be associated with an increased risk of developing disease and adverse outcomes, irrespective of their mutation status. The pathogenesis of ARVD/C ranges from a spectrum of exercise-induced cardiomyopathy to a pure familial disease. Index patients and family members inheriting a pathogenic mutation should be recommended to limit exercise participation. According to the current AHA guidelines, individuals with inherited cardiomyopathies such as ARVD/C are recommended to limit exercise participation to only a few recreational sports. Future studies are warranted, focusing on a "safe exercise dose" whereby ARVD/C patients can participate in and continue to gain the health benefits of exercise and maintain overall cardiovascular health. In addition, further research is needed to study the mechanisms by which exercise causes RV cardiomyopathy and to identify genes that may be involved in pathways influenced by exercise.

## ACKNOWLEDGMENTS

The authors wish to acknowledge funding from the Dr. Francis P. Chiaramonte Private Foundation, St. Jude Medical Inc, and Medtronic Inc. The authors are grateful to the ARVD/C patients and families who have made this work possible.

## REFERENCES

1. Marcus FI, Fontaine GH, Guiraudon G, et al. Right ventricular dysplasia: a report of 24 adult cases. Circulation 1982;65:384–98.
2. Basso C, Corrado D, Marcus FI, et al. Arrhythmogenic right ventricular cardiomyopathy. Lancet 2009;373:1289–300.
3. Thiene G, Nava A, Corrado D, et al. Right ventricular cardiomyopathy and sudden death in young people. N Engl J Med 1988;318:129–33.
4. Dalal D, Nasir K, Bomma C, et al. Arrhythmogenic right ventricular dysplasia: a United States experience. Circulation 2005;112:3823–32.
5. Saguner AM, Brunckhorst C, Duru F. Arrhythmogenic ventricular cardiomyopathy: a paradigm shift from right to biventricular disease. World J Cardiol 2014;6:154–74.
6. Gerull B, Heuser A, Wichter T, et al. Mutations in the desmosomal protein plakophilin-2 are common in arrhythmogenic right ventricular cardiomyopathy. Nat Genet 2004;36:1162–4.
7. Rampazzo A, Nava A, Malacrida S, et al. Mutation in human desmoplakin domain binding to plakoglobin causes a dominant form of arrhythmogenic right ventricular cardiomyopathy. Am J Hum Genet 2002;71:1200–6.
8. Syrris P, Ward D, Evans A, et al. Arrhythmogenic right ventricular dysplasia/cardiomyopathy associated with mutations in the desmosomal gene desmocollin-2. Am J Hum Genet 2006;79:978–84.
9. den Haan AD, Tan BY, Zikusoka MN, et al. Comprehensive desmosome mutation analysis in North Americans with arrhythmogenic right ventricular dysplasia/cardiomyopathy. Circ Cardiovasc Genet 2009;2:428–35.
10. Cox MG, van der Zwaag PA, van der Werf C, et al. Arrhythmogenic right ventricular dysplasia/cardiomyopathy: pathogenic desmosome mutations in index-patients predict outcome of family screening: Dutch arrhythmogenic right ventricular dysplasia/cardiomyopathy genotype-phenotype follow-up study. Circulation 2011;123:2690–700.
11. Pilichou K, Nava A, Basso C, et al. Mutations in desmoglein-2 gene are associated with arrhythmogenic right ventricular cardiomyopathy. Circulation 2006;113:1171–9.
12. Awad MM, Dalal D, Cho E, et al. DSG2 mutations contribute to arrhythmogenic right ventricular dysplasia/cardiomyopathy. Am J Hum Genet 2006; 79:136–42.
13. Quarta G, Syrris P, Ashworth M, et al. Mutations in the Lamin A/C gene mimic arrhythmogenic right ventricular cardiomyopathy. Eur Heart J 2012;33: 1128–36.
14. van der Zwaag PA, van Rijsingen IAW, Asimaki A, et al. Phospholamban R14del mutation in patients diagnosed with dilated cardiomyopathy or arrhythmogenic right ventricular cardiomyopathy: evidence supporting the concept of arrhythmogenic cardiomyopathy. Eur J Heart Fail 2012;14:1199–207.
15. Calore M, Lorenzon A, De Bortoli M, et al. Arrhythmogenic cardiomyopathy: a disease of intercalated discs. Cell Tissue Res 2014. [Epub ahead of print].
16. van Hengel J, Calore M, Bauce B, et al. Mutations in the area composita protein alphaT-catenin are associated with arrhythmogenic right ventricular cardiomyopathy. Eur Heart J 2013;34:201–10.
17. Peters S, Trummel M, Meyners W. Prevalence of right ventricular dysplasia-cardiomyopathy in a non-referral hospital. Int J Cardiol 2004;97:499–501.
18. Nava A, Thiene G, Canciani B, et al. Familial occurrence of right ventricular dysplasia: a study involving nine families. J Am Coll Cardiol 1988;12:1222–8.

19. Basso C, Corrado D, Thiene G. Cardiovascular causes of sudden death in young individuals including athletes. Cardiol Rev 1999;7:127–35.
20. Marcus FI, Zareba W, Calkins H, et al. Arrhythmogenic right ventricular cardiomyopathy/dysplasia clinical presentation and diagnostic evaluation: results from the North American Multidisciplinary Study. Heart Rhythm 2009;6:984–92.
21. Quarta G, Muir A, Pantazis A, et al. Familial evaluation in arrhythmogenic right ventricular cardiomyopathy: impact of genetics and revised task force criteria. Circulation 2011;123:2701–9.
22. te Riele AS, James CA, Rastegar N, et al. Yield of serial evaluation in at-risk family members of patients with ARVD/C. J Am Coll Cardiol 2014;64:293–301.
23. te Riele AS, Bhonsale A, James CA, et al. Incremental value of cardiac magnetic resonance imaging in arrhythmic risk stratification of arrhythmogenic right ventricular dysplasia/cardiomyopathy-associated desmosomal mutation carriers. J Am Coll Cardiol 2013;62:1761–9.
24. te Riele AS, Tandri H, Bluemke DA. Arrhythmogenic right ventricular cardiomyopathy (ARVC): cardiovascular magnetic resonance update. J Cardiovasc Magn Reson 2014;16:50.
25. Philips B, Madhavan S, James CA, et al. Arrhythmogenic right ventricular dysplasia/cardiomyopathy and cardiac sarcoidosis: distinguishing features when the diagnosis is unclear. Circ Arrhythm Electrophysiol 2014;7:230–6.
26. Groeneweg JA, Bhonsale A, James CA, et al. Clinical presentation, long-term follow-up, and disease penetrance of arrhythmogenic right ventricular dysplasia/cardiomyopathy in 1001 patients and family members [abstract]. Circulation 2014;130: A13189.
27. McKoy G, Protonotarios N, Crosby A, et al. Identification of a deletion in plakoglobin in arrhythmogenic right ventricular cardiomyopathy with palmoplantar keratoderma and woolly hair (Naxos disease). Lancet 2000;355:2119–24.
28. Protonotarios N, Tsatsopoulou A. Naxos disease and Carvajal syndrome: cardiocutaneous disorders that highlight the pathogenesis and broaden the spectrum of arrhythmogenic right ventricular cardiomyopathy. Cardiovasc Pathol 2004;13:185–94.
29. Bhonsale A, Groeneweg JA, James CA, et al. Impact of genotype on clinical course in arrhythmogenic right ventricular dysplasia/cardiomyopathy associated mutation carriers. Eur Heart J 2015. [Epub ahead of print].
30. Tandri H, Asimaki A, Dalal D, et al. Gap junction remodeling in a case of arrhythmogenic right ventricular dysplasia due to plakophilin-2 mutation. J Cardiovasc Electrophysiol 2008;19:1212–4.
31. Oxford EM, Musa H, Maass K, et al. Connexin43 remodeling caused by inhibition of plakophilin-2
expression in cardiac cells. Circ Res 2007;101: 703–11.
32. Merner ND, Hodgkinson KA, Haywood AF, et al. Arrhythmogenic right ventricular cardiomyopathy type 5 is a fully penetrant, lethal arrhythmic disorder caused by a missense mutation in the TMEM43 gene. Am J Hum Genet 2008;82:809–21.
33. Beffagna G, Occhi G, Nava A, et al. Regulatory mutations in transforming growth factor-beta3 gene cause arrhythmogenic right ventricular cardiomyopathy type 1. Cardiovasc Res 2005;65: 366–73.
34. Tiso N, Stephan DA, Nava A, et al. Identification of mutations in the cardiac ryanodine receptor gene in families affected with arrhythmogenic right ventricular cardiomyopathy type 2 (ARVD2). Hum Mol Genet 2001;10:189–94.
35. Klauke B, Kossmann S, Gaertner A, et al. De novo desmin-mutation N116S is associated with arrhythmogenic right ventricular cardiomyopathy. Hum Mol Genet 2010;19:4595–607.
36. Taylor M, Graw S, Sinagra G, et al. Genetic variation in titin in arrhythmogenic right ventricular cardiomyopathy-overlap syndromes. Circulation 2011;124:876–85.
37. Corrado D, Basso C, Rizzoli G, et al. Does sports activity enhance the risk of sudden death in adolescents and young adults? J Am Coll Cardiol 2003; 42:1959–63.
38. Xu T, Yang Z, Vatta M, et al. Compound and digenic heterozygosity contributes to arrhythmogenic right ventricular cardiomyopathy. J Am Coll Cardiol 2010;55:587–97.
39. Marcus FI, McKenna WJ, Sherrill D, et al. Diagnosis of arrhythmogenic right ventricular cardiomyopathy/ dysplasia: proposed modification of the task force criteria. Circulation 2010;121:1533–41.
40. Jain R, Dalal D, Daly A, et al. Electrocardiographic features of arrhythmogenic right ventricular dysplasia. Circulation 2009;120:477–87.
41. Wichter T, Paul M, Wollmann C, et al. Implantable cardioverter/defibrillator therapy in arrhythmogenic right ventricular cardiomyopathy: single-center experience of long-term follow-up and complications in 60 patients. Circulation 2004;109:1503–8.
42. Bhonsale A, James CA, Tichnell C, et al. Incidence and predictors of implantable cardioverter-defibrillator therapy in patients with arrhythmogenic right ventricular dysplasia/cardiomyopathy undergoing implantable cardioverter-defibrillator implantation for primary prevention. J Am Coll Cardiol 2011;58:1485–96.
43. te Riele AS, James CA, Sawant AC, et al. Systematic approach to arrhythmogenic right ventricular dysplasia/cardiomyopathy family screening in a large transatlantic cohort [abstract]. Circulation 2014;130:A16401.

44. James CA, Tichnell C, Murray B, et al. General and disease-specific psychosocial adjustment in patients with arrhythmogenic right ventricular dysplasia/cardiomyopathy with implantable cardioverter defibrillators: a large cohort study. Circ Cardiovasc Genet 2012;5:18–24.

45. Marcus GM, Glidden DV, Polonsky B, et al. Efficacy of antiarrhythmic drugs in arrhythmogenic right ventricular cardiomyopathy: a report from the North American ARVC Registry. J Am Coll Cardiol 2009; 54:609–15.

46. Philips B, te Riele AS, Sawant A, et al. Outcomes and ventricular tachycardia recurrence characteristics after epicardial ablation of ventricular tachycardia in arrhythmogenic right ventricular dysplasia/cardiomyopathy. Heart Rhythm 2015;12:716–25.

47. Tedford RJ, James C, Judge DP, et al. Cardiac transplantation in arrhythmogenic right ventricular dysplasia/cardiomyopathy. J Am Coll Cardiol 2012; 59:289–90.

48. Marcus FI, Fontaine G. Arrhythmogenic right ventricular dysplasia/cardiomyopathy: a review. Pacing Clin Electrophysiol 1995;18:1298–314.

49. Kirchhof P, Fabritz L, Zwiener M, et al. Age- and training-dependent development of arrhythmogenic right ventricular cardiomyopathy in heterozygous plakoglobin-deficient mice. Circulation 2006;114: 1799–806.

50. Fabritz L, Hoogendijk MG, Scicluna BP, et al. Load-reducing therapy prevents development of arrhythmogenic right ventricular cardiomyopathy in plakoglobin-deficient mice. J Am Coll Cardiol 2011;57:740–50.

51. James CA, Bhonsale A, Tichnell C, et al. Exercise increases age-related penetrance and arrhythmic risk in arrhythmogenic right ventricular dysplasia/cardiomyopathy-associated desmosomal mutation carriers. J Am Coll Cardiol 2013;62:1290–7.

52. Mitchell JH, Haskell W, Snell P, et al. Task force 8: classification of sports. J Am Coll Cardiol 2005;45: 1364–7.

53. Sawant AC, Murray B, Tichnell C, et al. Exercise influences penetrance and outcomes in family members of arrhythmogenic right ventricular dysplasia/cardiomyopathy patients carrying a pathogenic desmosomal mutation [abstract]. Circulation 2014; 130:A11215.

54. Sawant AC, Bhonsale A, Te Riele AS, et al. Exercise has a disproportionate role in the pathogenesis of arrhythmogenic right ventricular dysplasia/cardiomyopathy in patients without desmosomal mutations. J Am Heart Assoc 2014;3(6):e001471.

55. Vreeker A, van Stuijvenberg L, Hund TJ, et al. Assembly of the cardiac intercalated disk during pre- and postnatal development of the human heart. PLoS One 2014;9:e94722.

56. Wang Q, Lin JL, Chan SY, et al. The Xin repeat-containing protein, mXinβ, initiates the maturation of the intercalated discs during postnatal heart development. Dev Biol 2013;374:264–80.

57. Saberniak J, Hasselberg NE, Borgquist R, et al. Vigorous physical activity impairs myocardial function in patients with arrhythmogenic right ventricular cardiomyopathy and in mutation positive family members. Eur J Heart Fail 2014;16:1337–44.

58. Rojas A, Calkins H. Present understanding of the relationship between exercise and arrhythmogenic right ventricular dysplasia/cardiomyopathy. Trends Cardiovasc Med 2014. http://dx.doi.org/10.1016/j.tcm.2014.10.007.

59. Maron BJ, Ackerman MJ, Nishimura RA, et al. Task force 4: HCM and other cardiomyopathies, mitral valve prolapse, myocarditis, and Marfan syndrome. J Am Coll Cardiol 2005;45:1340–5.

60. Pelliccia A, Corrado D, Bjørnstad HH, et al. Recommendations for participation in competitive sport and leisure-time physical activity in individuals with cardiomyopathies, myocarditis and pericarditis. Eur J Cardiovasc Prev Rehabil 2006;13:876–85.

61. Maron BJ, Chaitman BR, Ackerman MJ, et al. Recommendations for physical activity and recreational sports participation for young patients with genetic cardiovascular diseases. Circulation 2004;109: 2807–16.

62. Heidbuchel H, Prior DL, La Gerche A. Ventricular arrhythmias associated with long-term endurance sports: what is the evidence? Br J Sports Med 2012;46(Suppl 1):i44–50.

63. La Gerche A, Heidbuchel H, Burns AT, et al. Disproportionate exercise load and remodeling of the athlete's right ventricle. Med Sci Sports Exerc 2011;43: 974–81.

64. Aaron CP, Tandri H, Barr RG, et al. Physical activity and right ventricular structure and function. The MESA-Right Ventricle Study. Am J Respir Crit Care Med 2011;183:396–404.

65. Breuckmann F, Mohlenkamp S, Nassenstein K, et al. Myocardial late gadolinium enhancement: prevalence, pattern, and prognostic relevance in marathon runners. Radiology 2009;251:50–7.

66. Benito B, Gay-Jordi G, Serrano-Mollar A, et al. Cardiac arrhythmogenic remodeling in a rat model of long-term intensive exercise training. Circulation 2011;123:13–22.

67. Heidbüchel H. High prevalence of right ventricular involvement in endurance athletes with ventricular arrhythmias: role of an electrophysiologic study in risk stratification. Eur Heart J 2003;24:1473–80.

68. La Gerche A, Robberecht C, Kuiperi C, et al. Lower than expected desmosomal gene mutation prevalence in endurance athletes with complex ventricular arrhythmias of right ventricular origin. Heart 2010;96: 1268–74.

# Left Ventricular Hypertrophy and Arrhythmogenesis

Mohammad Shenasa, MD[a,b,*], Hossein Shenasa, MD[a,b],
Nabil El-Sherif, MD[c,d]

## KEYWORDS

- Left ventricular hypertrophy • Ventricular arrhythmias • Atrial fibrillation • Hypertension
- Hypertensive heart disease • Arrhythmogenesis • Torsades de pointes

## KEY POINTS

- Left ventricular hypertrophy (LVH) is a common yet underdiagnosed condition with a heterogeneous cause; the most common cause is long-term hypertension and valvular heart disease.
- LVH diagnosis is based on electrocardiogram (ECG) and other cardiac imaging modalities, such as echocardiogram, cardiac magnetic resonance (CMR) imaging, and cardiac computed tomography (CCT).
- Aggressive management of specific causes of LVH such as hypertension control and appropriate management of valvular heart disease may reverse LVH and its consequences.
- Atrial and ventricular arrhythmias are common in moderate to severe LVH, are often underdiagnosed, and require specific management based on the cause.
- Mechanisms of atrial and ventricular arrhythmias in LVH are diverse and depend on specific causes, mostly related to dispersion of refractoriness that promotes reentry arrhythmias.
- LVH is no longer considered a benign condition and indeed is a silent killer; however, it is a treatable and preventable condition.

## INTRODUCTION

### Definition of Left Ventricular Hypertrophy

LVH is due to an increase in cardiomyocyte size (cell hypertrophy), which results in increased left ventricular (LV) mass and cavity size. The normal LV mass for men is 135 g and LV mass index is 71 g/m². For women, the normal values are 99 g and 62 g/m², respectively. LVH is then usually defined as 2 standard deviations more than the normal.[1–6]

LVH is a common and often underdiagnosed condition and remains silent in the early stages, eventually leading to congestive heart failure (CHF).[7] In patients with a definite ECG pattern of LVH, there is a 59% overall mortality at 12 years. LVH as an independent risk factor increases the risk of coronary artery disease (CAD) by 3-fold. It also increases the risk of sudden cardiac death (SCD) 6- to 8-fold in men and 3-fold in women. It increases the risk of CHF by 10-fold at 16 years. The LIFE (Losartan Intervention For Endpoint reduction in hypertension) study examined the presence of LVH and ST-T wave changes. LVH also increases the risk of myocardial infarction (MI) and other cardiovascular morbidity and mortality in patients with hypertension.[8]

The authors have nothing to disclose.
[a] Department of Cardiovascular Services, O'Connor Hospital, San Jose, CA 95128, USA; [b] Heart and Rhythm Medical Group, 105 North Bascom Avenue, San Jose, CA 92128, USA; [c] State University of New York, Downstate Medical Center, 450 Clarkson Avenue, Brooklyn, NY 11203, USA; [d] Cardiology Division, New York Harbor VA Healthcare System, 800 Poly Place, Brooklyn, NY 11209, USA
* Corresponding author. Heart and Rhythm Medical Group, 105 North Bascom Avenue, San Jose, CA 92128.
E-mail address: mohammad.shenasa@gmail.com

## ELECTROCARDIOGRAM CRITERIA OF LEFT VENTRICULAR HYPERTROPHY

The following are the 2 most used criteria[1–3]:

1. The Sokolow-Lyon voltage criteria: S wave in lead V1 + R wave in lead V5 or V6 greater than or equal to 3.50 mV or R wave in lead V5 or V6 greater than 2.60 mV
2. The Cornell voltage criteria: For women, R wave in lead aVL + S wave in lead V3 greater than 2.00 mV. For men, R wave in lead aVL + S wave in lead V3 greater than 2.80 mV[9]

## THE ELECTROCARDIOGRAPHIC MANIFESTATION OF LEFT VENTRICULAR HYPERTROPHY

Although ECG is easily accessible and cheap, the diagnostic yield of LVH by ECG is only 2.4%, with a low sensitivity and specificity (25%–60%) compared with echocardiography (Echo).[10–12] Furthermore, the diagnostic yield of LVH by ECG is affected by race, gender, medications, and so on. The following are the ECG abnormalities observed in patients with established LVH:

1. Left atrial (LA) abnormalities such as negative p-wave suggest an increase of the left atrial size.
2. There is increased QRS voltage.
3. There is increased QRS duration.
4. Left-axis deviation in hypertensive patients suggests presence of LVH.

5. Left bundle branch block (in advanced stages) is seen.
6. Repolarization abnormalities (ie, ST-T wave changes) are observed.

A slow R wave progression (V1-V3), although nonspecific, may be seen in patients with LVH (one has to exclude underlying anteroseptal MI). **Fig. 1** is an example of significant LVH and ST-T wave abnormalities in a patient with aortic stenosis.

## ECHOCARDIOGRAPHIC CRITERIA OF LEFT VENTRICULAR HYPERTROPHY

The diagnostic yield of LVH by Echo is 17.4%. The equation for LV mass is (g) $= 1.05[($left ventricular end-diastolic diameter (LVEDD) + IVS (interventricular septal thickness) + PW (posterior wall thickness)$)^3 - $ LVEDD$^3]$. LV mass was divided by body surface area to obtain the LV mass index. According to data from the Framingham Heart Study, LVH was defined as LVMI (left ventricular mass index) greater than or equal to 150 g/m$^2$.[5,13–18]

Echo indices that are usually measured during an Echo examination are listed below:

- LV geometry
- Wall thickness
- Motion
- LV systolic function
- LV diastolic function

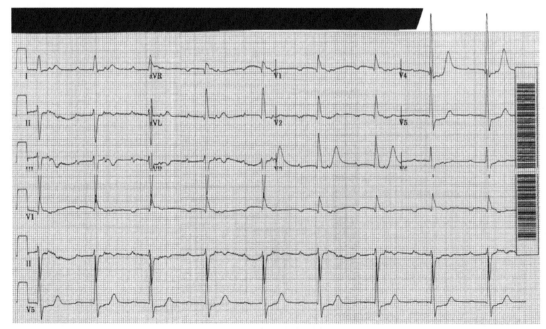

**Fig. 1.** Twelve-lead electrogram of an 85-year-old male with severe aortic stenosis, two-to-one A-V block with prolonged PR Interval of the conducted beats, incomplete right bundle branch block, left ventricular hypertrophy, and ST-T wave abnormalities.

- Diastolic filling abnormalities, Doppler transmitral that flow, that is, early and atrial wave ratio
- LV strain
- Stroke work
- Evidence of myocardial ischemia evaluated during stress Echo

Because LV mass is related to body size and is different in the female gender, this measurement should be corrected for body weight and gender. In general, Echo measurement of LVH and mass has a reasonable accuracy of 80% specificity and sensitivity.

### Anatomic and Structural Consideration

The myocardium has 3 main components[19]:

1. The muscular compartment consisting of myocytes that make up 30% of the myocardial cells and about 70% of cardiac tissue volume
2. The interstitial compartment formed by fibroblast and collagen compounds
3. The vasculature compartment

Cardiac myocytes and fibers play an important role in the pathogenesis of many conditions. Cardiac fiber orientation is often disarrayed in many pathologic conditions. Disarrayed fiber orientation increases anisotropic conduction, which provides a substrate for ventricular tachyarrhythmias (VT). **Fig. 2** shows an example of myocardial fiber disarray using diffusion-tensor MRI (DT-MRI).[20]

Both pressure and volume overload increase LV wall stress, which is a principle mechanical factor in the development of LVH. Multiple biochemical, cellular, and genetic factors (upregulation or downregulation of myocardial cell response to pressure overload and volume) are involved in this process that eventually leads to progression of heart failure and arrhythmias.[21] **Fig. 3** summarizes these pathophysiologic pathways of hypertension and LVH that lead to heart failure and arrhythmias.

### MOLECULAR BASIS AND GENETICS OF LEFT VENTRICULAR HYPERTROPHY AND LEFT VENTRICULAR REMODELING

Important molecular, ionic, and genetic pathways are involved in the genesis of LVH, arrhythmogenesis, and response to therapy. They are well discussed in the section LVH and Arrhythmogenesis and in the articles by Diez and Lips, and Kehat and Mokentin.[22–24]

### ETIOLOGY OF LEFT VENTRICULAR HYPERTROPHY

Three different patterns of LVH are recognized depending on its cause, which has 2 distinct geometric patterns as described later.[25] **Table 1** summarizes LV geometry in hypertension and LVH.

1. Concentric LVH, whereby there is an increase in the ratio of the wall thickness over chamber dimensions such as hypertension and aortic stenosis.

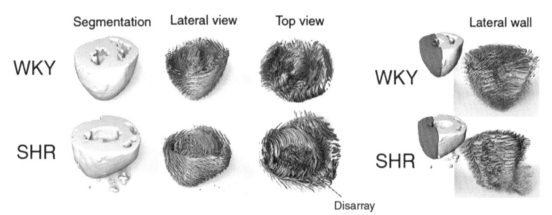

**Fig. 2.** Fiber tractography results from normal WKY (*top*) and diseased SHR (*bottom*) rats. First column: The MRI-based segmented myocardia, where the hypertrophied cardiac wall of the SHR may be seen. Second and third columns: Two different views of the fiber tracking results of the entire wall. Seen from the top, there is marked myofiber disarray in the lateral region of the SHR, as opposed to the WKY. Last column: A close-up, focusing on the free wall region where the disarray in the SHR is more noticeable. MRI, magnetic resonance imaging; SHR, spontaneously hypertensive rat; WKY, Wistar-Kyoto rat heart. (*From* Giannakidis A, Rohmer D, Veress A, et al. Diffusion tensor MRI-derived myocardial fiber disarray in hypertensive left ventricular hypertrophy; visualization, quantification and the effect on mechanical function. In: Shenasa M, Hindricks G, Borggrefe M, et al, editors. Cardiac Mapping. 4th edition. New York: Wiley-Blackwell; 2013. p. 579; with permission.)

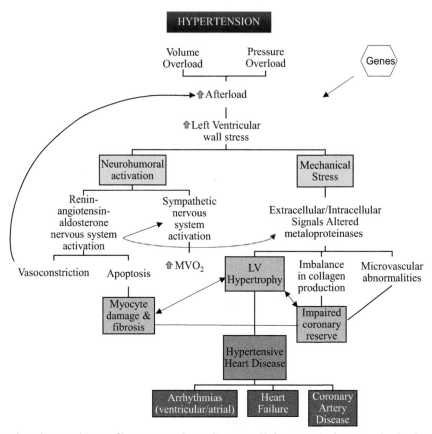

**Fig. 3.** Pathophysiologic pathways of hypertensive heart disease and left ventricular hypertrophy that lead to arrhythmias, heart failure, and coronary artery disease. LV, left ventricle; MV02, mixed venous oxygen saturation. (*Adapted from* Georgiopoulou VV, Kalogeropoulos AP, Raggi P, et al. Prevention, diagnosis, and treatment of hypertensive heart disease. Cardiol Clin 2010;28:677; with permission.)

2. Eccentric LVH, whereby there is a decrease in the ratio of wall thickness over chamber dimensions due to LV cavity dilatation such as mitral regurgitation, aortic insufficiency, and anemia.

In such cases, there is an increase in stroke volume.

1. Pressure overload: Pressure-overload LVH causes concentric hypertrophy.
   a. Hypertension, the most common cause of LVH
   b. Aortic stenosis
   c. Infiltrative myocardial disease
   d. Static exercise
2. Volume overload: Volume overload produces eccentric LVH.
   a. Mitral regurgitation
   b. Aortic regurgitation
   c. Anemia
   d. Heart failure
   e. Obesity[26]
3. Neurohormonal causes of LVH[27]
   Other causes that also have important differential diagnosis include the following:
   a. Physiologic adaptation to physical training in athletes[28,29]

| Table 1 Geometric patterns of LVH | |
|---|---|
| **Concentric** | **Eccentric** |
| • Pressure overload<br>  ○ Hypertension<br>  ○ Aortic stenosis<br>• Static exercise<br>• Infiltrative myocardial disease | • Volume overload<br>  ○ Aortic insufficiency<br>  ○ Mitral regurgitation<br>  ○ Anemia<br>• Dynamic exercise (may be a physiologic adaptation)<br>• Heart failure<br>• Obesity |

b. Primary infiltrative genetic cardiomyopathies, hypertrophic cardiomyopathy (HCM), or other infiltrative cardiomyopathies such as amyloidosis and hemochromatosis[12,30,31]

c. Remodeling following myocardial injury such as acute MI

It is important to differentiate physiologic from pathologic hypertrophy.[32,33]

## HYPERTENSION AND LEFT VENTRICULAR HYPERTROPHY

Long-standing hypertension is the most common cause of LVH. At some point during the natural history of hypertension, a compensatory increase in the LV mass as a response to increased pressure overload occurs.[34–36] LVH therefore has become a preclinical disease and poses an independent risk factor for ischemic heart disease, CHF, arrhythmias, stroke, and SCD. Other pathophysiologic factors that are involved in this process include obesity, metabolic syndrome, age, gender, race, and genetic and even environmental factors. Many neurohormonal factors, such as angiotensin II, lead to myocardial remodeling and fibrosis. Cardiac effects of angiotensin II relevant to hypertrophy and arrhythmogenesis include increased wall stress that facilitates local noradrenaline release and inhibits central vagal activity, fibrosis, decreased conduction velocity, disorganized cell-to-cell coupling, increased dispersion of action potential duration (APD), stimulated myocyte growth, and structural vascular changes.[23]

The multiple organ involvement of preclinical and eventually clinical hypertension leads to manifest LVH, heart failure, and death.

Hypertensive LVH is more evident in blacks than in whites. Similarly, heart failure, SCD, and stroke are more common in blacks than in whites for the same degree of LVH.[37,38]

Cardiovascular effects of hypertension are as follows:

1. LVH
2. Diastolic dysfunction
3. LV systolic dysfunction
4. Microvascular dysfunction
5. Atrial and ventricular arrhythmias
6. Peripheral vascular disease
7. CAD
8. Cerebrovascular disease

### Hypertensive Heart Disease

Hypertensive heart disease (HHD) is defined as changes in myocardial structure, function, coronary vasodilation, and conduction system of the heart as a result of prolonged high blood pressure, which contributes to increased morbidity and mortality.

HHD thus constitutes a spectrum of hemodynamic and structural changes in the cardiovascular system. In its early phases, HHD produces LVH, LA enlargement, and diastolic dysfunction and eventually leads to CHF at the other end of the spectrum.

The pathophysiology of HHD constitutes a complex interplay of hemodynamic structural, functional, neurohormonal, cellular, molecular and genetic factors. In addition, owing to a compensatory response to these changes, the cardiovascular system undergoes significant changes (remodeling) that lead to hypertrophy and eventually heart failure, fibrosis, and cell death.

### Left Ventricular Hypertrophy as an Independent Risk Factor

LVH increases the morbidity and mortality of cardiovascular disease, including CAD, CHF, atrial fibrillation (AF), supra and ventricular arrhythmias, stroke, and sudden death. It is often underdiagnosed and underestimated.

## RISK FACTORS FOR ARRHYTHMIAS IN HYPERTENSIVE PATIENTS

1. Age
2. Levels of diurnal and nocturnal systolic blood pressure during 24 hours
3. LA diameter
4. LV mass
5. Maximum duration and dispersion of the P-wave on the ECG
6. Alcohol
7. Other diseases

## HEMODYNAMIC CONSEQUENCES OF LEFT VENTRICULAR HYPERTROPHY

Risk factors for progression of LVH in patients with hypertension include the following:

1. Angiotensin II
2. Norepinephrine
3. Epinephrine
4. Increased peripheral and cardiac sympathetic drive[27]
5. Endothelial dysfunction[39]
6. Natriuretic peptides
7. Adrenomedullin[40]
8. Leptin
9. Other unknown factors

## Left Ventricular Hypertrophy and Sudden Cardiac Death

It has long been known that LVH is an independent risk factor for SCD, mostly because of ventricular arrhythmias, which is underrecognized. This factor is further discussed in the following section.[41–46]

## Left Ventricular Hypertrophy and Arrhythmias

LVH may produce a variety of arrhythmias alone, including atrial premature depolarization, with AF being the most common. Others include the following:

- Supraventricular arrhythmias
- Ventricular arrhythmias, including premature ventricular contractions (PVC), couplets, nonsustained VT, sustained VT, ventricular fibrillation, and sudden death

## Left Ventricular Hypertrophy and Arrhythmogenesis

LV geometric adaptation to hypertension is heterogeneous. An important consequence of hypertension and LVH in inherited cardiac fibrosis is that it promotes myocardial heterogeneity, which sets up ventricular arrhythmias and SCD.

LVH causes remodeling at several levels:

1. Ion channel remodeling
2. Gap junction remodeling
3. Remodeling of the cytoskeleton, proteins, and calcium hemostasis
4. Depolarization and repolarization change
5. Abnormal conduction
6. Electromechanical contraction disturbances

All these factors lead to arrhythmias and pump failure.

## Left Ventricular Hypertrophy and Atrial Arrhythmias

AF is the most common arrhythmia in patients with hypertension.[47–49] Risk factors for development of AF in patients with hypertension include age, level of diurnal and nocturnal systolic blood pressure during 24-hour blood pressure monitoring, LA diameter, LV mass, and maximum duration and dispersion of the P-wave of the ECG.[49,50]

# LEFT VENTRICULAR HYPERTROPHY AND VENTRICULAR ARRHYTHMIAS
## Arrhythmogenicity of the Hypertrophied Heart

A large body of evidence has shown the prevalence of ventricular arrhythmias in patients with LVH, and potential mechanisms have been evaluated in human, animal, and in vitro models.[44] In a recent meta-analysis, the incidence of ventricular arrhythmias was 5.5% compared with 1.2% in patients without LVH.[44] The occurrence of VT or fibrillation was 2.8-fold greater in the presence of LVH.[51] Furthermore, findings from the Oregon Sudden Unexpected Death Study (Oregon SUDS) confirmed the LVH–SCD association in the community, also showing that LVH and severe LV systolic dysfunction are independent predictors of SCD that may contribute to risk through distinct mechanistic pathways.[44]

## Electrophysiologic Mechanisms of Arrhythmogenicity of Hypertrophied Myocardium

### Remodeling of active membrane properties in left ventricular hypertrophy

LVH is accompanied by significant remodeling of the ventricular myocardium in both the cellular and interstitial compartments, which promotes ventricular arrhythmogenesis resulting from reentry and triggered activity. Myocardial electrical remodeling manifests as abnormalities of repolarization (prolonged QTc) and depolarization (prolonged QRS interval), both of which facilitate reentrant arrhythmias.[52,53] At a cellular level, there is decreased density of sodium and potassium pumps, which leads to decreased intracellular potassium concentrations and prolonged repolarization.[54] Along these lines, cellular studies have shown that adenosine triphosphate (ATP)-sensitive potassium channels are more likely to be open during ischemia in hypertrophied myocytes compared with normal myocytes[55]; this can also prolong ventricular repolarization, allowing for afterdepolarizations and triggered activity that initiate ventricular arrhythmias. In this regard, previous studies have shown that the hypertrophied myocardium is more prone to arrhythmia in response to known torsadogenic drugs.[56]

The link between abnormalities of myocardial electrical remodeling and ventricular arrhythmogenesis in LVH has been reported from a variety of in vivo animal models. An early study in a canine model of LVH reported that dogs that were administered calcium agonists had more early afterdepolarizations and ventricular arrhythmias than dogs without LVH.[57] Rials and colleagues[58] induced LVH with aortic banding in a feline model and observed increased susceptibility to inducible polymorphic VT. In a rabbit model, LVH created by renal artery ligation displayed increased dispersion of refractoriness, a lower ventricular fibrillation threshold, and action potential prolongation.[59]

## Remodeling of intracellular matrix in left ventricular hypertrophy

In addition to inhomogeneity of active membrane ionic properties, alterations in the passive electrical properties of hypertrophied myocardium due to interstitial fibrosis as well as specific quantitative and/or qualitative changes in gap-junction proteins have been reported. There is reduction in connexin 43 expression that slowed cell-to-cell conduction.[60] Increased myocardial interstitial fibrosis is a consistent finding in LVH, with significant effects on electrical conduction.[61] More recent studies indicate a potentially important role for myofibroblasts that proliferate in conditions of increased myocardial fibrosis, such as LVH. These cells contribute to enhancement of fibrosis by secreting more collagen and fibronectin, whereas myofibroblasts may promote reentry by acting as passive and delayed electrical conduits for excitatory current flow.[62] These collective alterations in myocardial interstitial remodeling can result in differential slowing of ventricular conduction, creating the conditions for microreentry and arrhythmogenesis in LVH.[63]

## The autonomic system and arrhythmogenicity of left ventricular hypertrophy

There is evidence for significant abnormalities in autonomic tone with LVH, which contribute further to ventricular arrhythmogenesis. It has long been recognized that increased LV mass in normotensive and hypertensive patients is coupled with increased cardiac sympathetic activity when measured using multiple techniques, including coronary venous plasma concentration of noradrenaline, pressor response to exogenous noradrenaline infusion, 24-hour urinary catecholamine levels, and pressure response to ergometric exercise.[64,65] Sympathetic activation has been shown to exert a direct proarrhythmic effect that may lead to VTs and SCD.[66]

## Other potential mechanisms of increased arrhythmogenicity of left ventricular hypertrophy

Other electrophysiologic mechanisms of arrhythmogenicity of hypertrophied myocardium include upregulation of Na/Ca exchange current and enhanced sarcoplasmic reticulum Ca release that create a more favorable setting for both early and delayed afterdepolarizations.[67] A genetic predisposition to LVH has been identified, which seems to be distinct from genetic transmission of hypertension.[68,69] A large number of novel genetic variants have been identified from human populations that could further expand the list of

distinct mechanistic processes leading to ventricular arrhythmogenesis. Genome-wide association studies identified 12 single-nucleotide polymorphisms associated with LVH. One of these is KCNB1, which encodes a voltage-gated potassium channel and is dephosphorylated by calcineurin, thus identified as a potential candidate gene related to arrhythmogenesis in LVH.[68]

## Cardiac Hypertrophy and Ischemia

The coexistence of cardiac hypertrophy and ischemia can create a particularly arrhythmogenic substrate.[70] Earlier studies using a canine model showed evidence that electrophysiology of ischemia in hypertrophied myocardium was altered compared with nonhypertrophied myocardium, with an increased incidence of VT.[71,72] However, most experimental studies investigated the effects of global ischemia/reperfusion on hypertrophy,[73,74] which is not a good experimental surrogate for the clinical setting in which regional ischemia is the norm. Furthermore, although most studies that investigated the effects of ischemia on hypertrophy showed evidence of increased dispersion of repolarization, conclusions were usually based on indirect or limited mapping of cardiac repolarization.[73–75] In contrast, Koshevnikov and colleagues[76] have designed a study to investigate the electrophysiologic effects of regional ischemia in a guinea pig model of hypertrophy using detailed optical mapping of membrane voltage. The study has shown 2 electrophysiologic mechanisms that can result in increased dispersion of repolarization when regional ischemia is superimposed on hypertrophy, an increased dispersion of repolarization at the border between the ischemic zone and nonischemic zone and a greater tendency to develop APD alternans. The increased dispersion of repolarization was primarily the result of more marked shortening of prolonged APD in the ischemic zone compared with the nonischemic zone (**Figs. 4** and **5**). These observations are consistent with previous reports.[75,77] Using conventional microelectrode studies, Kohya and colleagues[73] showed enhanced APD shortening induced by simulated ischemia in hypertrophied rat heart. Experiments in hypertrophied feline LV myocytes revealed that the open-state probability of ATP-sensitive K+ channel was significantly higher at various pH levels and depleted ATP conditions and that the magnitude of the ICa-L was significantly reduced during metabolic inhibition.[78] Both mechanisms can explain the greater degree of ischemia-induced APD shortening in

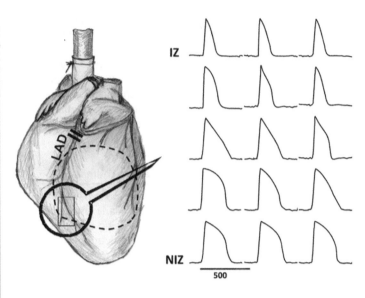

**Fig. 4.** Optical recordings of membrane voltage obtained from a perfused Langendorff preparation of a hypertrophied guinea pig heart during ischemia. The diagram on the left shows the site of left anterior descending artery ligation marked by the double bar and the outline of the ischemic zone (*dotted line*). The right panel illustrates action potentials from 3 horizontal and 5 vertical contiguous pixels across the border between the ischemic zone and nonischemic zone (*highlighted*). The recordings were obtained after 5 minutes of ischemia during pacing at cycle length 400 milliseconds. Note the development of varying degrees of shortening of APD in the ischemic zone (IZ) compared with the nonischemic zone (NIZ).

hypertrophy. Early observations of Janse and colleagues[79] have also shown that the initiating beat of VT in early ischemia is due to focal activity arising from the nonischemic side of the border zone possibly due to the flow of current between the ischemic zone and nonischemic zone.

## ISCHEMIA-INDUCED ACTION POTENTIAL DURATION ALTERNANS IN HYPERTROPHIED HEART

Rate-dependent APD alternans induced by global ischemia is ubiquitous.[80,81] By contrast, regional ischemia superimposed on hypertrophy more frequently resulted in rate-dependent APD alternans compared with nonhypertrophied myocardium (**Fig. 6**).[76] In a previous study, Lakireddy and

colleagues[81] showed that spatially heterogeneous shortening of APD during ischemia coupled with a more spatially homogeneous lengthening of CaiT duration played a major role in the development of APD alternans. The mechanism of the spatially heterogeneous shortening of APD during ischemia is related, among other factors, to the degree of local increase in the level of [K+]0. Several studies have shown inhomogeneities in [K+]0 during ischemia, which is more pronounced in hypertrophy[77]; this could possibly explain the greater incidence of ischemia-induced APD alternans in hypertrophy. In summary, regional ischemia superimposed on hypertrophied myocardium resulted in a greater degree of dispersion of repolarization, APD alternans, and higher incidence of VT. It is important to emphasize that increased dispersion of repolarization is

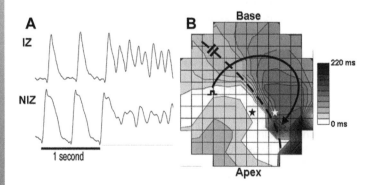

**Fig. 5.** Optical recordings of membrane voltage obtained from a hypertrophied guinea pig heart after 10 minutes of left anterior descending artery occlusion illustrates the onset of ventricular tachyarrhythmia (VT). (*A*) Action potential recordings from 2 sites 2 mm apart on each side of the border between the ischemic zone (IZ) and nonischemic zone (NIZ) (*asterisks*). The first 3 action potentials are paced at a cycle length of 500 milliseconds. Note the development of a 60-millisecond conduction delay between the 2 sites, the marked shortening of APD of the IZ site, and the onset of a non-self-terminating VT. (*B*) Epicardial isochronal activation map of the last paced beat before the onset of VT shows development of an arc of conduction block (represented by crowded isochrones) at the border between the IZ and NIZ. A wave front that started at the site of pacing in the right ventricle circulated around the arc of block in a pattern consistent with circus movement reentry.

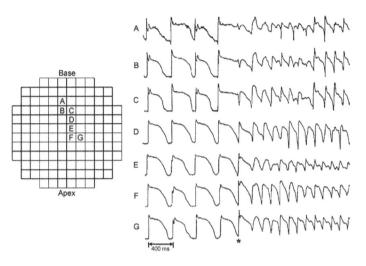

**Fig. 6.** Selected optical recordings of membrane voltage obtained after 8 minutes of ischemia in a guinea pig heart with hypertrophy. Seven action potential (AP) recordings labeled A to G are illustrated on the right, and their position on the epicardial surface of the ventricle is shown in the schematic photodiode array on the left. The first 4 APs at each recording represent paced APs at a cycle length of 400 milliseconds. The fifth AP was a spontaneous premature beat (*asterisk*) that initiated a non-self-terminating VT. Recordings A to C were from contiguous sites close to the basal region of the ventricle and showed APD alternans with the first AP with short duration followed by an AP with long duration (ABAB sequence). Recordings E to G were from contiguous sites toward the apical region of the ventricle and showed APD alternans with the first AP with long duration (BABA sequence). Recording D was obtained from a site between the 2 groups of discordant alternans, and it showed no discernible APD alternans. Because of the spatially discordant alternans, the premature focal excitation failed to activate sites with prolonged APD (sites A, B, and C which only showed a subthreshold potential), whereas it activated sites with shorter APD (sites E, F, and G). This spatial heterogeneity of activation provided the substrate for reentrant excitation.

only one of the substrates for reentrant VT during ischemia, besides impaired conduction, decreased excitability, and reduced cellular coupling.

### Prognostic Significance of Left Ventricular Hypertrophy

As said earlier, LVH, irrespective of cause and diagnostic method, poses an increased risk of cardiovascular overall morbidity and mortality. Adjusted for its comorbidity, LVH increases mortality rate by 1.5 to 3.5 per year.[6,82–85]

### Regression Left Ventricular Hypertrophy

LV mass can be decreased by different types of intervention, such as weight loss in obese patients. Most antihypertensive medications, notably angiotensin converting enzyme blockers and angiotensin receptor blocker, reverse (regress) the LVH.

Similarly, correction of other pressure and volume overload factors reverses LVH. The magnitude of LVH regression is directly affected not only by an optimal blood pressure control and related risk factors but also by genetic factors that determines the magnitude of LVH regression. Multiple studies have evaluated LVH regression in different substrates and interventions, which are beyond the purpose and scope of this review.[86–89]

**Fig. 7** demonstrates regression of LVH and ST-T wave changes after correction of severe aortic stenosis, from the same patient as in **Fig. 1**.

## IMAGING TECHNIQUES IN THE DIAGNOSIS AND RESPONSE TO THERAPY IN PATIENTS WITH LEFT VENTRICULAR HYPERTROPHY
### Cardiac MRI

CMR is considered the gold standard for the measurement of LV mass and volume. Advantages of CMR are as follows[20,50,90–92]:

1. Has high spatial and temporal resolution
2. Allows multiplane image acquisition
3. Is free of ionizing radiation
4. Has the highest reproducibility compared with other noninvasive imaging modalities

The disadvantages of CMR are artifact due to patient movement and arrhythmias, claustrophobia, not easily accessible (widely used), and high cost. Puntmann and colleagues[32] and Bacharova and colleagues[82] compared the diagnostic yield and value of MRI with ECG in patients with LVH. As expected, they reported that MRI is superior and provides important phenotypic information compared with ECG.

### Cardiac Computed Tomography

CCT provides high resolution and accurate information of LV mass, volume, and function. The important limitation is its ionizing radiation exposure. There exists a high correlation between CMR imaging and CCT for the measurement of LV mass and volume.[93]

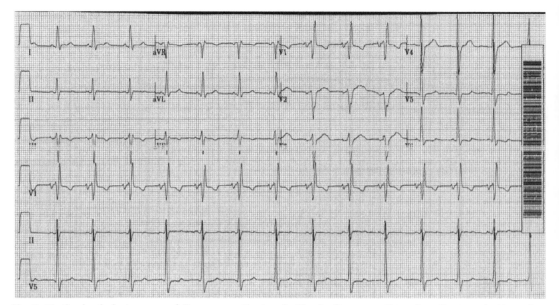

**Fig. 7.** Twelve-lead electrogram of the same patient as in **Fig. 1** after correction of aortic stenosis. Note sinus rhythm with normal PR interval, incomplete right bundle branch block, significant regression of left ventricular hypertrophy, and improvement in ST-T wave abnormalities.

### Single-Photon Emission Computed Tomography and PET

Single-photon emission computed tomography is also used in patients suspected or diagnosed with coronary disease and myocardial ischemia, and it provides accurate measurement of LV mass, volume, and function.

## MANAGEMENT OF LEFT VENTRICULAR HYPERTROPHY

Optimal and timely management of hypertension and other causes should reverse the LVH and decrease the potential consequences such as heart failure and arrhythmias. One should avoid hypokalemia, bradycardia, and medications that potentially prolong QT-interval.[94,95] Specific cause-based management, guideline adherence, and evidence-based management should be the center of approach to the management of LVH and its consequences; which is beyond the scope of this review and discussed elsewhere.[1,94] Risk stratification and reduction in cardiovascular risk should be the integral point of management. Regression of LVH and its benefits certainly improve the outcome and lower the risks increased by AF, ventricular arrhythmias, and SCD. In patients with hypertension, one needs to evaluate the LV geometry and function by Echo and other imaging modalities and recognize the magnitude of hypertension-induced LVH.[96–99]

## FUTURE DIRECTIONS

At present, angiotensin II and angiotensin receptor blocks are among the first-line therapy in patients with hypertension and HHD.

Advanced imaging technologies such as DT-MRI help us better understand the electromechanical basis of LVH in different substrates as well as the differential diagnosis of different forms of hypertrophy as discussed earlier in **Fig. 2**. Cardiac MRI will probably be used more often, when there is a question of differential diagnosis of LVH and ECG or Echo does not provide adequate answers for clinical management.

Advanced therapeutics such as renal denervation have been reported to improve the magnitude of LVH and diastolic dysfunction.[100–102]

## SUMMARY

- Hypertension is the most common cause of LVH.
- LVH has a wide spectrum of clinical course ranging from preclinical phase with impaired-filling ventricular remodeling and diastolic dysfunction to progression of LV dilatation, heart failure, CAD, myocardial ischemia, and infarction. LVH causes both atrial and ventricular arrhythmias and increases the risk of SCD.
- LVH is no longer considered a benign condition; it is a silent killer that is preventable.[103]

- An important differential diagnosis is HCM athlete's heart.
- Advanced imaging modalities may help to differentiate conditions.
- Appropriate management of the causes of LVH (ie, optimal blood pressure control and correction of valvular heart disease, such as aortic stenosis and mitral and aortic regurgitation) results in regression of LVH and lowers the risk of its complications including heart failure, atrial and ventricular arrhythmias, and SCD.

## ACKNOWLEDGMENTS

The authors thank Mariah Smith and Shayan Aminilari for their assistance in preparing this article.

## REFERENCES

1. Mirvis DM, Goldberger AL. Electrocardiography. Braunwald's heart disease: a textbook of cardiovascular medicine. 10th edition. Philadelphia: Elsevier; 2015. p. 114–54.
2. Sokolow M, Lyon TP. The ventricular complex in left ventricular hypertrophy as obtained by unipolar precordial and limb leads. Am Heart J 1949; 37(2):161–86.
3. Romhilt DW, Bove KE, Norris FJ, et al. A critical appraisal of the electrocardiographic criteria for the diagnosis of left ventricular hypertrophy. Circulation 1969;40(2):185–95.
4. Butler PM, Legget SI, Howe CM, et al. Identification of electrocardiographic criteria for diagnosis of right ventricular hypertrophy due to mitral stenosis. Am J Cardiol 1986;57(8):639–43.
5. Lorenz CH, Walker ES, Morgan VL, et al. Normal human right and left ventricular mass, systolic function, and gender differences by cine magnetic resonance imaging. J Cardiovasc Magn Reson 1999;1:7–21.
6. Lorell B, Carabello B. Left ventricular hypertrophy: pathogenesis, detection, and prognosis. Circulation 2000;102:470–9.
7. Chambers J. Left ventricular hypertrophy: an underappreciated coronary risk factor. BMJ 1995; 311:273–4.
8. Okin PM, Devereux RB, Nieminen MS, et al. Electrocardiographic strain pattern and prediction of cardiovascular morbidity and mortality in hypertensive patients. Hypertension 2004;44:48–54.
9. Levy D, Labib S, Anderson K, et al. Determinants of sensitivity and specificity of electrocardiographic criteria for left ventricular hypertrophy. Circulation 1990;81:815–20.
10. Macfarlane P. Is electrocardiography still useful in the diagnosis of cardiac chamber hypertrophy and dilatation? Cardiol Clin 2006;24:401–11.
11. Prisant M. Hypertensive heart disease. J Clin Hypertens 2005;7:231–8.
12. Shenasa M, Shenasa H. Electrocardiographic markers of sudden cardiac death in different substrates. The ECG handbook of contemporary challenges. Minneapolis, MN: Cardiotext; 2015. Chapter 6.
13. Levy D, Savage DD, Garrison RJ, et al. Echocardiographic criteria for left ventricular hypertrophy: the Framingham Heart Study. Am J Cardiol 1987; 59:956–60.
14. Levy D, Murabito JM, Anderson KM, et al. Echocardiographic left ventricular hypertrophy: clinical characteristics: the Framingham Heart Study. Clin Exp Hypertens 1992;14:85–97.
15. Kannel W, Gordon T, Castelli WP, et al. Electrocardiographic left ventricular hypertrophy and risk of coronary heart disease. The Framingham Study. Ann Intern Med 1970;72(6):813–22.
16. Solomon SD, Wu J, Gillam L. Echocardiography. Braunwald's heart disease: a textbook of cardiovascular medicine. 10th edition. Philadelphia: Elsevier; 2015.
17. Feingenbaum H, Armstrong W, Ryan T. Feigenbaum's echocardiography. 6th edition. Philadelphia: Lippincott William & Wilkins; 2005.
18. Oh JK, Seward JB, Tajik AJ. The Echo manual. 3rd edition. Philadelphia: Lippincott William & Wilkins; 2006.
19. Kahan T, Bergfeldt L. Left ventricular hypertrophy in hypertension: its arrhythmogenic potential. Heart 2005;91:250–6.
20. Giannakidis A, Rohmer D, Veress A, et al. Diffusion tensor magnetic resonance imaging-derived myocardial fiber disarray in hypertensive left ventricular hypertrophy; visualization, quantification and the effect on mechanical function. In: Shenasa M, Hindricks G, Borggrefe M, et al, editors. Cardiac mapping. 4th edition. Oxford, UK: Wiley-Blackwell; 2013. Chapter 53. p. 574–88.
21. Lacchini R, Luizon M, Gasparini S, et al. Effect of genetic polymorphisms of vascular endothelial growth factor on left ventricular hypertrophy in patients with systemic hypertension. Am J Cardiol 2014;113:491–6.
22. Diez J, Frohlich ED. A translational approach to hypertensive heart disease. Hypertension 2010;55:1–8.
23. Lips D, deWindt LJ, Kraaij D, et al. Molecular determinants of myocardial hypertrophy and failure: alternative pathways for beneficial and maladaptive hypertrophy. Eur Heart J 2003;24:883–96.
24. Kehat I, Molkentin JD. Molecular pathways underlying cardiac remodeling during pathophysiological stimulation. Circulation 2010;122:2727–35.

25. Yuda S, Khoury V, Marwick TH. Influence of wall stress and left ventricular geometry on the accuracy of dobutamine stress echocardiography. J Am Coll Cardiol 2002;40:1311–9.

26. Lavie CJ, McAuley PA, Church TS, et al. Obesity and cardiovascular diseases: implications regarding fitness, fatness, and severity in the obesity paradox. J Am Coll Cardiol 2014;63: 1345–54.

27. Schlaich MP, Kaye DM, Lambert E, et al. Relation between cardiac sympathetic activity and hypertensive left ventricular hypertrophy. Circulation 2003;108:560–5.

28. Zilinski J, Contursi M, Isaacs S, et al. Myocardial adaptation to recreational marathon training among middle-aged men. Circ Cardiovasc Imaging 2015;8:e002487.

29. Maron B, Pelliccia A. The heart of trained athletes: cardiac remodeling and the risks of sports including sudden death. Circulation 2006;114: 1633–44.

30. Yilmaz A, Sechtem U. Diagnostic approach and differential diagnosis in patients with hypertrophied left ventricles. Heart 2014;100:662–71.

31. Namdar M, Steffel J, Jetzer S, et al. Value of electrocardiogram in the differentiation of hypertensive heart disease, hypertrophic cardiomyopathy, aortic stenosis, amyloidosis, and Fabry disease. Am J Cardiol 2012;109:587–93.

32. Puntmann VO, Jahnke C, Gebker R, et al. Usefulness of magnetic resonance imaging to distinguish hypertensive and hypertrophic cardiomyopathy. Am J Cardiol 2010;106:1016–22.

33. Kobza R, Cuculi F, Abacherli R, et al. Twelve-lead electrocardiography in the young: physiologic and pathologic abnormalities. Heart Rhythm 2012;9(12):2018–22.

34. Drazner MH. The progression of hypertensive heart disease. Circulation 2011;123:327–34.

35. Frohlich ED, Apstein C, Chobanian AV, et al. The heart in hypertension. N Engl J Med 1992;327: 998–1008.

36. Schillaci G, Verdecchia P, Porcellati C, et al. Continuous relation between left ventricular mass and cardiovascular risk in essential hypertension. Hypertension 2000;35:580–6.

37. Fox E, Musani S, Samdarshi T, et al. Clinical correlates and prognostic significance of change in standardized left ventricular mass in a community-based cohort of African Americans. J Am Heart Assoc 2015;4:e001224.

38. Drazner MH, Dries DL, Peshock RM, et al. Left ventricular hypertrophy is more prevalent in blacks than whites in the general population: the Dallas Heart Study. Hypertension 2005;46:124–9.

39. Ichikawa KI, Hidai C, Okuda C, et al. Endogenous endothelin-1 mediates cardiac hypertrophy and switching of myosin heavy chain gene expression in rate ventricular myocardium. J Am Coll Cardiol 1996;27:1286.

40. Xin W, Toshio N, Kazumi A, et al. Upregulation of ligand, receptor system, and amidating activity of adrenomedullin in left ventricular hypertrophy of severely hypertensive rats: effects of angiotensin-converting enzyme inhibitors and diuretic. Hypertension 2003;21(6):1171–81.

41. Haider A, Larson M, Benjamin E, et al. Increased left ventricular mass and hypertrophy are associated with increased risk for sudden death. J Am Coll Cardiol 1998;32:1454–9.

42. Narayanan K, Reinier K, Teodorescu C, et al. Electrocardiographic versus echocardiographic left ventricular hypertrophy and sudden cardiac arrest in the community. Heart Rhythm 2014;11:1040–6.

43. Laukkanen J, Khan H, Kurl S, et al. Left ventricular mass and the risk of sudden cardiac death: a population-based study. J Am Heart Assoc 2014; 3:e001285.

44. Stevens S, Reinier K, Chugh S. Increased left ventricular mass as a predictor of sudden cardiac death: is it time to put it to the test? Circ Arrhythm Electrophysiol 2013;6:212–7.

45. Soliman E, Shah A, Boerkircher A, et al. Inter-relationship between electrocardiographic left ventricular hypertrophy and QT prolongation as predictors of increased risk of mortality in the general population. Circ Arrhythm Electrophysiol 2014;7:400–6.

46. Okin PM, Bang CN, Wachtell K, et al. Relationship of sudden cardiac death to new-onset atrial fibrillation in hypertensive patients with left ventricular hypertrophy. Circ Arrhythm Electrophysiol 2013;6: 243–51.

47. Raman SV. The hypertensive heart: an integrated understanding informed by imaging. J Am Coll Cardiol 2010;55:91–6.

48. Verdecchia P, Reboldi R, Bentivoglio M, et al. Atrial fibrillation in hypertension: predictors and outcome. Hypertension 2003;41:218–23.

49. Kannel WB, Abbott RD, Savage DD, et al. Epidemiologic features of chronic atrial fibrillation: the Framingham Study. N Engl J Med 1982;306:1018.

50. Chrispin J, Jain A, Soliman EZ, et al. Association of electrocardiographic and imaging surrogates of left ventricular hypertrophy with incident atrial fibrillation: MESA (Multi-Ethnic Study of Atherosclerosis). J Am Coll Cardiol 2014;63:2007–13.

51. Chatterjee S, Bavishi C, Sardar P, et al. Meta-Analysis of left ventricular hypertrophy and sustained arrhythmias. Am J Cardiol 2014;114:1049–52.

52. Gillis AM, Mathison HJ, Kulisz E, et al. Dispersion of ventricular repolarization and ventricular fibrillation in left ventricular hypertrophy: influence of selective potassium channel blockers. J Pharmacol Exp Ther 2000;292:381–6.

53. Kulan K, Ural D, Komsuoğlu B, et al. Significance of QTc prolongation on ventricular arrhythmias in patients with left ventricular hypertrophy secondary to essential hypertension. Int J Cardiol 1998;64:179–84.

54. Lee SW, Schwartz A, Adams RJ, et al. Decrease in Na+,K+-ATPase activity and [3H]ouabain binding sites in sarcolemma prepared from hearts of spontaneously hypertensive rats. Hypertension 1983;5:682–8.

55. Cameron JS, Kimura S, Jackson-Burns DA, et al. ATP-sensitive K+ channels are altered in hypertrophied ventricular myocytes. Am J Physiol 1988;255(5 Pt 2):H1254–8.

56. Panyasing Y, Kijtawornrat A, Del rio C, et al. Uni- or bi-ventricular hypertrophy and susceptibility to drug-induced torsades de pointes. J Pharmacol Toxicol Methods 2010;62:148–56.

57. Ben-David J, Zipes DP, Ayers GM, et al. Canine left ventricular hypertrophy predisposes to ventricular tachycardia induction by phase 2 early after depolarizations after administration of BAY K 8644. J Am Coll Cardiol 1992;20:1576–84.

58. Rials SJ, Wu Y, Ford N, et al. Effect of left ventricular hypertrophy and its regression on ventricular electrophysiology and vulnerability to inducible arrhythmia in the feline heart. Circulation 1995;91:426–30.

59. Rials SJ, Wu Y, Xu X, et al. Regression of left ventricular hypertrophy with captopril restores normal ventricular action potential duration, dispersion of refractoriness, and cardiac death after coronary artery occlusion in conscious dogs. Circulation 1982;65:1192–7.

60. Peters NS, Green CR, Poole-Wilson PA, et al. Reduced content of connexin43 gap junctions in ventricular myocardium from hypertrophied and ischemic human hearts. Circulation 1993;88:864–75.

61. Weber KT, Brilla CG. Pathological hypertrophy and cardiac interstitium. Fibrosis and rennin–angiotensin–aldosterone system. Circulation 1991;83:1849–65.

62. Gaudesius G, Miragoli M, Thomas SP, et al. Coupling of cardiac electrical activity over extended distances by fibroblasts of cardiac origin. Circ Res 2003;93:421–8.

63. Wolk R. Arrhythmogenic mechanisms in left ventricular hypertrophy. Europace 2000;2:216–23.

64. Ferrara LA, Mancini M, de Simone G, et al. Adrenergic nervous system and left ventricular mass in primary hypertension. Eur Heart J 1989;10:1036–40.

65. Kelm M, Schäfer S, Mingers S, et al. Left ventricular mass is linked to cardiac noradrenaline in normotensive and hypertensive patients. J Hypertens 1996;14:1357–64.

66. Barron HV, Lesh MD. Autonomic nervous system and sudden cardiac death. J Am Coll Cardiol 1996;27:1053–60.

67. Antoons G, Oros A, Bito V, et al. Cellular basis for triggered ventricular arrhythmias that occur in the setting of compensated hypertrophy and heart failure: consideration for diagnosis and management. J Electrocardiol 2007;40:S8–14.

68. Arnett DK, Li N, Tang W, et al. Genome-wide association study identifies single-nucleotide polymorphism in KCNB1 associated with left ventricular mass in humans: the HyperGEN Study. BMC Med Genet 2009;10:43.

69. Arnett DK, de las Fuentes L, Broeckel U. Genes for left ventricular hypertrophy. Curr Hypertens Rep 2004;6:36–41.

70. Levy D, Anderson KM, Savage DD, et al. Risk of ventricular arrhythmia in left ventricular hypertrophy: the Framingham Heart Study. Am J Cardiol 1987;60:560–5.

71. Koyanagi S, Eastham C, Marcus ML. Effects of chronic hypertension and left ventricular hypertrophy on the incidence of sudden cardiac death after coronary artery occlusion in conscious dogs. Circulation 1982;55:1192–7.

72. Martins JB, Kim W, Marcus ML. Chronic hypertension and left ventricular hypertrophy facilitate induction of sustained ventricular tachycardia in dogs three hours after left circumflex coronary artery disease. J Am Coll Cardiol 1989;14:365–73.

73. Kohya T, Kimura S, Myerburg RJ, et al. Susceptibility of hypertrophied rat hearts to ventricular fibrillation during acute ischemia. J Mol Cell Cardiol 1988;20:159–68.

74. Nguyen T, Salibi EE, Rouleau JL. Post infarction survival and inducibility of ventricular arrhythmias in the spontaneously hypertensive rat. Effects of ramipril and hydralazine. Circulation 1998;98:2074–80.

75. Wolk R, Sneddon KP, Dempster J, et al. Regional electrophysiological effects of left ventricular hypertrophy in isolated rabbit hearts under normal and ischemic conditions. Cardiovasc Res 2000;48:120–8.

76. Koshevnikov D, Caref EB, El-Sherif N. Mechanisms of enhanced arrhythmogenecity of regional ischemia in the hypertrophied heart. Heart Rhythm 2009;6:522–7.

77. Vermeulen JT, Hanno TL, Rademaker H. Electrophysiologic and cellular ionic changes during acute ischemia in failing and normal rabbit myocardium. J Mol Cell Cardiol 1996;28:123–31.

78. Furukawa T, Myerburg RJ, Furukawa N, et al. Metabolic inhibition of ICa-L and IK differs in feline left ventricular hypertrophy. Am J Physiol 1994;266:H1121–31.

79. Janse J, Van capelle FJ, Morsink H, et al. Flow of "injury" current and pattern of excitation during early ventricular arrhythmias in acute regional myocardial ischemia in isolated porcine and canine hearts. Circ Res 1980;47:151–65.

80. Choi BR, Salama G. Simultaneous maps of optical action potentials and calcium transients in guinea-pig hearts: mechanisms underlying concordant alternans. J Physiol (London) 2000;529:171–88.

81. Lakireddy V, Baweja P, Syed A, et al. Contrasting effects of ischemia on the kinetics of membrane voltage and intracellular calcium transient underlie electrical alternans. Am J Physiol Heart Circ Physiol 2005;288:H400–7.

82. Bacharova L, Chen H, Estes H, et al. Determinants of discrepancies in detection and comparison of the prognostic significance of left ventricular hypertrophy by electrocardiogram and cardiac magnetic resonance imaging. Am J Cardiol 2015;115(4): 515–22.

83. Levy D, Garrison RJ, Savage DD, et al. Prognostic implications of echocardiographically determined left ventricular mass in the Framingham Heart Study. N Engl J Med 1990;322:1561–6.

84. Vakili BA, Okin PM, Devereux RB. Prognostic implications of left ventricular hypertrophy. Am Heart J 2001;141:334–41.

85. Krumholtz HM, Larson M, Levy D. Prognosis of left ventricular geometric patterns in the Framingham Heart Study. J Am Coll Cardiol 1995;25:879–84.

86. Devereux RB, Wachtell K, Gerdts E, et al. Prognostic significance of left ventricular mass change during treatment of hypertension. JAMA 2004; 292:2350–6.

87. Okin PM, Wachtell K, Devereux RB, et al. Regression of electrocardiographic left ventricular hypertrophy and decreased incidence of new-onset atrial fibrillation in patients with hypertension. JAMA 2006;296:1242–8.

88. Okin PM, Devereux RB, Jern S, et al. Regression of electrocardiographic left ventricular hypertrophy during antihypertensive treatment and the prediction of major cardiovascular events. JAMA 2004; 292:2343–9.

89. Artham SM, Lavie CJ, Milani RV, et al. Clinical impact of left ventricular hypertrophy and implications for regression. Prog Cardiovasc Dis 2009; 52:153–67.

90. Wachtell K, Greve A. Structural and functional cardiac changes are target organ damage that increases risk of atrial fibrillation. J Am Coll Cardiol 2014;63(19):2014–5.

91. Kuruvilla S, Janardhann R, Antokowiak P, et al. Increased extracellular volume and altered mechanics are associated with LVH in hypertensive heart disease, not hypertension alone. J Am Coll Cardiol 2015;8:172–80.

92. Gaasch W, Aurigemma G. CMR imaging of extracellular volume and myocardial strain in hypertensive heart disease. J Am Coll Cardiol 2015;8:181–3.

93. Raman SV, Shah M, McCarthy B, et al. Multi-detector row cardiac computed tomography accurately quantifies right and left ventricular size and function compared with cardiac magnetic resonance. Am Heart J 2006;151(3):736–44.

94. Gradman AH, Alfayoumi F. From left ventricular hypertrophy to congestive heart failure: management of hypertensive heart disease. Prog Cardiovasc Dis 2006;48:326–41.

95. Moser M, Herbert PR. Prevention of disease progression, left ventricular hypertrophy and congestive heart failure in hypertension treatment trials. J Am Coll Cardiol 1996;27(5):1214–8.

96. Rials S, Wu Y, Xu X, et al. Regression of left ventricular hypertrophy with captopril restores normal ventricular action potential duration, dispersion of refractoriness, and vulnerability to inducible ventricular fibrillation. Circulation 1997;96:1330–6.

97. Solomon SD, Appelbaum E, Manning WJ, et al. Effect of the direct renin inhibitor aliskiren, the angiotensin receptor block losartan, or both on left ventricular mass in patients with hypertension and left ventricular hypertrophy. Circulation 2009; 119:530.

98. Pierdomenico SD, Lappennda D, Cuccurollo F. Regression of echocardiographic left ventricular hypertrophy after 2 years of therapy reduces cardiovascular risk in patients with essential hypertension. Am J Hypertens 2008;21:464.

99. Ang DS, Fahey TP, Wright GA, et al. Development and validation of a clinical score to identify echocardiographic left ventricular hypertrophy in patients with cardiovascular disease. Am J Hypertens 2008;21:1011.

100. Schirmer S, Sayed M, Reil J, et al. Improvements in left ventricular hypertrophy and diastolic function following renal denervation. J Am Coll Cardiol 2014;63:1916–23.

101. Bakris G, Nathan S. Renal denervation and left ventricular mass regression: a benefit beyond blood pressure reduction? J Am Coll Cardiol 2014;63: 1924–5.

102. Takeuchi M, Borden WB, Nakai H, et al. Reduced and delayed untwisting of the left ventricle in patients with hypertension and left ventricular hypertrophy: a study using two-dimensional speckle tracking imaging. Eur Heart J 2007;28:2756–62.

103. Gardin JM, Lauer MS. Left ventricular hypertrophy: the next treatable, silent killer? JAMA 2004;292: 2396–8.

# Arrhythmias in Dilated Cardiomyopathy

Saurabh Kumar, BSc (Med), MBBS, William G. Stevenson, MD, Roy M. John, MD, PhD*

## KEYWORDS

- Dilated cardiomyopathy • Atrial fibrillation • Atrial flutter • Ventricular tachycardia
- Catheter ablation • Atrioventricular block • Lamin A/C cardiomyopathy

## KEY POINTS

- Dilated cardiomyopathy is characterized by the presence of left ventricular dilatation and systolic dysfunction in the absence of abnormal loading conditions or coronary artery disease, and can be of familial origin in one-third of patients.
- Patients with dilated cardiomyopathies can develop a spectrum of bradyarrhythmias and tachyarrhythmias including sinus node dysfunction, various degrees of atrioventricular block, interventricular conduction delay, and atrial and ventricular arrhythmias.
- Device implantation is recommended for bradyarrhythmias, but requires the consideration of implantable defibrillators for associated left ventricular dysfunction or conditions that carry a high risk of malignant ventricular arrhythmias before the onset of left ventricular dysfunction such as lamin A/C cardiomyopathy. Cardiac resynchronization therapy should also be considered if there is concomitant left bundle branch block.
- In general, tachyarrhythmias are poorly tolerated because of left ventricular dysfunction, which also limits antiarrhythmic drug options owing to the risk of ventricular proarrhythmia. Catheter ablation is generally more effective than drugs for the control of supraventricular arrhythmias.
- Sustained ventricular arrhythmias in dilated cardiomyopathy are generally due to scar-mediated reentry or bundle branch reentry; catheter ablation is moderately effective for the management of ventricular arrhythmias.

## INTRODUCTION

Dilated cardiomyopathy (DCM) is defined by the presence of left ventricular (LV) dilatation and systolic dysfunction in the absence of abnormal loading conditions (eg, hypertension or valve disease) or coronary artery disease sufficient to explain global systolic impairment.[1] The prevalence of DCM remains unknown but can be familial or nonfamilial. It is estimated that 25% to 40% of patients in the Western population may have familial disease.[1,2] A family history of premature sudden cardiac death, conduction system disease, or skeletal myopathy may accompany the presence of a cardiomyopathy. Familial forms of DCM can be due to mutations in cytoskeletal, sarcomeric protein/Z-band, nuclear membrane, and intercalated disc protein genes. Most are autosomal dominant, but recessive and X-linked patterns of inheritance have also been described. Familial

Dr S. Kumar is a recipient of the Neil Hamilton Fairley Overseas Research scholarship cofunded by the National Health and Medical Research Council and the National Heart Foundation of Australia; and the Bushell Traveling Fellowship funded by the Royal Australasian College of Physicians. Dr W.G. Stevenson is coholder of a patent for needle ablation that is consigned to Brigham and Women's Hospital. Dr R.M. John receives consulting fees/honoraria from St. Jude Medical, Medtronic, and Boston Scientific.
Department of Medicine, Brigham and Women's Hospital, Harvard Medical School, 75 Francis Street, Boston, MA 02115, USA
* Corresponding author. Cardiovascular Division, Brigham and Women's Hospital, 75 Francis Street, Boston, MA 02115.
E-mail address: Rjohn2@partners.org

forms of DCM associated with atrial arrhythmias have been reported with mutation in the sodium channel gene, SCN5A, and lamin A/C genes.[3] DCM may also occur in X-linked disorders such as the muscular dystrophies (eg, Becker and Duchenne muscular dystrophy). Mitochondrial cytopathies and inherited metabolic disorders such as hemochromatosis can also be associated with DCM. Acquired causes include sequelae from inflammatory disorders such as vasculitides including Kawasaki disease and Churg-Strauss syndrome, abnormality related to pregnancy (postpartum cardiomyopathy), hypothyroidism, toxins such as alcohol, anthracyclines, tyrosine kinase inhibitors, other chemotherapeutic agents, and nutritional deficiencies (eg, thiamine).[1] Persistent tachycardias and frequent premature ventricular contractions (PVCs) can provoke a reversible cardiomyopathy or worsening of preexisting cardiac dysfunction.

The risk of life-threatening arrhythmias leading to sudden death is largely determined by the cause and severity of the DCM. Inflammatory processes such as giant cell myocarditis and sarcoidosis, and some familial cardiomyopathies (eg, Lamin mutations) may present with malignant arrhythmias early in the course of the disease.

## BRADYARRHYTHMIAS AND CONDUCTION ABNORMALITIES IN DILATED CARDIOMYOPATHIES

Conduction system disease can occur with virtually all cardiomyopathies, but is particularly prevalent in some familial forms of DCM such as the cardiolaminopathies (lamin A/C mutations),[4] mitochondrial diseases (eg, Kearns-Sayre syndrome),[4] storage disorders (Fabry disease), and infiltrative diseases such as cardiac amyloidosis.[1] Patients with DCM can thus manifest sinus node dysfunction, various degrees of atrioventricular (AV) block, interventricular conduction delay, and bundle branch block. Progressive His-Purkinje conduction disease can result in paroxysmal heart block and sudden cardiac death.

The presence of intraventricular conduction delay has been associated with regional mechanical delay within the left ventricle (dyssynchrony), resulting in reduced ventricular systolic function, altered myocardial metabolism, functional mitral regurgitation, and adverse remodeling accompanied by ventricular dilatation. The presence of ventricular dyssynchrony resulting from left bundle branch block is associated with worsening heart failure, sudden cardiac death, and increased mortality.[5]

The onset of AV conduction defects in middle age or earlier should prompt an evaluation for inflammatory or familial cardiomyopathy. In a review of unexplained heart block in patients younger than 55 years, cardiac sarcoidosis or giant cell myocarditis accounted for 25% of cases; both diagnoses were associated with a higher incidence of sudden death from ventricular arrhythmias or the need for cardiac transplantation.[6] As some of these disorders are also associated with a risk of ventricular arrhythmias and sudden death, patients who require a pacemaker for bradyarrhythmias may also warrant consideration of an implantable cardioverter-defibrillator (ICD) and/or cardiac resynchronization therapy (CRT)-defibrillator device. CRT is recommended for DCM patients with an LV ejection fraction (LVEF) of 35% or less, sinus rhythm, left bundle branch block (LBBB) with a QRS duration of at least 150 milliseconds, and New York Heart Association (NYHA) class II, III, or ambulatory IV heart failure symptoms despite guideline-driven optimal medical therapy.[5] CRT-defibrillator implantation significantly reduces the risk of death or heart failure in comparison with ICD alone in patients with these clinical characteristics.[5]

## SUPRAVENTRICULAR TACHYARRHYTHMIAS IN DILATED CARDIOMYOPATHY

Patients with DCM can develop atrial ectopy, atrial tachycardia, atrial flutter, and atrial fibrillation (AF). Of particular note is that the presence of AV block, sinus node dysfunction, atrial ectopy, or atrial arrhythmias in dilated cardiomyopathy should prompt investigation for familial lamin A/C cardiomyopathy.[7] In such patients, conduction disease or supraventricular or ventricular arrhythmias may precede the development of ventricular dilatation and dysfunction.[7] AV node–dependent sustained SVTs such as AV nodal reentry and accessory pathway–mediated arrhythmia can occur unrelated to the DCM. Ventricular preexcitation has been described in association with mutations in the PRKAG2 gene that also cause conduction defects, increased ventricular wall thickness, and progressive LV dysfunction.[8]

In some patients, incessant atrial tachycardia may cause tachycardia-mediated cardiomyopathy that can reverse after successful catheter ablation. In one series, atrial tachycardia from the left and right atrial appendage sites was associated with a high incidence of incessant tachycardia and LV dysfunction. After successful ablation, LV function was restored in 97% of patients at a mean of 3 months.[9] However, in long-term follow-up, despite recovery of ventricular function, patients who had atrial tachycardia–mediated cardiomyopathy continued to manifest differences in LV structure and function including diffuse fibrosis long after arrhythmia cure, indicating that recovery is often incomplete.[10] Rapid ventricular rates can lead to development or exacerbation of heart failure in patients with DCM. Antiarrhythmic drugs may provide suppression but do not lead to cure. Owing to the presence of structural heart disease, commonly used antiarrhythmic drugs that are effective when used in patients with normal ventricular function (eg, flecainide, sotalol) may have a greater risk of ventricular proarrhythmia in patients with DCM. Hence, options are limited to drugs such as amiodarone, which is associated with significant cardiac and noncardiac end organ toxicities. Many of these arrhythmias can be treated with catheter ablation with success rates of greater than 90% and complication rates of less than 5%.[11]

## ATRIAL FLUTTER AND ATRIAL TACHYCARDIA IN DILATED CARDIOMYOPATHIES

Atrial flutter is also a common arrhythmia in patients with DCM. The most common form is typical right atrial flutter characterized by the presence of classic saw-tooth flutter waves in the inferior leads of the electrocardiogram (ECG). The presence of atrial flutter usually suggests an underlying predisposition to AF, which will eventually be identified in most of these patients.[12] Indeed, electrophysiologic and electroanatomic evaluation of patients with atrial flutter, remote from their episodes of flutter, have shown larger atrial volumes, prolonged P-wave duration, slowed atrial conduction, higher incidence of fractionated electrograms, and lower atrial voltage when compared with healthy subjects. These diffuse atrial abnormalities may be associated with structural changes and sinus node dysfunction. All of these factors may promote the subsequent development of AF.[13]

The circuit for typical right atrial flutter is characterized by broad activation wavefront rotation along the tricuspid annulus anteriorly, with the crista terminalis acting as a functional posterior conduction barrier.[14] A critical isthmus of this circuit is at the floor of the right atrium between the inferior tricuspid annulus and the inferior vena cava, termed the cavo-tricuspid isthmus. A reverse typical atrial flutter also exists with clockwise activation around the tricuspid annulus. Atrial flutter is usually poorly tolerated in patients with DCM, tends to be associated with rapid heart rates, and has a higher incidence of recurrence after cardioversion and antiarrhythmic drugs in comparison with catheter ablation. Typical cavo-tricuspid isthmus–dependent atrial flutter is

amenable to cure with catheter ablation, with a greater than 90% chance of success.[14] Most patients will, however, eventually develop AF.

Atypical forms of atrial flutter are unusual unless there has been scar from prior cardiac surgery or catheter or surgical ablation of AF. Atypical flutters may be due to macro-reentry around the pulmonary veins, the mitral annulus, or in the left atrial roof. Dual or multiloop reentry circuits may also occur involving, for example, the roof and mitral annulus.[15] In general, these atypical flutters are poorly hemodynamically tolerated, antiarrhythmic drugs are often ineffective, and catheter ablation may be necessary to restore sinus rhythm. In patients in whom ablation fails or heart failure status is precarious, AV nodal ablation with AV sequential pacing may be a therapeutic option and can be associated with improvement in heart failure, with some pooled observational data suggesting an improvement in all-cause and cardiovascular mortality.[16] In the presence of significant LV dysfunction, biventricular pacing may be warranted to prevent deterioration caused by dyssynchrony created by right ventricular (RV)-only pacing.

## ATRIAL FIBRILLATION IN DILATED CARDIOMYOPATHIES

AF is more common than atrial flutter in patients with DCM. Epidemiologic studies have shown that 30% to 40% of patients with congestive heart failure from any cause will develop AF during the course of their disease and that when present, AF is associated with increased morbidity and mortality.[17–19] In experimental models the increased propensity of AF is associated with atrial structural abnormalities, with increased atrial fibrosis associated with conduction slowing and conduction heterogeneity.[20] In humans, Sanders and colleagues[21] also showed that AF in patients with congestive heart failure is associated with widespread areas of low voltage and electrical silence consistent with scar, and with regional atrial conduction slowing with prolongation of the P-wave duration, in addition to altered sinus node function. Although focal drivers originating from within atrial muscular extensions along the pulmonary veins mediate paroxysmal AF, the mechanisms in persistent AF are less clear.[22] Pulmonary vein foci might be important for arrhythmia initiation in a subset of patients, although mechanisms that maintain rather than initiate the arrhythmia likely play the dominant role. Atrial electrical and structural remodeling outside the pulmonary veins is likely of importance to the persistence of AF.[14] Rotors, or high-frequency sources within the atrium, have been recently proposed as mechanisms for both initiation and maintenance of persistent AF.[23]

Heart failure is associated with an increased risk of thromboemboli and stroke in patients with AF, and anticoagulation is warranted. Further management focuses on rate control and consideration of whether to attempt to restore and maintain sinus rhythm. Although AF is associated with increased heart failure and mortality, attempts to maintain sinus rhythm with antiarrhythmic drug therapy, including amiodarone, have not been shown to be beneficial in comparison with a rate-control strategy in randomized trials.[20,24,25] Inability to maintain sinus rhythm may be a marker of more advanced disease. One post hoc on-treatment analysis suggested that the presence of sinus rhythm was associated with a reduction in mortality, but that the use of antiarrhythmic drugs increased mortality by 49%, implying that the beneficial of sinus rhythm might be offset by adverse effects of antiarrhythmic drugs.[24] A post hoc analysis of the AF-CHF trial, in which amiodarone was the major antiarrhythmic drug, did not find any benefit of sinus rhythm.[25] It should also be recognized that trials of rate control versus rhythm control are likely affected by a bias introduced by acceptance of the patient and physician for staying in AF if the patient is randomized to a rate-control approach. Patients agreeing to that strategy may be less likely to be symptomatic from AF. In addition, some proponents of rhythm control argue that sinus rhythm may be preferred over rate control if it could be achieved by a method other than drug therapy.[26] Recently, a small randomized trial showed improvement in LV function, functional capacity, and heart failure symptoms in patients with LV systolic dysfunction and heart failure randomized to catheter ablation in comparison with rate control.[27] Meta-analyses of catheter ablation for AF in patients with LV systolic dysfunction suggested benefit on ventricular function, especially when performed early rather than later after development of AF and heart failure.[28]

Although the benefit of maintaining sinus rhythm remains controversial, many patients experience deterioration in heart failure with the emergence of AF and many are symptomatic with the arrhythmia. These factors often motivate attempts to maintain sinus rhythm in selected patients. Because of the aforementioned risks of proarrhythmia, amiodarone is the major drug option when ventricular function is severely depressed.[29] Sotalol and dofetilide are may be considered for patients with acceptable ventricular function and preserved renal function. The risks of these therapies must be carefully considered, and patients require close follow-up for toxicities and potential proarrhythmia. Proarrhythmia risks are mitigated to some extent by an ICD when present. However, if drugs slow the sinus rate or suppress AV nodal conduction such that RV pacing results, this may have an adverse hemodynamic effect (see earlier discussion).

Achieving adequate rate control of AF is extremely important. Rapid rates by themselves can lead to tachycardia-induced cardiomyopathy, and likely aggravate heart failure and ventricular dysfunction in other forms of cardiomyopathy. Although a lenient rate-control strategy allowing resting rates up to 110 beats per minute in patients without symptoms who have preserved ventricular function has been described,[30] this is not acceptable in patients with depressed ventricular function. β-Adrenergic blockers are first-line therapy. Calcium-channel blockers are avoided because of their negative inotropic effects. Digoxin is also often helpful, particularly when combined with a β-adrenergic blocker. Digoxin use, however, has been associated with increased mortality, which does not seem to be explained by greater severity of heart failure in the digoxin-treated patients.[31] If digoxin is used, serum levels should be monitored and kept below 1 ng/dL.[29]

## VENTRICULAR ARRHYTHMIAS AND SUDDEN DEATH IN DILATED CARDIOMYOPATHIES

Patients with DCM can develop any variety of ventricular arrhythmias including PVCs, sustained monomorphic ventricular tachycardia (SMVT), polymorphic ventricular tachycardia (VT), and ventricular fibrillation (VF). Holter monitoring studies have demonstrated that PVCs (often multifocal) are present in up to 90% of patients with DCM, and nonsustained VT is seen in 40% to 60% of patients.[32,33] The frequency of arrhythmias increases with the severity of heart failure. Arrhythmia mechanisms are not well defined, but triggered activity is a likely cause of ventricular ectopy. Sustained monomorphic VT is less common in DCM than in patients with prior myocardial infarction. When it does occur, it is most commonly related to reentry around scar in 80%, with the remaining 20% attributable to other mechanisms caused by bundle branch reentry or enhanced automaticity.[34] Cardiac arrest can be due to polymorphic VT or monomorphic VT degenerating to VF. Asystolic arrest and pulseless electric activity are common modes of death, particularly in end-stage heart failure.[35] Several other causes contribute to arrhythmic deaths and are important considerations in patients who are resuscitated. Arrhythmias can also occur as a consequence of myocardial ischemia or infarction in patients with concomitant coronary artery disease. Antagonists of the renin-angiotensin-aldosterone system, β-adrenergic blockers, and renal dysfunction reduce potassium excretion predisposing to fatal sinusoidal VT or bradyarrhythmias due to hyperkalemia.

## Anatomic Substrate for Ventricular Arrhythmias in Dilated Cardiomyopathy

DCM is characterized by reduction in the number of contractile myocytes, hypertrophy, interstitial and perivascular fibrosis, and foci of myocyte necrosis and replacement fibrosis, all of which contribute to the arrhythmic substrate.[35,36] The scar patterns observed in DCM are fundamentally different from those from myocardial infarction caused by coronary occlusion. Postinfarction scars tend to be large, governed by coronary artery distribution, and are subendocardial or transmural. In DCM, necropsy studies have shown that only 14% of subjects have grossly visible scars. Multiple patchy areas of replacement fibrosis were far more common, being evident histologically in 35% of sections of the right ventricle and in 57% of sections of the left ventricle.[37] Scars were small in the majority (64%) of patients and were involved the ventricular septum in nearly all (91%) patients.[37] Other features observed include hypertrophied and atrophic myocytes, myofiber disarray, nuclear changes, and cytoskeletal disorganization.[38] Unlike postinfarction substrate whereby fibrosis is not progressive, the anatomic changes in DCM may be continuous and progressive, with an increasing amount of mid-myocardial or epicardial scarring observed over time.[39] In a human study, Liuba and colleagues[39] examined the endocardial voltage maps of 13 patients with nonischemic cardiomyopathy and recurrent SMVT 32 months apart. Nearly half of the patients studied had an increase in endocardial scar of 16%; inferred mid-myocardial or epicardial scar (based on unipolar voltage abnormality) increase was between 6.5% and 46.2% of the LV surface. Scar progression was accompanied by a significant decline in LVEF.

Gadolinium-enhanced cardiac magnetic resonance (CMR) imaging studies provide a noninvasive method of detecting scars.[40] Fibrosis detected by magnetic resonance imaging (MRI) is evident in 40% to 50% of DCM patients.[15,41] Unique to DCM, the regions of hyperenhancement may be patchy or show longitudinal striae of enhancement in the mid wall, and do not follow a coronary arterial distribution.[15,41] On average, regions of hyperenhancement account for up to 10% to 12% of the ventricular mass.[42,43] Fibrosis was found to most commonly affect the basal segments of the left ventricle, and was distributed predominantly in the mid-myocardium and epicardium.[43–47]

Evidence for the critical interdependence of fibrosis and ventricular arrhythmias in DCM patients comes from studies showing that the pattern and extent of myocardial fibrosis is a predictor of both inducible[45] and spontaneous VT independent of LVEF.[41,42] The location of scar (endocardial, mid-myocardial, epicardial) can also impact on ablation success for ventricular arrhythmias, with mid-myocardial scarring less amenable to successful ablation.[44] Scar has also been associated with an increased risk for sudden death.[48] Approximately 5% to 10% of monomorphic VT in DCM are related to the His-Purkinje system, most commonly bundle branch reentry.

## Electrophysiologic Substrate for Ventricular Tachycardia in Dilated Cardiomyopathy

The electrophysiologic milieu is created by poorly coupled surviving muscle bundles within regions of interstitial fibrosis.[49] In addition to fibrosis, other factors, such as altered expression and distribution of connexin proteins and increased sympathetic activity, can further enhance the susceptibility to arrhythmias in DCM patients.[50,51] Poor cell-to-cell coupling promotes regions of conduction slowing, leading to functional and anatomic conduction block and causing reentrant excitation. In some scar regions an isthmus of slow conduction may have a complex 3-dimensional path for propagation within and/or across all 3 myocardial layers that causes sustained VT.[52]

Much of our understanding of SMVT in DCM comes from studies of mapping and ablation in which scar is detected from evidence of low voltage (<1.5 mV in bipolar recordings) and abnormal electrograms. Electrophysiologic mapping in patients with DCM generally have shown fewer abnormal electrograms (eg, low-voltage, long-duration, or fractionated electrograms) than in patients with VT caused by coronary disease.[53] Patients with DCM and SMVT had a greater percentage of abnormal electrograms than those with no VT.[53] Hsia and colleagues[54] characterized the electrophysiologic substrate in 9 patients with VT and nonischemic cardiomyopathy, showing that: (1) confluent regions of abnormal electrograms existed in all of the patients; (2) the regions were typically confined to the basal and lateral aspects of the LV, adjacent to the mitral valve annulus; (3) the low-voltage regions involved less

**A**

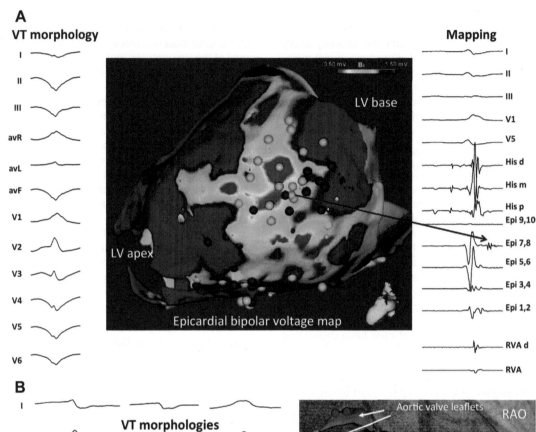

**VT morphology**

I, II, III, avR, avL, avF, V1, V2, V3, V4, V5, V6

LV base

LV apex

Epicardial bipolar voltage map

0.50 mV    Bi    1.50 mV

**Mapping**

I, II, III, V1, V5, His d, His m, His p, Epi 9,10, Epi 7,8, Epi 5,6, Epi 3,4, Epi 1,2, RVA d, RVA

**B**

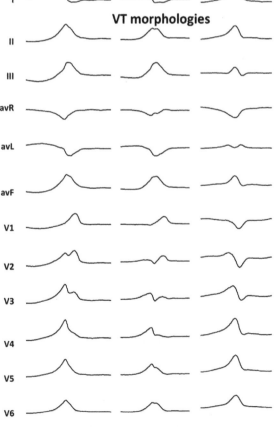

**VT morphologies**

I, II, III, avR, avL, avF, V1, V2, V3, V4, V5, V6

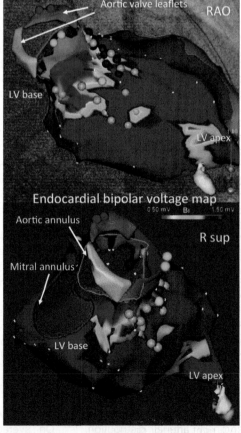

Aortic valve leaflets    RAO

LV base

LV apex

Endocardial bipolar voltage map

0.50 mV    Bi    1.50 mV

Aortic annulus    R sup

Mitral annulus

LV base

LV apex

than 25% of the total surface area of the left ventricle; (4) VTs originated in the abnormal voltage areas; and (5) despite the small region of scar, it was capable of supporting multiple reentrant VTs. This study supported the important role of the anatomic substrate for VT in DCM.

Soejima and colleagues[55] studied 28 patients with VT and DCM, and performed epicardial mapping in 8 patients, demonstrating that: (1) VTs in DCM were most commonly the result of myocardial reentry associated with scar; (2) the scar, although most commonly adjacent to a valve annulus, may be deep in the endocardium and could be greater in extent on the epicardium than on the endocardium; and (3) epicardial mapping and ablation is likely to improve success in DCM substrate.

Haqqani and colleagues[56] showed in some patients with DCM (11.6% in their series referred for catheter ablation) that there might be isolated intramural substrate confined to the septum capable of supporting multiple unmappable VTs. The scar might remain undetected during bipolar voltage mapping, and its delineation would rely on cardiac MRI and abnormal unipolar voltage.[56] The presence of isolated septal scar may be detected by the presence apically displaced transmural breakthrough in combination with the presence of delayed transmural conduction time (>40 milliseconds) and fractionated, late, split, and wide (>95 milliseconds) bipolar electrograms during RV basal pacing while recording from an adjacently placed catheter on the LV endocardial side.[57]

More recently, investigators have examined the relationship between anatomic sites of scar, associated electrophysiologic abnormalities, and typical ECG patterns of monomorphic VT in DCM patients. Piers and colleagues[46] showed that DCM patients exhibit 2 predominant scar patterns (anteroseptal and inferolateral) that count for 89% of arrhythmogenic substrate in such patients (Fig. 1). Three distinct VT morphologies were highly suggestive of the presence of these scars. The presence of right bundle branch block (RBBB),

left/right inferior axis with positive concordance or LBBB, left/right inferior axis, and early (≤V3) precordial transition were characteristic of anteroseptal scar. By contrast, an RBBB right inferior/superior axis and late (≥V5) precordial transition was characteristic of inferolateral scar.[46]

Oloriz and colleagues[58] also found that anteroseptal and inferolateral scar accounted for most arrhythmogenic substrate in DCM patients. The presence of an LBBB pattern inferior-axis VT was predictive of anteroseptal scar (positive predictive value, 100%). An RBBB pattern with superior axis had a positive predictive value of 89% for an inferolateral scar. In this series, VT originating from the inferolateral scar often required epicardial ablation, in contrast to VT originating from an anteroseptal scar that more frequently seemed to have an intramural origin requiring ablation from the aortic root or the anteroseptal LV endocardium, but not from the epicardium.[46,58] Furthermore, anteroseptal scars were less frequently associated with the presence of late potentials. By contrast, inferolateral scar subtypes had a higher frequency of epicardial late potentials. VT recurrence was noted be higher with anteroseptal scar attributable to the intramural location of the circuits.[58]

Haqqani and colleagues[56] also found that in DCM with isolated septal substrate, the morphology of VT may exhibit a precordial transition pattern break in V2 with qR/Rs morphology in V1 and V3 but reversal of this in V2, usually in the presence of an inferior-axis RBBB configuration. This morphology was mapped to the superior LV septum with exit in the preaortic LV summit region, and was ablated from several locations in this vicinity (superior LV septum, basal preaortic epicardium, anterior interventricular vein, and left coronary cusp). Valles and colleagues[59] combined several ECG criteria into a 4-step algorithm that predicted the site of origin of VTs from the basal-superior/lateral epicardium in patients with nonischemic cardiomyopathy. The criteria included, in a stepwise fashion: the absence of Q waves in inferior leads; a pseudo-delta wave greater than or equal to 75 milliseconds; maximum deflection

Fig. 1. Examples of 2 patients with idiopathic dilated cardiomyopathies and inferolateral epicardial scar (A) and anteroseptal endocardial scar (B). In A, clinical ventricular tachycardia (VT) of right bundle superior axis with an inducible lateral exit that originated from within a dense network of late potentials (arrow) over the epicardial lateral left ventricle (LV) (blue dots on the mapping image). Radiofrequency ablation was performed through this area to render the clinical VT noninducible, taking care to avoid ablation to sites overlying the epicardial coronary arteries. In B, multiple basal septal VTs were inducible, originating from within anteroseptal endocardial left ventricular scar confined to the periaortic region that was targeted with radiofrequency ablation. Although the clinical VT was abolished, not all inducible VTs were abolished, owing to the origin being in the septal aspect of the scar involving the His-Purkinje system. Ablation was avoided in this region to prevent complete heart block. RAO, right anterior oblique view; R sup, right superior view.

index greater than or equal to 0.59; and the presence of a Q wave in lead I. This 4-step algorithm had a 95% specificity and at least 20% sensitivity for identifying basal-superior/lateral epicardial origin of VTs in nonischemic cardiomyopathy.

### Preventing Sudden Death in Dilated Cardiomyopathy

The ICD remains the most effective form of therapy in the prevention of sudden cardiac death in patients with DCM. Its role in the treatment of survivors of sudden death with a meaningful life expectancy greater than 12 months is undisputed. The role of the ICD in primary prevention is less well established unless there is evidence of systolic LV dysfunction with LVEF of 35% or less.[60] The DEFINITE trial, a randomized controlled trial of standard medical therapy versus standard medical therapy plus a single-chamber ICD in 458 patients with DCM, LVEF 35% or less, and PVCs or nonsustained VT, showed an 80% reduction in sudden cardiac death in patients randomized to ICDs, although the difference in total mortality (annual rate of 7% vs 7.9%) did not reach statistical significance.[61] The SCD-HeFT trial showed a 23% reduction in all-cause mortality in more than 2500 patients (half with DCM) with an LVEF less than 35% who were randomized to an ICD versus placebo or amiodarone.[62]

Present guidelines recommend ICDs for DCM patients with sustained VT, heart failure and LVEF 35% or less, or syncope, and state that ICDs may be considered under several other situations, including for patients with familial cardiomyopathy associated with sudden death and those with depressed LV function without heart failure symptoms.[63] For patients with a new diagnosis of DCM, it is usual to treat with optimal heart failure medications for 6 months and reassess for recovery of ventricular function before consideration of an ICD for primary prevention, unless there are high-risk features such as sarcoidosis, giant cell myocarditis, or familial cardiomyopathy known to be associated with ventricular arrhythmias.

Markers of specific arrhythmia risk have yet to be shown to be of clinical value in selecting patients for ICDs. For many years programmed ventricular stimulation has been thought to have no utility in predicting the risk of sudden cardiac death among DCM patients, which is somewhat surprising given the recognition that monomorphic VT is often due to scar-related reentry in this population.[35] Recently, Gatzoulis and colleagues[64] reported outcomes of 158 patients with idiopathic dilated cardiomyopathy without a history of sustained ventricular arrhythmias who underwent programmed ventricular stimulation. Sustained monomorphic VT was induced in 13%, ventricular flutter in 6%, and polymorphic VT/VF in 9%. ICDs were implanted in 41 of 44 patients with inducible arrhythmias and in 28 of the noninducible group. During a median follow-up of 42 months, 73% of patients with inducible VT and an ICD had a VT terminated by the ICD, compared with 18% of patients who received an ICD but did not have inducible VT. Overall there were only 4 sudden arrhythmic deaths, occurring in 3 of the 44 patients with inducible VT and 1 of the 114 patients without inducible VT. Total mortality was 15%, most of which was due to progressive heart failure.[64]

Fibrosis detected by CMR has been shown to be related to arrhythmia substrate and risk, but its utility for selecting patients to receive an ICD has yet to be demonstrated.[48,65] In 472 patients with DCM reported by Gulati and colleagues,[48] mid-wall fibrosis was present in 30%. Presence of fibrosis was associated with a history of arrhythmia, more ICD implants, and a 4.6-fold increase in sudden death or sustained ventricular arrhythmia after adjustment for a history of malignant ventricular arrhythmia and LVEF.[48,65]

Some familial forms of DCM are associated with a particularly high risk of arrhythmias and sudden death, including some SCN5A mutations and lamin A/C cardiomyopathies. Early prophylactic ICD implantation should be considered in high-risk individuals with these diseases, as ventricular arrhythmias may occur early in the course of disease, in the presence of normal ventricular function with little or no ventricular dilatation.[35]

### Management of Recurrent Ventricular Arrhythmias in Dilated Cardiomyopathies

Suppression of ambient ventricular ectopy has not been shown to reduce the risk of sudden death. In the SCD-HeFT trial, amiodarone therapy, which is a potent suppressor of ambient ectopy, did not improve survival.[62] Frequent and repetitive monomorphic VT comprising in excess of 10% to 20% of heart beats can lead to a cardiomyopathy and worsening of preexisting LV dysfunction.[66] These PVCs may be idiopathic, a diagnosis that is often made retrospectively after complete recovery of LV function after arrhythmia suppression. Occasionally an underlying cardiomyopathy manifests with progressive LV dysfunction. Catheter ablation is successful in achieving greater than 80% reduction in ectopic activity in 70% to 90% of patients, with highest success rates for arrhythmia arising in the RV outflow tract.[66] Suppression with amiodarone is also a consideration.

Therapy for arrhythmias is also needed for recurrent arrhythmias that cause symptoms, most commonly recurrent ICD shocks. Amiodarone is the major antiarrhythmic agent, particularly when ventricular function is severely depressed. In patients with compensated heart failure, sotalol is an option. Other antiarrhythmic drugs such as quinidine and mexiletine are also potential candidates, especially when catheter ablation is unsuccessful or not an option. For patients with recurrent sustained monomorphic VT, catheter ablation is a consideration.

## CATHETER ABLATION FOR VENTRICULAR TACHYCARDIA
### Scar-Related Ventricular Tachycardia

Experience with catheter ablation of SMVT in DCM is limited in comparison with that for VTs that occur in patients with coronary artery disease. Success rates depend on VT substrate location, which can be endocardial, intramural, or epicardial. Endocardial VTs can generally be ablated. An epicardial approach is necessary in one-third of patients and is associated with higher complication rates. Those that require ablation in the epicardium most commonly are related to scar extending along the lateral basal portion of the LV, as discussed earlier. Delivery of ablation lesions may be limited by the proximity to overlying coronary arteries. The left phrenic nerve can also be in close proximity, requiring techniques to reduce the risk of phrenic nerve injury. Intramural substrate is particularly common for scars involving the basal septum and periaortic region. Ablation from both sides of the scar can be successful, but in some cases standard radiofrequency ablation fails.

However, sustained monomorphic VT that triggers frequent ICD shocks or electrical storms can be controlled with ablation and adjunctive antiarrhythmic medications in the majority. Experienced centers performing catheter ablation in patients with nonischemic cardiomyopathy have reported that complete absence of inducible VT can be achieved in 38% to 67% of patients.[67–69] Persistent inducibility is strongly associated with future recurrence.[67,68] Patients found to have apical VTs have a worse prognosis than those with nonapical VTs, thought to be due to a larger scar volume extending from the base toward the apex.[70]

The success rate for catheter ablation of VT in DCM is lower than that for ischemic VT. VT recurs in 50% to 60% during short-term follow-up (up to 1 year), although VT burden can be significantly reduced.[54,55,59,67,68] In the authors' experience, transcoronary ethanol ablation, surgical cryoablation, or both are sometimes required to control VT when antiarrhythmic drugs or endocardial and epicardial catheter ablation fails or is not possible. Sequential ablation on both sides of the septum (for septal VTs) or both endocardial and epicardial aspects of the ventricular free wall is required in some cases. Bipolar ablation may also be used to create deeper lesions than is possible with sequential unipolar ablation.[71] Transcoronary alcohol ablation is particularly useful in targeting basal septal substrate or intramural substrate, and may abolish VT storms and reduce arrhythmia burden. It cannot be used, however, if there are no accessible coronary arterial branches supplying the target region.[72,73] Surgical cryoablation is usually reserved for patients in whom all nonsurgical efforts fail to control VT.[74,75] The use of a novel ablation catheter with a retractable needle may help target intramural substrate, and initial human feasibility studies are promising.[76]

### Bundle Branch Reentry

Ablation is highly successful for a unique form of sustained monomorphic VT that utilizes the conduction system, known as bundle branch reentry (BBRVT). In one series, BBRVT was inducible in 17% to 41% of patients with nonischemic cardiomyopathy, but other series document it in approximately 5% of DCM patients with monomorphic VT.[77] BBRVT is due to a circuit in which the reentry wavefront most commonly propagates anterogradely over the right bundle, through the septum and then retrogradely over the left bundle. Activation of the ventricles via the terminal right bundle fibers produces VT that has a typical LBBB QRS pattern. The reverse sequence of conduction can also occur, leading to an RBBB-configuration QRS.

Presentation is usually with rapid VT (rates often >200 beats/min) resulting in syncope or cardiac arrest. Evidence of slow conduction in the His-Purkinje system is usually present during sinus rhythm, manifesting as interventricular conduction delay or LBBB. Catheter ablation of the right bundle is highly effective in abolishing BBRVT. However, other, scar-related VTs are also present in up to 60% to 70% of patients who remain at high risk for sudden death.[55,78] An ICD is usually warranted. Although ablation of the left bundle can also be effective, it is usually avoided because of possible adverse effects on cardiac synchrony and ventricular function.

## SUMMARY

Cardiomyopathies are associated with atrial and ventricular arrhythmias. The management of AF is evolving, and further trials will help clarify the role of catheter ablation in this population. ICDs are the major therapy for patients with sustained VT or at significant risk of life-threatening ventricular arrhythmias. Antiarrhythmic drugs and ablation are important for controlling recurrent arrhythmias. Ongoing studies defining the arrhythmia substrate with MRI and relating genotype to arrhythmia phenotype in genetic cardiomyopathies are advancing our understanding of the disease.

## REFERENCES

1. Elliott P, Andersson B, Arbustini E, et al. Classification of the cardiomyopathies: a position statement from the European Society of Cardiology Working Group on Myocardial and Pericardial Diseases. Eur Heart J 2008;29:270–6.
2. Pugh TJ, Kelly MA, Gowrisankar S, et al. The landscape of genetic variation in dilated cardiomyopathy as surveyed by clinical DNA sequencing. Genet Med 2014;16:601–8.
3. Remme CA. Cardiac sodium channelopathy associated with SCN5A mutations: electrophysiological, molecular and genetic aspects. J Physiol 2013;591:4099–116.
4. Rapezzi C, Arbustini E, Caforio AL, et al. Diagnostic work-up in cardiomyopathies: bridging the gap between clinical phenotypes and final diagnosis. A position statement from the ESC working group on myocardial and pericardial diseases. Eur Heart J 2013;34:1448–58.
5. Tracy CM, Epstein AE, Darbar D, et al. 2012 ACCF/AHA/HRS focused update of the 2008 guidelines for device-based therapy of cardiac rhythm abnormalities: a report of the American College of Cardiology Foundation/American Heart Association Task Force on practice guidelines. Heart Rhythm 2012;9:1737–53.
6. Kandolin R, Lehtonen J, Kupari M. Cardiac sarcoidosis and giant cell myocarditis as causes of atrioventricular block in young and middle-aged adults. Circ Arrhythm Electrophysiol 2011;4:303–9.
7. Lakdawala NK, Givertz MM. Dilated cardiomyopathy with conduction disease and arrhythmia. Circulation 2010;122:527–34.
8. Gollob MH, Seger JJ, Gollob TN, et al. Novel PRKAG2 mutation responsible for the genetic syndrome of ventricular preexcitation and conduction system disease with childhood onset and absence of cardiac hypertrophy. Circulation 2001;104:3030–3.
9. Medi C, Kalman JM, Haqqani H, et al. Tachycardia-mediated cardiomyopathy secondary to focal atrial tachycardia: long-term outcome after catheter ablation. J Am Coll Cardiol 2009;53:1791–7.
10. Ling LH, Kalman JM, Ellims AH, et al. Diffuse ventricular fibrosis is a late outcome of tachycardia-mediated cardiomyopathy after successful ablation. Circ Arrhythm Electrophysiol 2013;6:697–704.
11. Spector P, Reynolds MR, Calkins H, et al. Meta-analysis of ablation of atrial flutter and supraventricular tachycardia. Am J Cardiol 2009;104:671–7.
12. Waldo AL, Feld GK. Inter-relationships of atrial fibrillation and atrial flutter mechanisms and clinical implications. J Am Coll Cardiol 2008;51:779–86.
13. Stiles MK, Wong CX, John B, et al. Characterization of atrial remodeling studied remote from episodes of typical atrial flutter. Am J Cardiol 2010;106:528–34.
14. Lee G, Sanders P, Kalman JM. Catheter ablation of atrial arrhythmias: state of the art. Lancet 2012;380:1509–19.
15. McCrohon JA, Moon JC, Prasad SK, et al. Differentiation of heart failure related to dilated cardiomyopathy and coronary artery disease using gadolinium-enhanced cardiovascular magnetic resonance. Circulation 2003;108:54–9.
16. Ganesan AN, Brooks AG, Roberts-Thomson KC, et al. Role of AV nodal ablation in cardiac resynchronization in patients with coexistent atrial fibrillation and heart failure a systematic review. J Am Coll Cardiol 2012;59:719–26.
17. Stevenson WG, Stevenson LW. Atrial fibrillation in heart failure. N Engl J Med 1999;341:910–1.
18. Middlekauff HR, Stevenson WG, Stevenson LW. Prognostic significance of atrial fibrillation in advanced heart failure. A study of 390 patients. Circulation 1991;84:40–8.
19. Wang TJ, Larson MG, Levy D, et al. Temporal relations of atrial fibrillation and congestive heart failure and their joint influence on mortality: the Framingham heart study. Circulation 2003;107:2920–5.
20. Roy D, Talajic M, Nattel S, et al. Rhythm control versus rate control for atrial fibrillation and heart failure. N Engl J Med 2008;358:2667–77.
21. Sanders P, Morton JB, Davidson NC, et al. Electrical remodeling of the atria in congestive heart failure: electrophysiological and electroanatomic mapping in humans. Circulation 2003;108:1461–8.
22. Haissaguerre M, Jais P, Shah DC, et al. Spontaneous initiation of atrial fibrillation by ectopic beats originating in the pulmonary veins. N Engl J Med 1998;339:659–66.
23. Narayan SM, Krummen DE, Shivkumar K, et al. Treatment of atrial fibrillation by the ablation of localized sources: CONFIRM (Conventional Ablation for Atrial Fibrillation with or without Focal Impulse and Rotor Modulation) trial. J Am Coll Cardiol 2012;60:628–36.
24. Wyse DG, Waldo AL, DiMarco JP, et al. A comparison of rate control and rhythm control in patients with atrial fibrillation. N Engl J Med 2002;347:1825–33.

25. Talajic M, Khairy P, Levesque S, et al. Maintenance of sinus rhythm and survival in patients with heart failure and atrial fibrillation. J Am Coll Cardiol 2010; 55:1796–802.
26. Corley SD, Epstein AE, DiMarco JP, et al. Relationships between sinus rhythm, treatment, and survival in the Atrial Fibrillation Follow-Up Investigation of Rhythm Management (AFFIRM) study. Circulation 2004;109:1509–13.
27. Hunter RJ, Berriman TJ, Diab I, et al. A randomized controlled trial of catheter ablation versus medical treatment of atrial fibrillation in heart failure (the CAMTAF trial). Circ Arrhythm Electrophysiol 2014; 7:31–8.
28. Anselmino M, Matta M, D'Ascenzo F, et al. Catheter ablation of atrial fibrillation in patients with left ventricular systolic dysfunction: a systematic review and meta-analysis. Circ Arrhythm Electrophysiol 2014;7(6):1011–8.
29. January CT, Wann LS, Alpert JS, et al. 2014 AHA/ACC/HRS guideline for the management of patients with atrial fibrillation: executive summary: a report of the American College of Cardiology/American Heart Association Task Force on Practice Guidelines and the Heart Rhythm Society. Circulation 2014;130: 2071–104.
30. Van Gelder IC, Groenveld HF, Crijns HJ, et al. Lenient versus strict rate control in patients with atrial fibrillation. N Engl J Med 2010;362:1363–73.
31. Freeman JV, Reynolds K, Fang M, et al. Digoxin and risk of death in adults with atrial fibrillation: the ATRIA-CVRN study. Circ Arrhythm Electrophysiol 2014;8(1):49–58.
32. von Olshausen K, Schafer A, Mehmel HC, et al. Ventricular arrhythmias in idiopathic dilated cardiomyopathy. Br Heart J 1984;51:195–201.
33. Meinertz T, Hofmann T, Kasper W, et al. Significance of ventricular arrhythmias in idiopathic dilated cardiomyopathy. Am J Cardiol 1984;53:902–7.
34. Stevenson WG, Soejima K. Catheter ablation for ventricular tachycardia. Circulation 2007;115: 2750–60.
35. Sen-Chowdhry S, McKenna WJ. Sudden death from genetic and acquired cardiomyopathies. Circulation 2012;125:1563–76.
36. de Jong S, van Veen TA, van Rijen HV, et al. Fibrosis and cardiac arrhythmias. J Cardiovasc Pharmacol 2011;57:630–8.
37. Roberts WC, Siegel RJ, McManus BM. Idiopathic dilated cardiomyopathy: analysis of 152 necropsy patients. Am J Cardiol 1987;60:1340–55.
38. de Leeuw N, Ruiter DJ, Balk AH, et al. Histopathologic findings in explanted heart tissue from patients with end-stage idiopathic dilated cardiomyopathy. Transpl Int 2001;14:299–306.
39. Liuba I, Frankel DS, Riley MP, et al. Scar progression in patients with nonischemic cardiomyopathy and ventricular arrhythmias. Heart Rhythm 2014;11: 755–62.
40. Moon JC, Reed E, Sheppard MN, et al. The histologic basis of late gadolinium enhancement cardiovascular magnetic resonance in hypertrophic cardiomyopathy. J Am Coll Cardiol 2004;43:2260–4.
41. Iles L, Pfluger H, Lefkovits L, et al. Myocardial fibrosis predicts appropriate device therapy in patients with implantable cardioverter-defibrillators for primary prevention of sudden cardiac death. J Am Coll Cardiol 2011;57:821–8.
42. Wu KC, Weiss RG, Thiemann DR, et al. Late gadolinium enhancement by cardiovascular magnetic resonance heralds an adverse prognosis in nonischemic cardiomyopathy. J Am Coll Cardiol 2008; 51:2414–21.
43. Masci PG, Barison A, Aquaro GD, et al. Myocardial delayed enhancement in paucisymptomatic nonischemic dilated cardiomyopathy. Int J Cardiol 2012;157:43–7.
44. Bogun FM, Desjardins B, Good E, et al. Delayed-enhanced magnetic resonance imaging in nonischemic cardiomyopathy: utility for identifying the ventricular arrhythmia substrate. J Am Coll Cardiol 2009;53:1138–45.
45. Nazarian S, Bluemke DA, Lardo AC, et al. Magnetic resonance assessment of the substrate for inducible ventricular tachycardia in nonischemic cardiomyopathy. Circulation 2005;112:2821–5.
46. Piers SR, Tao Q, van Huls van Taxis CF, et al. Contrast-enhanced MRI-derived scar patterns and associated ventricular tachycardias in nonischemic cardiomyopathy: implications for the ablation strategy. Circ Arrhythm Electrophysiol 2013;6:875–83.
47. Bluemke DA. MRI of nonischemic cardiomyopathy. AJR Am J Roentgenol 2010;195:935–40.
48. Gulati A, Jabbour A, Ismail TF, et al. Association of fibrosis with mortality and sudden cardiac death in patients with nonischemic dilated cardiomyopathy. JAMA 2013;309:896–908.
49. de Bakker JM, van Capelle FJ, Janse MJ, et al. Fractionated electrograms in dilated cardiomyopathy: origin and relation to abnormal conduction. J Am Coll Cardiol 1996;27:1071–8.
50. Chauhan VS, Downar E, Nanthakumar K, et al. Increased ventricular repolarization heterogeneity in patients with ventricular arrhythmia vulnerability and cardiomyopathy: a human in vivo study. Am J Physiol Heart Circ Physiol 2006;290:H79–86.
51. Stein M, Noorman M, van Veen TA, et al. Dominant arrhythmia vulnerability of the right ventricle in senescent mice. Heart Rhythm 2008;5:438–48.
52. de Bakker JM, van Capelle FJ, Janse MJ, et al. Slow conduction in the infarcted human heart. 'Zigzag' course of activation. Circulation 1993;88:915–26.
53. Cassidy DM, Vassallo JA, Miller JM, et al. Endocardial catheter mapping in patients in sinus rhythm:

relationship to underlying heart disease and ventricular arrhythmias. Circulation 1986;73:645–52.

54. Hsia HH, Callans DJ, Marchlinski FE. Characterization of endocardial electrophysiological substrate in patients with nonischemic cardiomyopathy and monomorphic ventricular tachycardia. Circulation 2003;108:704–10.

55. Soejima K, Stevenson WG, Sapp JL, et al. Endocardial and epicardial radiofrequency ablation of ventricular tachycardia associated with dilated cardiomyopathy: the importance of low-voltage scars. J Am Coll Cardiol 2004;43:1834–42.

56. Haqqani HM, Tschabrunn CM, Tzou WS, et al. Isolated septal substrate for ventricular tachycardia in nonischemic dilated cardiomyopathy: incidence, characterization, and implications. Heart Rhythm 2011;8:1169–76.

57. Betensky BP, Kapa S, Desjardins B, et al. Characterization of trans-septal activation during septal pacing: criteria for identification of intramural ventricular tachycardia substrate in nonischemic cardiomyopathy. Circ Arrhythm Electrophysiol 2013;6:1123–30.

58. Oloriz T, Silberbauer J, Maccabelli G, et al. Catheter ablation of ventricular arrhythmia in nonischemic cardiomyopathy: anteroseptal versus inferolateral scar sub-types. Circ Arrhythm Electrophysiol 2014; 7:414–23.

59. Valles E, Bazan V, Marchlinski FE. ECG criteria to identify epicardial ventricular tachycardia in nonischemic cardiomyopathy. Circ Arrhythm Electrophysiol 2010;3:63–71.

60. Russo AM, Stainback RF, Bailey SR, et al. ACCF/HRS/AHA/ASE/HFSA/SCAI/SCCT/SCMR 2013 appropriate use criteria for implantable cardioverter-defibrillators and cardiac resynchronization therapy: a report of the American College of Cardiology Foundation appropriate use criteria task force, Heart Rhythm Society, American Heart Association, American Society of Echocardiography, Heart Failure Society of America, Society for Cardiovascular Angiography and Interventions, Society of Cardiovascular Computed Tomography, and Society for Cardiovascular Magnetic Resonance. J Am Coll Cardiol 2013;61:1318–68.

61. Kadish A, Dyer A, Daubert JP, et al. Prophylactic defibrillator implantation in patients with nonischemic dilated cardiomyopathy. N Engl J Med 2004; 350:2151–8.

62. Bardy GH, Lee KL, Mark DB, et al. Amiodarone or an implantable cardioverter-defibrillator for congestive heart failure. N Engl J Med 2005;352:225–37.

63. Epstein AE, DiMarco JP, Ellenbogen KA, et al. 2012 ACCF/AHA/HRS focused update incorporated into the ACCF/AHA/HRS 2008 guidelines for device-based therapy of cardiac rhythm abnormalities: a report of the American College of Cardiology Foundation/American Heart Association Task Force on Practice Guidelines and the Heart Rhythm Society. Circulation 2013;127:e283–352.

64. Gatzoulis KA, Vouliotis AI, Tsiachris D, et al. Primary prevention of sudden cardiac death in a nonischemic dilated cardiomyopathy population: reappraisal of the role of programmed ventricular stimulation. Circ Arrhythm Electrophysiol 2013;6:504–12.

65. Assomull RG, Prasad SK, Lyne J, et al. Cardiovascular magnetic resonance, fibrosis, and prognosis in dilated cardiomyopathy. J Am Coll Cardiol 2006; 48:1977–85.

66. Lee GK, Klarich KW, Grogan M, et al. Premature ventricular contraction-induced cardiomyopathy: a treatable condition. Circ Arrhythm Electrophysiol 2012;5:229–36.

67. Piers SR, Leong DP, van Huls van Taxis CF, et al. Outcome of ventricular tachycardia ablation in patients with nonischemic cardiomyopathy: the impact of noninducibility. Circ Arrhythm Electrophysiol 2013;6:513–21.

68. Dinov B, Fiedler L, Schonbauer R, et al. Outcomes in catheter ablation of ventricular tachycardia in dilated nonischemic cardiomyopathy compared with ischemic cardiomyopathy: results from the prospective heart centre of Leipzig VT (HELP-VT) study. Circulation 2014;129:728–36.

69. Tokuda M, Tedrow UB, Kojodjojo P, et al. Catheter ablation of ventricular tachycardia in nonischemic heart disease. Circ Arrhythm Electrophysiol 2012;5: 992–1000.

70. Frankel DS, Tschabrunn CM, Cooper JM, et al. Apical ventricular tachycardia morphology in left ventricular nonischemic cardiomyopathy predicts poor transplant-free survival. Heart Rhythm 2013;10: 621–6.

71. Koruth JS, Dukkipati S, Miller MA, et al. Bipolar irrigated radiofrequency ablation: a therapeutic option for refractory intramural atrial and ventricular tachycardia circuits. Heart Rhythm 2012;9: 1932–41.

72. Tokuda M, Kojodjojo P, Tung S, et al. Acute failure of catheter ablation for ventricular tachycardia due to structural heart disease: causes and significance. J Am Heart Assoc 2013;2:e000072.

73. Tokuda M, Sobieszczyk P, Eisenhauer AC, et al. Transcoronary ethanol ablation for recurrent ventricular tachycardia after failed catheter ablation: an update. Circ Arrhythm Electrophysiol 2011;4:889–96.

74. Anter E, Hutchinson MD, Deo R, et al. Surgical ablation of refractory ventricular tachycardia in patients with nonischemic cardiomyopathy. Circ Arrhythm Electrophysiol 2011;4:494–500.

75. Sarkozy A, Tokuda M, Tedrow UB, et al. Epicardial ablation of ventricular tachycardia in ischemic heart disease. Circ Arrhythm Electrophysiol 2013; 6:1115–22.

76. Sapp JL, Beeckler C, Pike R, et al. Initial human feasibility of infusion needle catheter ablation for refractory ventricular tachycardia. Circulation 2013; 128:2289–95.

77. Blanck Z, Dhala A, Deshpande S, et al. Bundle branch reentrant ventricular tachycardia: cumulative experience in 48 patients. J Cardiovasc Electrophysiol 1993;4:253–62.

78. Lopera G, Stevenson WG, Soejima K, et al. Identification and ablation of three types of ventricular tachycardia involving the His-Purkinje system in patients with heart disease. J Cardiovasc Electrophysiol 2004;15:52–8.

# Cardiac Sarcoidosis and Consequent Arrhythmias

Matthew M. Zipse, MD, William H. Sauer, MD*

## KEYWORDS

- Cardiac sarcoidosis • Ventricular arrhythmias • Sudden cardiac death • Atrioventricular block

## KEY POINTS

- A cardiac electrophysiologist is an integral part of the multidisciplinary team taking care of patients with sarcoidosis because arrhythmias and electrocardiographic changes are the most common presentations indicating cardiac involvement.
- Inflammation and granulomatous infiltration of myocardium is the cause of electrocardiographic abnormalities, conduction disturbances, atrial arrhythmias, ventricular arrhythmias, and sudden death.
- Immunosuppression and catheter ablation can reduce arrhythmic burden in patients with cardiac sarcoidosis.
- An implanted cardiac defibrillator is indicated in most patients with cardiac involvement according to expert consensus based on observational research.

## INTRODUCTION

Sarcoidosis is a systemic inflammatory disease of unknown cause, characterized by the formation of noncaseating granulomas and resultant scarring of affected organs. Myocardial involvement occurs in 20% to 30% of cases, though only roughly one-quarter of these patients are diagnosed antemortem.[1,2] This discrepancy is partly caused by the inherent difficulties in making the diagnosis of cardiac sarcoidosis (CS) and partly caused by the potential for the presenting manifestation of CS to be sudden cardiac death.[3]

Electrophysiologic (EP) findings are underrecognized in CS and are more common than congestive heart failure (Table 1). Electrocardiography and invasive EP testing are important components in the evaluation and diagnosis of CS. After myocardial involvement has been established, an implantable cardiac defibrillator (ICD) may be indicated. Many patients with CS will also have a pacing indication, given a high incidence of atrioventricular (AV) block in this population. Atrial

and ventricular tachyarrhythmias are also common manifestations of CS and require management with antiarrhythmic therapy, immunosuppression, and/or catheter ablation. This article focuses on the EP manifestations of CS and the role of the cardiac electrophysiologist in the multidisciplinary team essential for screening, risk stratification, and management of patients with this rare disease.

## ROLE OF THE CARDIAC ELECTROPHYSIOLOGIST IN DIAGNOSING CARDIAC SARCOIDOSIS
### Electrophysiology Study

In patients with extracardiac sarcoidosis and unexplained palpitations and/or syncope, an EP study can identify an arrhythmic cause and potentially suggest cardiac involvement, particularly when imaging studies are inconclusive (Box 1). Inducible monomorphic ventricular tachycardia (VT) in these patients is a major diagnostic criterion for establishing cardiac involvement in the revised JMH (Japanese Ministry of Health) criteria and is

Disclosure: Dr. Sauer receives educational grant support from manufacturers of defibrillators.

Section of Cardiac Electrophysiology, Division of Cardiology, University of Colorado, 12401 East 17th Avenue, B132, Aurora, CO 80045, USA

* Corresponding author. Section of Cardiac Electrophysiology, University of Colorado Hospital, 12401 East 17th Avenue, B132, Aurora, CO 80045.

E-mail address: william.sauer@ucdenver.edu

cardiacEP.theclinics.com

**Table 1**
**Incident arrhythmic presentation of CS**

| Arrhythmia | Prevalence in Study Series (%) |
|---|---|
| Atrioventricular block | 26–67 |
| Bundle branch block | 12–61 |
| Atrial arrhythmias | 23–25 |
| Ventricular arrhythmias | 11–73 |
| Sudden cardiac death | 12–65 |
| Congestive heart failure | 10–30 |

*Data from* Refs.[1,14,15,26,27,39]

among the Heart Rhythm Society (HRS)/American College of Cardiology (ACC)/World Association for Sarcoidosis and Other Granulomatous Disorders' criteria for probable CS in the recently released consensus statement (**Box 2**).[4,5] Accordingly, ventricular stimulation with inducible VT is both a risk factor for sudden death and a potential path for the diagnosis of a CS in the absence of other criteria.[6,7]

### Electroanatomical Mapping

Three-dimensional electroanatomical mapping (EAM) systems have proven to be invaluable tools in the mapping and ablation of complex arrhythmias. These systems are also able to reconstruct chamber dimension and demonstrate the presence or absence of viable myocardium by the recording of voltage with a roving mapping catheter. EAM has been used in arrhythmogenic right ventricular (RV) cardiomyopathy (ARVC) with excellent correlation to cardiac MRI[8] and likely has similar utility for CS.

In cases of isolated CS or when sarcoidosis is suspected despite negative-yield extracardiac biopsy, endomyocardial biopsy may be required to confirm the diagnosis. In these cases, there may also be a role for EAM. The yield of the endomyocardial biopsy may be improved when performed with the guidance of voltage mapping in the EP laboratory, where the bioptome is directed to the areas of reduced voltage (ie, abnormal myocardium) and biopsies taken at these sites (**Fig. 1**).[9,10]

**Box 1**
**Indications for EP study in patients with sarcoidosis**

- Rare unexplained palpitations
- Risk stratification for sudden death in patients with known CS
- Unexplained syncope
- Evaluation of His-Purkinje system disease

### Clinical Overlap with Arrhythmogenic Right Ventricular Cardiomyopathy

CS can present with features that mimic ARVC, including repolarization and depolarization abnormalities on electrocardiogram (ECG) (including even the presence of an epsilon wave[11]), left bundle branch block morphology VT, abnormal signal-averaged ECG, and RV dilatation, among others. Taken together, CS can satisfy task force diagnostic criteria for ARVC.[9,11–13] Physicians should be aware that the conditions have overlapping clinical features and consider investigating for CS in the patients referred with possible ARVC in the appropriate clinical context.

### Conduction system disease and sinus node dysfunction

In CS, granulomatous infiltration of the basal interventricular septum can cause injury to the various elements of the cardiac conduction system, resulting in a variety of conduction disturbances leading to bundle branch block or any level of AV block. Because of the progressive nature of CS, the level and severity of conduction block may also progress in untreated CS (**Fig. 2**).

Bundle branch block (right bundle branch block in particular) has been observed on surface ECGs in 12% to 61% of cases of CS, depending on study series.[1,14–16] Although neither sensitive nor specific, both right and left bundle branch block are seen more commonly in patients with CS than those with sarcoidosis without myocardial involvement[16] and should prompt further investigations.

Complete AV block (CAVB) is one of the most common findings in patients with clinically evident CS, with a prevalence of 25% in one retrospective analysis.[1] Although usually thought to be related to infiltration of the conduction system itself, granulomatous involvement of the AV nodal artery has also been described as a cause of AV block in CS.[15] CAVB often occurs at a younger age in patients with sarcoidosis than in individuals with complete heart block from other causes.

Treatment of patients with high-grade AV block with permanent pacing should be performed in accordance with published guidelines.[17] However, the presence of AV block likely signifies extensive myocardial involvement from sarcoid granuloma and portends a higher risk of future ventricular arrhythmias (VAs).[18] For this reason, the recently published HRS' expert consensus statement gives a class IIa recommendation for ICD implantation (regardless of left ventricular ejection fraction [LVEF]) for the primary prevention of sudden cardiac death in CS if patients meet an indication for pacing.[4]

---

**Box 2**
**HRS' expert consensus statement diagnostic criteria for CS**

Diagnosis can be made by either histologic OR clinical diagnosis.

*Histologic Diagnosis Group*

Histologic presence of noncaseating granuloma on myocardial tissue biopsy with no alternative cause identified (including negative organismal stain, if applicable)

OR

*Clinical Diagnosis Group*

Probable cardiac involvement is adequate to establish the clinical diagnosis of CS if

1. There is histologically proven diagnosis of extracardiac sarcoidosis.

And

2. One or more of the following is present:

    a. Steroid/immunosuppressant-responsive cardiomyopathy or heart block

    b. Unexplained reduction in left ventricular ejection fraction less than 40%

    c. Unexplained sustained VT (spontaneous or induced)

    d. Second-degree, Mobitz type II heart block

    e. Third-degree heart block

    f. Patchy uptake on cardiac PET scan

    g. Late gadolinium enhancement on cardiac magnetic resonance

    h. Positive gallium uptake

And

3. Other causes of cardiac manifestations have been reasonably excluded.

*Adapted from* Birnie DH, Sauer W, Bogun F, et al. Heart Rhythm Society expert consensus statement on the diagnosis and management of arrhythmias associated with cardiac sarcoidosis. Heart Rhythm 2014;11(7):1–24; with permission.

---

If CAVB in CS is a result of granulomatous infiltration of the interventricular septum and inflammation that has not yet progressed to scar, then it may be reversible with immunosuppression therapy. Kato and colleagues[19] described their experience with 20 patients with CAVB and preserved LV function. CAVB resolved in 4 of 7 patients treated with corticosteroids (57%) but did not improve in any of the untreated patients. In another study, AV conduction improved to normal in 4 of 8 patients with CAVB with relatively preserved LV function but in none of the 4 patients with advanced LV dysfunction when given steroid treatment.[20] Several other studies have reported some success in the reversal of CAVB with steroid therapy (**Table 2**). Accordingly, current guidelines state (with a class IIa recommendation) that immunosuppression can be useful in patients with CS with Mobitz type II or third-degree heart block.

Lastly, it should be noted that CAVB in young patients (less than 60 years of age) should prompt evaluation for sarcoidosis, even in those who do not carry a previous diagnosis of extracardiac sarcoidosis. CAVB can be the initial manifestation of cardiac involvement in patients with a prior diagnosis of systemic sarcoidosis as well as the first clinical manifestation of sarcoidosis from any organ. This situation was the case in a Japanese study of 89 consecutive patients with no known history of sarcoidosis with high-grade AV block requiring permanent dual-chamber pacemaker implantation who were prospectively evaluated for CS. Ten cases (11.2%) of CS were diagnosed, most frequently in young women aged 40 to 69 years (32%).[21] Kandolin and colleagues[22] investigated 72 patients (aged <55 years) with unexplained AV block and found biopsy-verified CS in 14 (19%) and probable CS in 4 (6%) of the 72 patients. Patients with sarcoidosis had a significantly more adverse prognosis when compared with patients with idiopathic AV block in this series. Nery and colleagues[23] also found that patients with CAVB secondary to sarcoidosis were more likely to have adverse outcomes (VT and heart failure) than those with idiopathic CAVB. In their study, 32 patients with unexplained CAVB were

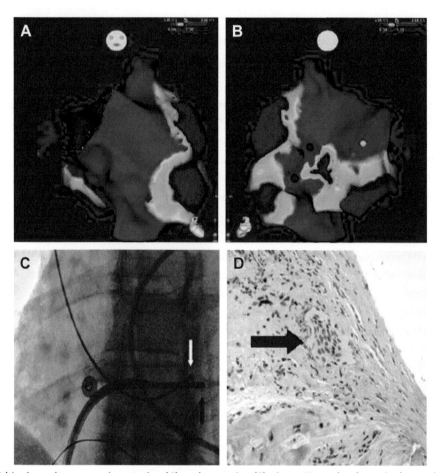

**Fig. 1.** RV bipolar voltage map in anterior (A) and posterior (B) views. Normal voltage is denoted in purple, whereas green, yellow, and red indicate low-voltage regions (<1.5 mV). (C) A bioptome (white arrow) is shown targeting the low-voltage region adjacent to the mapping catheter (black arrow) in a left anterior oblique 25° fluoroscopic projection. (D) A microscopic view of an endomyocardial biopsy specimen obtained from the RV septum showing noncaseating granuloma (arrow) (hematoxylin-eosin, original magnification × 200). (From Nery PB, Keren A, Healey J, et al. Isolated cardiac sarcoidosis: establishing the diagnosis with electroanatomic mapping-guided endomyocardial biopsy. Can J Cardiol 2013;29:1015e3; with permission.)

prospectively evaluated for CS, and 11 of 32 (34%) subjects were found to have CS and 11 of 11 were subsequently diagnosed with extracardiac sarcoidosis. Notably, major adverse cardiac events were observed in 3 subjects with CS but none with idiopathic AVB.[23]

Extensive granulomatous lesions in the sinoatrial node subendocardium have previously been described in autopsy series,[24,25] and sinus node dysfunction may be an underrecognized manifestation of CS. **Fig. 3** shows an ECG of a patient with sinus node dysfunction and CS, who ultimately had sinus arrest leading to a polymorphic VT arrest. Patients with sinus node dysfunction may have an indication for permanent pacing; if this is the case, dual-chamber ICD implantation may be reasonable, as with those patients requiring pacing for CAVB.

## Atrial Arrhythmias

Supraventricular arrhythmias and atrial fibrillation (AF) are common in CS, with a prevalence ranging from 23% to 36% (**Fig. 4**).[26,27] AF was the most common supraventricular arrhythmia reported, accounting for more than half of the atrial arrhythmias described in a study in which 32 of 100 patients with CS had atrial arrhythmias. After multivariate analysis in this study, left-atrial enlargement was the only parameter significantly associated with supraventricular arrhythmias (hazard ratio [HR] 6.12, 2.2–17.1, P<.01).[26]

A similar prevalence of atrial arrhythmias was described in a separate retrospective series, in which 16 of 44 (36%) patients with evidence of CS had documented atrial arrhythmias, the most common of which was atrial tachycardia (18%). In the 26 patients with ICDs in this cohort, 11.5% received

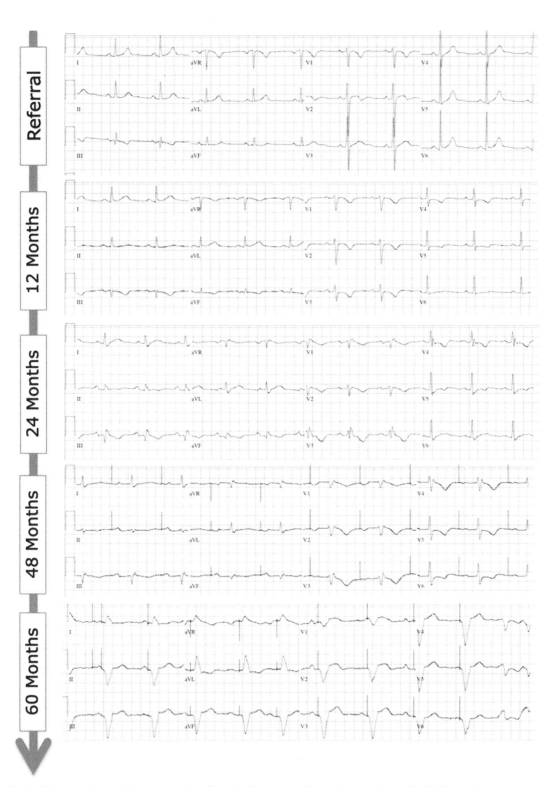

**Fig. 2.** Electrocardiographic progression of conduction system disease in a patient with CS. Shown here is the progression (sequential ECGs, from top to bottom) in one patient over a period of 5 years from sinus rhythm with a narrow QRS complex (referral), to first degree AV delay (12 months), to right bundle branch block (24 months), to sinus node dysfunction with need for atrial pacing (48 months), to complete heart block with ventricular pacing (60 months).

Table 2
Studies evaluating the efficacy of corticosteroids for recovery of AV conduction in CS patients

| Study | AVN Recovery, n/N (%) |
|---|---|
| Okamoto et al,[55] 1999 | 3/3 (100%) |
| Kato et al,[19] 2003 | 4/7 (57%) |
| Chapelon-Abric et al,[1] 2004 | 7/9 (78%) |
| Banba et al,[34] 2007 | 5/9 (56%) |
| Yodogawa et al,[56] 2013 | 4/12 (33%) |
| Kandolin et al,[22] 2011 | 4/17 (24%) |
| Total | 27/57 (47%) |

*Abbreviation:* AVN, AV node.

inappropriate ICD therapies for atrial arrhythmias.[27] This finding was similar to the 12% incidence of inappropriate therapies in a separate study.[28]

Atrial arrhythmias arise from a variety of mechanisms in CS, as evidenced in a series in which 15 of 65 patients (23%) with CS experienced 28 symptomatic supraventricular arrhythmias (9 AF, 3 atrial flutter, 16 atrial tachycardia). The mechanism of atrial arrhythmias was determined by EP testing to be from triggered activity in 11%, abnormal automaticity in 47%, and reentrant in 42% of the non-AF atrial arrhythmias.[29] Inflammation and edema associated with the initial infiltrative stage and scar that manifests as the disease progresses

to the fibrotic stage likely independently account for the differing mechanisms observed.

The variety of mechanisms and differing substrate for atrial arrhythmias in CS suggests that management of atrial arrhythmias may require a multifaceted approach of immunosuppression, antiarrhythmic therapy, and catheter ablation for arrhythmia control. In one of the series, the overall burden of AF seemed to decrease with immunosuppression.[29] Antiarrhythmic therapy can include the use of class IC agents, class III agents, or beta-blockers. The efficacy of these drugs for the control of atrial arrhythmias has not been specifically studied in CS.

Lastly, catheter ablation seems to be safe and effective in patients with CS. In a recent study reporting on a single-center experience of catheter ablation of atrial arrhythmias in 9 patients with CS with 10 different atrial arrhythmias, 2 patients had recurrences requiring repeat procedures; but all ultimately became arrhythmia free over a limited 1.8-year mean follow-up period. There were no complications reported in this small case series.[30]

## Ventricular Arrhythmias

Inflammation and fibrosis in CS can lead not only to atrial arrhythmias but also to VA by similar triggered, automatic, and reentrant mechanisms.[31–35] Sudden death secondary to VAs accounted for 25% to 65% of deaths caused by CS[14,15,36] before the routine use of ICDs. VAs have frequently been described as the sentinel presentation of CS.[3]

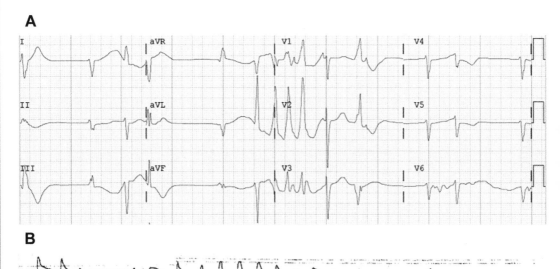

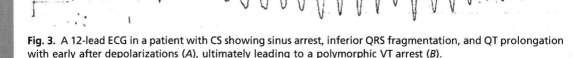

**Fig. 3.** A 12-lead ECG in a patient with CS showing sinus arrest, inferior QRS fragmentation, and QT prolongation with early after depolarizations (*A*), ultimately leading to a polymorphic VT arrest (*B*).

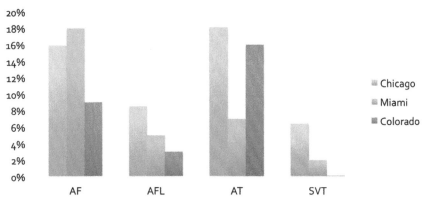

**Fig. 4.** Prevalence of atrial arrhythmias in 3 retrospective studies of cohorts of patients with CS. AFL, atrial flutter; AT, atrial tachycardia; SVT, other supraventricular tachycardia. (*Data from* Refs.[26,27,29])

Furthermore, it has been reported that CS may represent the underlying substrate in 28% of cases of monomorphic VT of unexplained cause.[37]

Inflammation associated with granuloma infiltration can play a significant role in the exacerbation of electrical storm in CS patients. Schuller and colleagues[28] found the incidence of ICD storm, defined as 3 or more appropriate ICD therapies in 24 hours, to be particularly high: 11% (16 of 112 patients) in their cohort. Predictors of ICD storm included LV dysfunction (odds ratio [OR] 6.71 [95% confidence interval (CI) 1.45–31.2], $P = .015$) and RV dysfunction (OR 3.86 [95% CI 1.16–12.8], $P = .03$), suggesting that more extensive myocardial involvement is a predisposing factor to electrical storm.

Because corticosteroids can play an integral role in arrhythmia suppression, treatment in new presentations of VAs should begin with assessment for active inflammatory sarcoid myocarditis and therapy with immunosuppression as indicated.[33,38,39] In other cases of VT in CS, the disease has already progressed to the fibrotic stage and generated scar. As in patients with other cardiomyopathies and VT, scar serves as substrate for reentry by creating both a zone of slow conduction and an anatomic barrier around which a circuit may propagate.[35]

### Antiarrhythmic Drugs for Ventricular Arrhythmias

Corticosteroids alone can be ineffective at preventing monomorphic VT,[31,33,34] as disease progression through the inflammatory stage has sometimes already progressed to scar formation creating an arrhythmic substrate, which is unlikely to be reversed with immunosuppression. Antiarrhythmic drug use varies widely and can include beta-blockers and class IA, IB, IC, and III agents—

used in isolation or in combination, each with variable outcome.[33,35,40] Mohsen and colleagues[40] reported that of the 21 patients in their series requiring antiarrhythmic drugs, 9 patients continued to have VAs and appropriate ICD therapies (with a mean of 8.7 shocks per patient over a mean 4-year follow-up period).

### Catheter Ablation of Ventricular Arrhythmias

When medical therapy is ineffective at complete arrhythmia suppression, catheter ablation is indicated (**Fig. 5**). VAs in sarcoid patients can be more difficult to ablate than in patients with other cardiomyopathies because ventricular involvement is frequently more diffuse and heterogeneous (**Table 3**). The complicated pattern of scarring that occurs with CS can provide substrate for circuits involving not only the endocardium but also the epicardium and midmyocardium, which may limit the efficacy of catheter ablation (**Table 4**).

Jefic and colleagues[33] have reported on 9 patients with CS and VT who underwent radiofrequency ablation, resulting in elimination of 31 of 44 (70%) inducible VTs and a subsequent decrease (n = 4) or complete elimination (n = 5) of VT over a mean follow-up period of 20 months. Most of the VTs were reentrant in mechanism, and VTs were found to be both endocardial and epicardial in origin as well as left and right sided, though the most prevalent location of reentry (7 of 21 VTs) was the tricuspid annulus.

Koplan and colleagues[32] reported their experience of VT ablation in patients with CS, with contrasting results to Jefic and colleagues.[33] In their case series, half of the patients were referred for heart transplantation for recurrent VTs postablation, and most patients (6 of 8) had recurrent VT. In this series, patients tended to have more severe

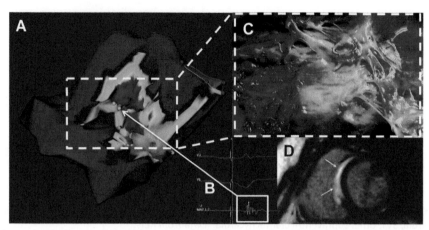

Fig. 5. Electroanatomical map of the RV septum obtained at the time of VT ablation (A). This area of reduced voltage with heterogeneous distribution of low-amplitude electrograms corresponds to the myocardial scar caused by sarcoidosis-related granuloma seen in the pathologic examination, and the arrow indicates the area of successful ablation at the critical isthmus between 2 larger areas of dense scar. The intracardiac electrogram recorded at this border zone site is shown in (B), and the RV endocardial and midmyocardial septal scar (arrows) is shown by cardiac magnetic resonance in (D). This patient ultimately died of systemic infection, potentially as a complication of immunosuppression 2 years after undergoing ablation; gross examination of the explanted heart at autopsy (C) reveals the granulomatous myocardial scarring of the RV septum correlating to the electroanatomical map from (A).

LV dysfunction, suggesting that arrhythmic substrate in the former series may have been more localized and amenable to radiofrequency ablation. Ultimately, with the varied severity of disease burden, a combination approach including immunosuppression, antiarrhythmic therapy, and catheter ablation may be required for arrhythmia control in CS.

**Table 3**
**EP characteristics of VTs in studies of catheter ablation of VT in patients with CS**

|  | Naruse et al,[41] 2014 | Jefic et al,[33] 2009 | Koplan et al,[32] 2006 | Dechering et al,[57] 2013 |
|---|---|---|---|---|
| Patients (n) | 14 | 9 | 8 | 8 |
| Average VTs Targeted/Patient (n) | 2.6 | 4.9 | 4.0 | 3.7 |
| VT cycle length (ms) | 400 ± 97 | 353 ± 72 | — | 326 ± 88 |
| **Morphology (n)** | | | | |
| LBBB inferior axis | 13 | 19 | — | — |
| LBBB superior axis | 8 | 8 | — | — |
| RBBB inferior axis | 5 | 12 | — | — |
| RBBB superior axis | 11 | 5 | — | — |
| **Sites of successful ablation (n)** | | | | |
| LV free wall | 5 | 4 | — | 0 |
| Perimitral valve | 6 | 3 | — | 2 |
| LV septum | 9 | 0 | — | 0 |
| RVOT | 0 | 5 | — | 2 |
| RV free wall | 2 | 0 | — | 0 |
| Peritricuspid valve | 5 | 7 | — | 0 |
| RV apex | 0 | 2 | — | 9 |
| RV septum | 10 | 0 | — | 0 |
| Epicardial ablation | 0 | 3 (33%) | 2 (25%) | 1 (13%) |

Abbreviations: LBBB, left bundle branch block; RBBB, right bundle branch block; RVOT, Right ventricular outflow tract.

**Table 4**
**Studies evaluating the efficacy of radiofrequency catheter ablation for VT in patients with CS**

| Study | n | LVEF (%) | Noninducible Postablation, n/N (%) | Recurrence, n/N (%) | Follow-Up (mo) |
|---|---|---|---|---|---|
| Koplan et al,[32] 2006 | 8 | 34 | 2/8 (25%) | 6/8 (75%) | 6–84 |
| Jefic et al,[33] 2009 | 9 | 42 | 5/9 (56%) | 4/9 (44%) | 19.8 |
| Dechering et al,[57] 2013 | 8 | 36 | 5/8 (63%) | — | — |
| Naruse et al,[41] 2014 | 14 | 40 | 27/35[a] (77%) | 6/14 (43%) | 39 |

[a] Represents reported number of VTs targeted in 14 patients.

Ultimately, a combination of management strategies, with medications and catheter ablation, may be necessary for control of VAs in CS. Naruse and colleagues[41] recently proposed such an approach to VT in CS; their systematic method resulted in 84% of patients free of recurrent VT over a median 33-month follow-up period. All 37 patients prospectively studied received antiarrhythmic therapy (usually amiodarone) and corticosteroid therapy, unless they refused. Twenty-three of 37 (62%) patients were free from any recurrent VT with medical therapy; the remainder subsequently underwent catheter ablation, during which 27 of 35 (77%) of scar-mediated and Purkinje-related VTs were successfully ablated in 14 patients. Ultimately, following VT ablation, all consenting patients in this study also underwent ICD implantation.

## THE ROLE OF THE IMPLANTABLE CARDIAC DEFIBRILLATOR FOR PREVENTION OF SUDDEN DEATH IN CARDIAC SARCOIDOSIS

As sudden cardiac death (SCD) accounts for 30% to 65% of deaths in CS,[14,15,36] after the diagnosis of CS is made, an ICD may be indicated as part of the management of SCD risk.[4]

### Risk Stratification

Most will agree that further risk stratification is needed to discern which patients with CS may benefit from the ICD, as some patients with CS seem to follow a fairly benign clinical course. In the most recent expert consensus guidelines, the ICD is contraindicated (class III recommendation) in patients with no history of syncope, normal ventricular function, no evidence of delayed contrast enhancement on cardiac magnetic resonance (CMR), a negative EP study, and with no indication for pacing.[4] Ultimately, risk stratification may be guided by a combination of CMR and PET findings, EP testing with programmed electrical stimulation, or by other high-risk clinical features, such as AV block, systolic dysfunction, or a history of syncope. Current guidelines recognize the paucity

of randomized prospective data and cite the limitations of retrospectively analyzed series; ultimately, further research is needed to better advise practice.

### Sudden death risk stratification by left ventricular and right ventricular systolic function

Because of both the element of active granulomatous inflammation and also the heterogeneous involvement of the LV and/or RV, CS may behave differently than other cardiomyopathies when it comes to risk of VAs and SCD. Accordingly, a different set of rules may govern SCD risk and ICD indications than the standard LVEF less than 35% that is often used for nonsarcoid cardiomyopathies. Although patients with CS with EF less than 35% should receive a primary prevention ICD in accordance with accepted device guidelines,[17] many patients with CS with EF greater than 35% may also be candidates for primary prevention ICD implantation.

Although a lower LVEF is associated with appropriate ICD therapy in several retrospective studies, many patients with only mildly impaired LV function also had substantial risk of VAs and resultant appropriate ICD shocks and antitachycardia pacing.[18,42,43] In fact, in the study by Kron and colleagues,[42] most primary and secondary prevention patients who received appropriate ICD therapies had an LVEF greater than 35%, suggesting that patients with CS with mild or moderately reduced LVEF may still be at substantial risk for VAs. Furthermore, in the study by Betensky and colleagues,[18] 7 of the 17 patients (41%) with appropriate ICD therapy had an LVEF greater than 35%. Although these studies noted that several patients with mild and moderately reduced EF received appropriate ICD therapies for VT/VF, Schuller and colleagues[28] reported that in their primary prevention cohort, no patient with normal right and LV function received an appropriate therapy. It is from these data that a class IIa recommendation for consideration of ICD implantation in patients with an LVEF of 36% to 49% and/or RVEF less than 40% after optimal medical therapy and initiation of immunosuppression if indicated was based.

### Sudden death risk stratification with cardiac imaging

CMR and PET are the imaging modalities with the highest sensitivity and specificity in the detection of CS.[5,44–46] CMR, in particular, has emerged as the test of choice at many centers in the evaluation of CS, owing in part to a lower false-positive rate. CMR uses T-2 weighted signal and early gadolinium images to detect acute inflammation and late gadolinium enhancement (LGE, also known as delayed contrast enhancement) to assess for fibrosis or scar. Preliminary data also suggest that surveillance with CMR can assess the efficacy of steroid therapy.[47,48]

Importantly, CMR has a role in risk stratification and prognosis. In a recent study of 155 consecutive patients with systemic sarcoidosis who underwent CMR for workup of suspected CS, LGE was present in 39 patients (25.5%); its presence was associated with a Cox HR of 31.6 for death, aborted sudden cardiac death, or appropriate ICD discharge[49] over a median 2.6-year follow-up period. Of the 12 patients with sudden cardiac death or appropriate ICD discharge in this study, all had LGE present on CMR. Sarcoid patients without LGE, even those with LV dilatation and severely impaired LVEF, did not experience SCD, suggesting CMR may provide prognostic data beyond that conferred by EF alone.

Although CMR may have a higher specificity, [18]F-fluoro-2-deoxyglucose PET ([18]F-FDG PET) seems to detect active inflammation in CS with a slightly higher sensitivity. However, as the uptake of [18]F-FDG is seen in other inflammatory myocardial diseases, PET is nonspecific for CS and must be interpreted in the appropriate clinical context. Like CMR, PET carries prognostic value: In a study of 118 patients with suspected CS, 60% had abnormal cardiac PET findings. Over a median follow-up of 1.5 years, abnormal PET findings were associated with an HR of 3.9 for death or VT, and an abnormal PET remained a significant predictor of death or VT even after multivariate analysis to adjust for EF and other clinical variables,[45] indicating PET offers prognostic value beyond EF alone.

### Sudden death risk stratification with electrophysiologic testing

There have also been limited studies investigating the role for programmed electrical stimulation (PES) for the inducibility of sustained monomorphic VT as a means of risk stratification of sudden cardiac death in patients with CS. One such study of 76 patients with CS undergoing PES showed that 6 of 8 patients (75%) with inducible VT went on to have VAs and ICD therapies, compared with 1 patient with sudden cardiac death among the 68 patients (1.5%) who had been noninducible by PES. In another study of 32 patients with CS, 4 of 6 patients (67%) with inducible VT went on to have appropriate ICD therapies, whereas 2 of 20 patients (10%) who were noninducible went on to have VAs or sudden cardiac death.[7] Although these studies suggest a potential role for EP testing in risk stratification, these data ultimately need to be replicated in larger cohorts. Furthermore, these studies are limited by mean follow-up periods of 5.0 years and 2.6 years, respectively; in light of CS as a progressive disease, the long-term prognostic value of a single negative EP study is unclear.

### Indications for Implantable Cardiac Defibrillator Therapy

The 2008 guidelines from the ACC/American Heart Association/HRS give a class IIA recommendation (level of evidence C) for ICD therapy in patients with sarcoidosis with evidence of myocardial involvement, regardless of symptoms or presentation.[50] As previously discussed, the HRS released an expert consensus statement in 2014 further refining the specific recommendations for ICD therapy as they pertain to patients with CS (**Box 3**).[4] Class I indications stand for secondary prevention devices and for those with severe LV dysfunction despite a period of optimal medical therapy as per recommendations for patients with other cardiomyopathies. These guidelines also give class II recommendations for ICD implantation in CS if there are other features considered to be higher risk (eg, need for permanent pacing, mild to moderately reduced LV [ie, EF 36%–49%]) or RV (ie, <40%) systolic function, or inducible VT by EP study.

Practice patterns, as surveyed before the release of the HRS' guidelines, are varied,[51] with some centers tending to implant ICDs in patients with CS only with class I indications (prior VAs or LVEF ≤35%), whereas other centers are offering ICDs to all patients with CS (in accordance with the IIA recommendation from the 2008 guidelines). Although the type of patient for which the primary prevention ICD will benefit does remain controversial in CS, what is becoming evident from several observational studies is that among those patients with CS who do receive ICDs, both appropriate and inappropriate ICD therapies are common.

### Studies of Defibrillator Therapies in Cardiac Sarcoidosis

Four observational studies have been published that report on ICD therapies in patients with CS.

---

**Box 3**
**HRS' expert consensus recommendations for ICD in patients with CS**

*Class I Recommendation*

ICD implantation *is recommended* in patients with CS and one or more of the following:

1. There is spontaneous sustained ventricular arrhythmias, including prior cardiac arrest.

2. The LVEF is 35% or less, despite optimal medical therapy and a period of immunosuppression (if there is active inflammation).

*Class IIa Recommendation*

ICD implantation *can be useful* in patients with CS, independent of ventricular function and one or more of the following:

1. An indication for permanent pacemaker implantation

2. Unexplained syncope or near-syncope, thought to be arrhythmic in cause

3. Inducible sustained VAs (>30 seconds of monomorphic VT or polymorphic VT) or clinically relevant ventricular fibrillation[a]

*Class IIb Recommendation*

ICD implantation *may be considered* in patients with an LVEF of 36% to 49% and/or an RVEF less than 40%, despite optimal medical therapy and a period of immunosuppression (if there is active inflammation).

*Class III Recommendations*

ICD implantation *is not recommended* in patients with no history of syncope, normal LVEF/RVEF, no LGE on CMR, a negative EP study, and no indication for permanent pacing. However, these patients should be closely followed for deterioration in ventricular function.

ICD implantation *is not recommended* in patients with one or more of the following:

1. Incessant ventricular arrhythmias

2. Severe New York Heart Association class IV heart failure

---

[a] Ventricular fibrillation with triple premature beats of less than 220 ms is considered a nonspecific response.
*From* Birnie DH, Sauer W, Bogun F, et al. Heart Rhythm Society expert consensus statement on the diagnosis and management of arrhythmias associated with cardiac sarcoidosis. Heart Rhythm 2014;11(7):1–24; with permission.

---

Betensky and colleagues[18] reviewed 45 patients (64% primary prevention, 2.6-year mean follow-up period) and found a high annualized appropriate therapy (shock and/or antitachycardia pacing) rate of 14.5%. Predictors of appropriate therapies included lower LVEF and complete heart block, signifying more advanced disease. Schuller and colleagues[28] reported on 112 patients (74% primary prevention, 2.8-year mean follow-up period) and found a similarly high annualized therapy rate of 13.2% (**Fig. 6**). In this cohort, no primary prevention patients with normal RV and LV function received an appropriate therapy, though there were many patients with only mild systolic dysfunction who received shocks and antitachycardia pacing. Mohsen and colleagues[40] found an annualized therapy rate of 9.6% in their mixed cohort of patients with primary and secondary prevention CS. The rate of inappropriate ICD therapies was quite high (30% over a 3.75-year mean follow-up duration). Kron and colleagues[42] published a multicenter retrospective review of 235 patients (99 of which were included in the aforementioned studies) and found male sex, syncope, lower LVEF, and high proportion of ventricular pacing each to be independent risk factors for appropriate therapies (with an annualized incidence of 8.6% in this study). Altogether, the rates of appropriate therapies in these 3 studies are notably higher than that observed in large primary prevention ICD trials, such as SCD-HeFT (Sudden Cardiac Death in Heart Failure Trial), whereby the incidence was approximately 5% per year.[52]

## Special Considerations for Postimplant Implantable Cardiac Defibrillator Management in Patients with Cardiac Sarcoidosis

Experience taking care of patients with CS with ICDs has brought some special considerations to light. Firstly, as highlighted by the 4 aforementioned studies, the burden of VAs, annualized

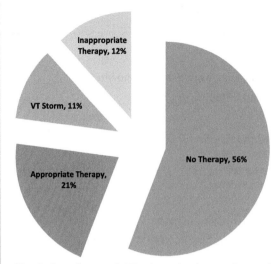

Fig. 6. Prevalence of ICD therapies in a cohort of patients with CS. (*From* Schuller JL, Zipse M, Crawford T, et al. Implantable cardioverter defibrillator therapy in patients with cardiac sarcoidosis. J Cardiovasc Electrophysiol 2012;23:925–9; with permission.)

rate of appropriate therapies, and prevalence of electrical storm[28] are all substantial. Also noteworthy is the high rate of inappropriate therapies (30% of patients in the study by Moshen and colleagues,[40] for example) caused in part by the high burden of atrial arrhythmias in CS.

Patients with CS and ICDs also have a high incidence of late reduction of sensed R waves. A case-control study on a cohort of 46 patients with CS and ICDs compared with 117 controls with other cardiomyopathies showed that patients with CS have a high incidence of significant (greater than 50%) reduction in measured electrograms (HR 9.10, 95% CI 2.50–33.06).[53] It is possible that local characteristics at the lead tip to tissue interface over time (eg, inflammation from local granuloma formation) could lead to these reductions in sensing, though the mechanism is unknown. Nonetheless, reductions in sensing can lead to significant clinical consequences, such as undersensing of VF and failure to deliver appropriate therapies and oversensing of T waves with the delivery of inappropriate therapies (**Fig. 7**). Measured R waves by the ICD should be followed over time and should prompt defibrillation threshold (DFT) testing if reductions

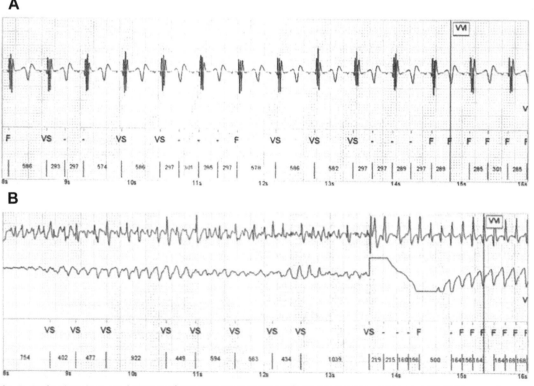

Fig. 7. Reductions in sensed R waves from ICDs in patients with CS can lead to ventricular fibrillation undersensing and failure to deliver appropriate shocks (A) as well as T-wave oversensing (B) and the potential delivery of inappropriate shocks.

in R waves are significant and may require lead revision if DFT testing fails.

Lastly, because patients with CS have a high incidence of AV block, many may either meet an indication for a biventricular ICD at the time of initial implant or may meet an indication for upgrade at the time of generator change if the burden of RV pacing is considerable, as supported by data from the BLOCK HF clinical trial.[54]

## SUMMARY

CS can present in the setting of advanced systemic disease or in clinical isolation. The manifestations of CS are highly variable: Myocardial involvement can be subclinical or it may lead to AV block, heart failure, atrial and VAs, or sudden cardiac death.

Because the overall burden of arrhythmia and conduction disease is high in patients with CS and management is complex and multifaceted, the cardiac electrophysiologist plays an important role in the multidisciplinary care of these patients. Ultimately, early referral of patients with a suspicion of CS to an electrophysiologist is necessary to aid in the initial diagnosis and risk assessment, in addition to providing ongoing follow-up for arrhythmia and implanted device management.

## REFERENCES

1. Chapelon-Abric C, de Zuttere D, Duhaut P, et al. Cardiac sarcoidosis: a retrospective study of 41 cases. Medicine 2004;83:315–34.
2. Silverman KJ, Hutchins GM, Bulkley BH. Cardiac sarcoid: a clinicopathologic study of 84 unselected patients with systemic sarcoidosis. Circulation 1978;58:1204–11.
3. Uusimaa P, Ylitalo K, Anttonen O, et al. Ventricular tachyarrhythmia as a primary presentation of sarcoidosis. Europace 2008;10:760–6.
4. Birnie DH, Sauer W, Bogun F, et al. Heart Rhythm Society expert consensus statement on the diagnosis and management of arrhythmias associated with cardiac sarcoidosis. Heart Rhythm 2014;11(7):1–24.
5. Soejima K, Yada H. The work-up and management of patients with apparent or subclinical cardiac sarcoidosis: with emphasis on the associated heart rhythm abnormalities. J Cardiovasc Electrophysiol 2009;20:578–83.
6. Mehta D, Mori N, Goldbarg SH, et al. Primary prevention of sudden cardiac death in silent cardiac sarcoidosis: role of programmed ventricular stimulation. Circ Arrhythm Electrophysiol 2011;4:43–8.
7. Aizer A, Stern EH, Gomes JA, et al. Usefulness of programmed ventricular stimulation in predicting future arrhythmic events in patients with cardiac sarcoidosis. Am J Cardiol 2005;96:276–82.
8. Boulos M, Lashevsky I, Reisner S, et al. Electroanatomic mapping of arrhythmogenic right ventricular dysplasia. JAC. J Am Coll Cardiol 2001;38:2020–7.
9. Nery PB, Keren A, Healey J, et al. Isolated cardiac sarcoidosis: establishing the diagnosis with electroanatomic mapping-guided endomyocardial biopsy. Can J Cardiol 2013;29:1015.e1–3.
10. Pieroni M, Russo Dello A, Marzo F, et al. High prevalence of myocarditis mimicking arrhythmogenic right ventricular cardiomyopathy. J Am Coll Cardiol 2009;53:681–9.
11. Vasaiwala SC, Finn C, Delpriore J, et al. Prospective study of cardiac sarcoid mimicking arrhythmogenic right ventricular dysplasia. J Cardiovasc Electrophysiol 2009;20:473–6.
12. Santucci PA, Morton JB, Picken MM, et al. Electroanatomic mapping of the right ventricle in a patient with a giant epsilon wave, ventricular tachycardia, and cardiac sarcoidosis. J Cardiovasc Electrophysiol 2004; 15:1091–4.
13. Vakil K, Minami E, Fishbein DP. Right ventricular sarcoidosis: is it time for updated diagnostic criteria? Tex Heart Inst J 2014;41:203–7.
14. Matsui Y, Iwai K, Tachibana T, et al. Clinicopathological study of fatal myocardial sarcoidosis. Ann N Y Acad Sci 1976;278:455–69.
15. Roberts WC, McAllister HA, Ferrans VJ. Sarcoidosis of the heart. A clinicopathologic study of 35 necropsy patients (group 1) and review of 78 previously described necropsy patients (group 11). Am J Med 1977;63:86–108.
16. Schuller JL, OLSON MD, Zipse MM, et al. Electrocardiographic characteristics in patients with pulmonary sarcoidosis indicating cardiac involvement. J Cardiovasc Electrophysiol 2011;22:1243–8.
17. Epstein AE, DiMarco JP, Ellenbogen KA, et al. 2012 ACCF/AHA/HRS focused update incorporated into the ACCF/AHA/HRS 2008 guidelines for device-based therapy of cardiac rhythm abnormalities: a report of the American College of Cardiology Foundation/American Heart Association Task Force on Practice Guidelines and the Heart Rhythm Society. Circulation 2013;127:e283–352.
18. Betensky BP, Tschabrunn CM, Zado ES, et al. Long-term follow-up of patients with cardiac sarcoidosis and implantable cardioverter-defibrillators. Heart Rhythm 2012;9:884–91.
19. Kato Y, Morimoto S-I, Uemura A, et al. Efficacy of corticosteroids in sarcoidosis presenting with atrioventricular block. Sarcoidosis Vasc Diffuse Lung Dis 2003;20:133–7.
20. Yodogawa K, Seino Y, Ohara T, et al. Effect of corticosteroid therapy on ventricular arrhythmias in patients with cardiac sarcoidosis. Ann Noninvasive Electrocardiol 2011;16:140–7.

21. Yoshida Y, Morimoto S, Hiramitsu S, et al. Incidence of cardiac sarcoidosis in Japanese patients with high-degree atrioventricular block. Am Heart J 1997;134:382–6.

22. Kandolin R, Lehtonen J, Kupari M. Cardiac sarcoidosis and giant cell myocarditis as causes of atrioventricular block in young and middle-aged adults. Circ Arrhythm Electrophysiol 2011;4:303–9.

23. Nery PB, Beanlands RS, Nair GM, et al. Atrioventricular block as the initial manifestation of cardiac sarcoidosis in middle-aged adults. J Cardiovasc Electrophysiol 2014;25(8):875–81.

24. Gozo EG, Cosnow I, Cohen HC, et al. The heart in sarcoidosis. Chest 1971;60:379–88.

25. Abeler V. Sarcoidosis of the cardiac conducting system. Am Heart J 1979;97:701–7.

26. Viles-Gonzalez JF, Pastori L, Fischer A, et al. Supraventricular arrhythmias in patients with cardiac sarcoidosis prevalence, predictors, and clinical implications. Chest 2013;143:1085–90.

27. Cain MA, Metzl MD, Patel AR, et al. Cardiac sarcoidosis detected by late gadolinium enhancement and prevalence of atrial arrhythmias. Am J Cardiol 2014; 113:1556–60.

28. Schuller JL, Zipse M, Crawford T, et al. Implantable cardioverter defibrillator therapy in patients with cardiac sarcoidosis. J Cardiovasc Electrophysiol 2012; 23:925–9.

29. Zipse MM, Schuller JL, Katz DF, et al. Atrial arrhythmias are common and arise from diverse mechanisms in patients with cardiac sarcoidosis. Heart Rhythm 2013;2013:1–2.

30. Willner JM, Viles-Gonzalez JF, Coffey JO, et al. Catheter ablation of atrial arrhythmias in cardiac sarcoidosis. J Cardiovasc Electrophysiol 2014; 25(9):958–63.

31. Winters SL, Cohen M, Greenberg S, et al. Sustained ventricular tachycardia associated with sarcoidosis: assessment of the underlying cardiac anatomy and the prospective utility of programmed ventricular stimulation, drug therapy and an implantable antitachycardia device. J Am Coll Cardiol 1991;18:937–43.

32. Koplan BA, Soejima K, Baughman K, et al. Refractory ventricular tachycardia secondary to cardiac sarcoid: electrophysiologic characteristics, mapping, and ablation. Heart Rhythm 2006;3:924–9.

33. Jefic D, Joel B, Good E, et al. Role of radiofrequency catheter ablation of ventricular tachycardia in cardiac sarcoidosis: report from a multicenter registry. Heart Rhythm 2009;6:189–95.

34. Banba K, Kusano KF, Nakamura K, et al. Relationship between arrhythmogenesis and disease activity in cardiac sarcoidosis. Heart Rhythm 2007;4: 1292–9.

35. Furushima H, Chinushi M, Sugiura H, et al. Ventricular tachyarrhythmia associated with cardiac sarcoidosis: its mechanisms and outcome. Clin Cardiol 2004;27: 217–22.

36. Fleming HA, Bailey SM. Sarcoid heart disease. J R Coll Physicians Lond 1981;15:245.

37. Nery PB, Mc Ardle BA, Redpath CJ, et al. Prevalence of cardiac sarcoidosis in patients presenting with monomorphic ventricular tachycardia. Pacing Clin Electrophysiol 2014;37:364–74.

38. Stees CS, Khoo MS, Lowery CM, et al. Ventricular tachycardia storm successfully treated with immunosuppression and catheter ablation in a patient with cardiac sarcoidosis. J Cardiovasc Electrophysiol 2011;22:210–3.

39. Yazaki Y, Isobe M, Hiroe M, et al. Prognostic determinants of long-term survival in Japanese patients with cardiac sarcoidosis treated with prednisone. Am J Cardiol 2001;88:1006–10.

40. Mohsen A, Jimenez A, Hood RE, et al. Cardiac sarcoidosis: electrophysiological outcomes on long-term follow-up and the role of the implantable cardioverter-defibrillator. J Cardiovasc Electrophysiol 2013;25(2):171–6.

41. Naruse Y, Sekiguchi Y, Nogami A, et al. Systematic treatment approach to ventricular tachycardia in cardiac sarcoidosis. Circ Arrhythm Electrophysiol 2014; 7:407–13.

42. Kron J, Sauer W, Schuller J, et al. Efficacy and safety of implantable cardiac defibrillators for treatment of ventricular arrhythmias in patients with cardiac sarcoidosis. Europace 2013;15:347–54.

43. Schuller JL, Lowery CM, Zipse M, et al. Diagnostic utility of signal-averaged electrocardiography for detection of cardiac sarcoidosis. Ann Noninvasive Electrocardiol 2011;16:70–6.

44. Youssef G, Beanlands RSB, Birnie DH, et al. Cardiac sarcoidosis: applications of imaging in diagnosis and directing treatment. Heart 2011;97:2078–87.

45. Blankstein R, Osborne M, Naya M, et al. Cardiac positron emission tomography enhances prognostic assessments of patients with suspected cardiac sarcoidosis. J Am Coll Cardiol 2014;63:329–36.

46. Ohira H, Tsujino I, Ishimaru S, et al. Myocardial imaging with 18F-fluoro-2-deoxyglucose positron emission tomography and magnetic resonance imaging in sarcoidosis. Eur J Nucl Med Mol Imaging 2008;35:933–41.

47. Vignaux O, Dhote R, Duboc D, et al. Clinical significance of myocardial magnetic resonance abnormalities in patients with sarcoidosis: a 1-year follow-up study. Chest 2002;122:1895–901.

48. Sekiguchi M, Yazaki Y, Isobe M, et al. Cardiac sarcoidosis: diagnostic, prognostic, and therapeutic considerations. Cardiovasc Drugs Ther 1996;10:495–510.

49. Greulich S, Deluigi CC, Gloekler S, et al. CMR imaging predicts death and other adverse events in suspected cardiac sarcoidosis. JACC Cardiovasc Imaging 2013;6:501–11.

50. Writing Committee Members, Epstein AE, DiMarco JP, et al. ACC/AHA/HRS 2008 guidelines for device-based therapy of cardiac rhythm abnormalities: executive summary: a report of the American College of Cardiology/American Heart Association Task Force on Practice Guidelines (Writing Committee to Revise the ACC/AHA/NASPE 2002 Guideline Update for implantation of cardiac pacemakers and Antiarrhythmia devices): developed in collaboration with the American Association for Thoracic Surgery and Society of Thoracic Surgeons. Circulation 2008;117:2820–40.

51. Hamzeh NY. Management of cardiac sarcoidosis in the United States. Chest 2012;141:154.

52. Bardy GH, Lee KL, Mark DB, et al. Amiodarone or an implantable cardioverter–defibrillator for congestive heart failure. N Engl J Med 2005;352:225–37.

53. Zipse MM, Varosy PD, Schuller JL, et al. Patients with cardiac sarcoidosis and ICDs have a high incidence of late reduction of measured electrograms. Heart Rhythm 2013;2013:1–2.

54. Curtis AB, Worley SJ, Adamson PB, et al. Biventricular pacing for atrioventricular block and systolic dysfunction. N Engl J Med 2013;368:1585–93.

55. Okamoto H, Mizuno K, Ohtoshi E. Cutaneous sarcoidosis with cardiac involvement. Eur J Dermatol 1999;9:466–9.

56. Yodogawa K, Seino Y, Shiomura R, et al. Recovery of atrioventricular block following steroid therapy in patients with cardiac sarcoidosis. J Cardiol 2013; 62:320–5.

57. Dechering DG, Kochhäuser S, Wasmer K, et al. Electrophysiological characteristics of ventricular tachyarrhythmias in cardiac sarcoidosis versus arrhythmogenic right ventricular cardiomyopathy. Heart Rhythm 2013;10:158–64.

# Arrhythmias in Chagasic Cardiomyopathy

 CrossMark

Chris Healy, MD[a], Juan F. Viles-Gonzalez, MD[a], Luis C. Sáenz, MD[b], Mariana Soto, MD[b], Juan D. Ramírez, MD[b], Andre d'Avila, MD, PhD[c],*

## KEYWORDS

- Chagas disease • *Trypanosoma cruzi* • Ventricular tachycardia • Sudden cardiac death
- Epicardial ablation

## KEY POINTS

- Chagasic cardiomyopathy is a common, but often under-recognized, cause of heart failure and ventricular arrhythmias.
- Arrhythmic risk often precedes left ventricular dysfunction in chagasic cardiomyopathy.
- Catheter ablation is a useful technique for the management of recurrent ventricular tachycardia in patients with chagasic cardiomyopathy, but epicardial access is frequently required to achieve optimal clinical outcomes.

## INTRODUCTION

Chagas disease (ChD) was discovered and described in 1909 by the Brazilian physician Carlos Chagas. More than a century after its original description, trypanosomiasis still causes significant morbidity and mortality and is classified as a neglected tropical disease that is prevalent in underdeveloped countries, particularly in South America[1] ChD causes several cardiovascular problems, including ventricular arrhythmias and sudden death. This article addresses the available evidence on the epidemiology, pathophysiology, clinical characteristics, and management of ventricular arrhythmias in chagasic cardiomyopathy.

## EPIDEMIOLOGY AND CAUSE

ChD is a chronic parasitosis that affects the heart and other organs and is caused by the protozoan parasite *Trypanosoma cruzi*. *T cruzi* is transmitted to humans mainly through parasite-laden feces from a hematophagous insect vector (*Triatoma*

*infestans* in American Southern Cone countries and *Rhodnius prolixus* in the Andean region and Central America). The triatomine vectors are only found in the Americas, where the disease in considered endemic (also called American trypanosomiasis). The prevalence of ChD is in the range of 1% to 6% in endemic areas based on estimations from the World Health Organization (WHO).[2,3] In addition, 8 million to 10 million people are infected worldwide (most concentrated in Latin American countries), 100 million people are at risk of infection, and 300,000 new cases are reported each year.[2–7] The triatomine vectors live in the walls and roofs of houses built with vegetable materials, a practice that is common many poor, rural areas of Latin America. For this reason, Chagas has been traditionally considered a disease of poverty. However, the epidemiologic pattern of ChD has shifted in recent decades because of urban migration from rural Latin American areas to cities in endemic countries and throughout the world. It is common for patients infected during

Conflicts of interest: None of the authors have any conflicts of interest to disclose.
[a] Department of Cardiac Electrophysiology, University of Miami Miller School of Medicine, 1295 NW 14th Street, South Building, Suite A, Miami, FL 33125, USA; [b] Cardiólogo-Electrofisiólogo, Fundación Cardio Infantil-Instituto de Cardiología, Calle 163A No 13B-60, Bogotá, Colombia; [c] Hospital Cardiologico, Rodovia SC 401, 121, Itacorubi, Florianopolis, Santa Catarina, Brazil, CEP: 88030-000
* Corresponding author.
*E-mail address:* andredavila@mac.com

Card Electrophysiol Clin 7 (2015) 251–268
http://dx.doi.org/10.1016/j.ccep.2015.03.016

cardiacEP.theclinics.com

childhood before moving from an endemic area to present as adults with clinical manifestations of the disease in nonendemic areas, leading to delays in timely diagnosis and treatment. The US Centers for Disease Control and Prevention have reported more than 300,000 immigrants living in the United States infected with *T cruzi*.[8] Similarly, approximately 30,000 to 45,000 individuals likely have undiagnosed chagasic cardiomyopathy with clinical manifestations that are confused with idiopathic cardiomyopathy by general practitioners working in nonendemic countries.

Undiagnosed infected patients who are not aware of their condition can become transmitters of the parasite after blood or organ donation, which is the most frequent mode of transmission in nonendemic countries.[9] Despite the association of ChD with poverty and its classification by the WHO as a neglected tropical disease, its economic burden is huge. The WHO estimates 50,000 deaths per year related to chagasic cardiomyopathy. Of these, 60%, 25%, and 15% are related to sudden cardiac death (SCD), heart failure, and stroke, respectively.[4–7] The high rate of sudden death associated with ChD frequently affects young and economically productive people, which can be shocking in what appear to be healthy young people, and also results in significant economic loss. In addition, patients with chagasic cardiomyopathy require long-term treatment, including medications and costly interventional procedures (pacemakers, implantable cardioverter-defibrillators [ICDs], cardiac resynchronization devices, ablations, and heart transplantation), imposing a large economic burden on the health care system. Recent estimations put the global cost associated with ChD at $7.19 billion per year, with more than 10% of this spent in the United States and Canada.[10]

## CHRONIC CARDIOMYOPATHY

Primary *T cruzi* infection is acquired most commonly during childhood and young adulthood through vector transmission in endemic areas. The acute phase (**Fig. 1**) of ChD is associated with local tissue inflammation at the parasite entry site and symptoms similar to other types of myocarditis, including malaise, fever, hepatomegaly, and splenomegaly. The acute phase is associated with death in 5% of cases secondary to acute myocarditis, pericardial effusion, and/or meningoencephalitis.[9–11] The electrocardiogram (ECG) in the acute phase can show sinus tachycardia, low voltage of the QRS complex, prolongation of the PR and/or QT intervals, and changes in ventricular repolarization.[11] Ventricular arrhythmias, atrial fibrillation, and right bundle branch block can also develop and are associated with a worse prognosis.[11] The clinical manifestations during the acute phase resolve spontaneously after 6 to 8 weeks in 90% of infected patients.[9,10] After the acute phase of the infection, most patients enter into the chronic

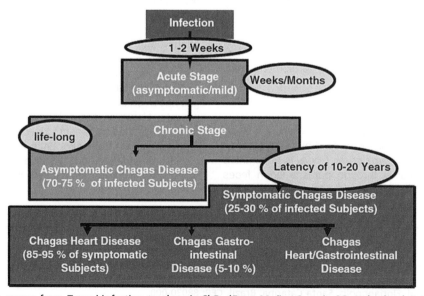

**Fig. 1.** Time course from *T cruzi* infection to chronic ChD. (*From* Muñoz-Saravia SG, Haberland A, Wallukat G, et al. Chronic Chagas' heart disease: a disease on its way to becoming a worldwide health problem: epidemiology, etiopathology, treatment, pathogenesis and laboratory medicine. Heart Fail Rev 2012;17(1):45–64; with permission.)

phase. The so-called indeterminate form[9,10] (see **Fig. 1**) is typically marked by positive serologic tests but no symptoms, ECG abnormalities, or other evidence of heart or visceral involvement.[9,10] Between 40% and 60% of infected patients remain in the indeterminate form throughout their lives with an excellent prognosis and a life expectancy similar to that of people without ChD.[9,10,12] However, 30% to 40% of infected patients develop determinate forms - cardiac, digestive (megaesophagus, megacolon), or mixed - that typically develop 30 to 40 years after the acute infection (see **Fig. 1**).[9,13] A direct progression from acute infection to any clinical form of ChD occurs in just 5% of cases.[13]

## CARDIAC INVOLVEMENT

Cardiac involvement is considered the most frequent and serious manifestation of chronic ChD.[14] Chagasic cardiomyopathy is a chronic myocarditis that affects all chambers of the heart, the parasympathetic cardiac nerves, and all levels of the conduction system.[15] The pathogenesis of cardiac damage is complex and not completely understood (**Fig. 2**). At least 4 possible mechanisms have been suggested: cardiac parasympathetic neuronal depopulation, immune-mediated myocardial injury, parasite persistence in cardiac tissue with secondary antigenic stimulation, and coronary microvascular abnormalities causing myocardial ischemia.[9,11,15]

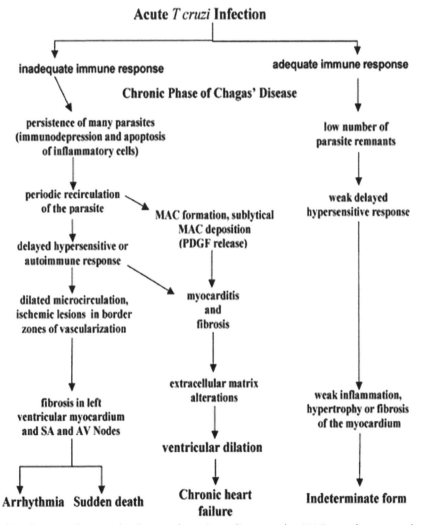

**Fig. 2.** Pathophysiologic mechanisms leading to chagasic cardiomyopathy. MAC, membrane attack complex of the complement cascade; PDGF, platelet-derived growth factor; SA, sinoatrial. (*From* Higuchi Mde L, Benvenuti LA, Martins Reis M, et al. Pathophysiology of the heart in Chagas' disease: current status and new developments. Cardiovasc Res 2003;60(1):96–107; with permission.)

### Cardiac Parasympathetic Neuronal Depopulation

Autopsy and animal studies of *T cruzi* infection have consistently shown parasympathetic neuronal depopulation and autonomic denervation occurring during the acute phase of the infection related to direct neuronal parasitism, as well as degeneration caused by periganglionic inflammation and an antineuronal autoimmune reaction.[9,15] In addition, cardiac parasympathetic denervation has been correlated with abnormal cardiac autonomic heart rate regulation shown by pharmacologic and physiologic testing, suggesting that patients with ChD are deprived of normal inhibitory parasympathetic tone in the sinus node.[9] This autonomic imbalance in chagasic patients could over time lead to catecholamine-induced cardiomyopathy. Recent studies have shown circulating antibodies that bind to myocardial adrenergic and cholinergic receptors triggering physiologic, molecular, and morphologic changes with the potential to cause myocardial damage.[16] Despite these findings, correlations between morphologic and functional changes in the cardiac autonomic system and degree of ventricular dysfunction have been inconsistent, and not enough evidence exists to prove that chagasic autonomic dysfunction results in myocyte damage.[11,15]

### Immune-mediated Myocardial Injury

Experimental evidence suggests that, after parasitemia, tissue parasitosis and intense myocarditis (in the acute phase) are controlled by immune mechanisms. Mild, focal inflammation persists during the indeterminate form of ChD.[17] This process is composed mainly of mononuclear cells and is associated with immunoglobulin and complement deposition in myocardial tissue, implicating immunologic factors in the genesis of cardiac tissue damage.[18] It is not clear why, after the acute phase, some patients are able to control their infection with a mild inflammatory response and no manifestations of significant cardiac damage, whereas others develop progressive cardiomyopathy with intense inflammation, necrosis, and reactive fibrosis. Some factors have been associated with stability or instability of this process: parasite load, parasite strain or tissue tropism, duration of infection, reinfection, and genetic and molecular mechanisms of host and parasite.[11,15] One of the mechanisms linking cardiac inflammatory lesions and immune response in ChD is autoimmune injury to cardiac structures. Experimental studies in mice infected with *T cruzi* have detected autoantibodies specific for structural proteins including cardiac myosin, desmin, and actin.[19] In addition, cross-reactive antibodies between human cardiac myosin heavy chain and the *T cruzi* protein B13 are more frequently found in the sera from chagasic patients with manifestations of cardiomyopathy than in patients with the indeterminate form of the disease.[20]

### Parasite Persistence in Cardiac Tissue with Secondary Antigenic Stimulation

Animal and human studies have identified *T cruzi* antigens and/or genomic material in inflammatory foci in cardiac and neuronal tissue.[21–24] Some studies have reported that reduction (by trypanocidal treatment) or enhancement of parasite load is related to attenuation or exacerbation of cardiomyopathy, suggesting that persistence of the parasite is important in the pathogenesis of chagasic cardiomyopathy.[25,26] Moreover, reactivation of the infection after years of the indeterminate form in patients with virally acquired immune deficiency syndromes supports this theory.[27] The mechanisms relating persistence of parasites to cardiac damage remain poorly understood, but continuous antigenic stimulation and inflammation have been suggested.[28]

### Coronary Microvascular Abnormalities

Pathologic studies as well as some clinical evidence suggest an important role of myocardial ischemia in the pathogenesis of chagasic cardiomyopathy. Several necroscopic studies have reported abnormalities of the microcirculation causing myocardial ischemia, which is responsible for the focal diffuse myocytolysis and subsequent reparative interstitial fibrosis characteristically found in chagasic hearts.[29,30] This observation seems to be confirmed by the microcirculatory and extracellular matrix findings on three-dimensional (3D) microscopy in chagasic cardiomyopathy. Severe and diffuse arteriolar dilatation associated with microvessel tortuosity has been found in chagasic cardiomyopathy but not in normal hearts or those with idiopathic dilated cardiomyopathy. It has been hypothesized that this diffuse arteriolar dilatation may cause deviation of blood flow from epicardial coronary arteries with high blood pressure to dilated arterioles with low blood pressure that are next to the coronaries branches, producing low perfusion pressure in the distal microvasculature supplying susceptible areas distal to the coronary branches (a steal phenomenon). The watershed areas between main coronary artery branches would be the most susceptible to this steal phenomenon, causing low perfusion pressure, secondary ischemia, microinfarctions, and reparative fibrosis.[29] The most frequently seen areas of myocardial scarring in chagasic cardiomyopathy are the posterolateral left ventricle (LV) and the left ventricular apex, the watershed zones between the right coronary and circumflex arteries, and the anterior descending and posterior descending coronary arteries, respectively.[31] In addition, histologic studies have consistently reported fibrotic segmental lesions in the conduction system supplied by the septal perforating arteries and atrioventricular (AV) nodal artery originating from the dominant coronary artery at the crux cordis. In addition, a decrease in the cross-sectional luminal areas of the epicardial coronary arteries supplying segments of dysfunctional LV wall in chagasic cardiomyopathy has been reported.[31]

The sum of diminished cross-sectional luminal area of the epicardial coronary arteries and dilatation of the related arterioles promotes the steal phenomenon in watershed regions distal to the coronary artery branches with secondary ischemia and coalescent microinfarctions, which could be one of the factors leading to the development of aneurysms in patients with ChD. Complimentarily, autonomic denervation and endothelial dysfunction related to the inflammatory process and/or induced by the parasite may explain the arteriolar dilatation seen in chagasic cardiomyopathy. Although attractive, chronic myocardial ischemia secondary to microvascular blood flow abnormalities is just a hypothesis and remains to be conclusively proved in the experimental and clinical settings.

## HISTOPATHOLOGY OF CHAGASIC CARDIOMYOPATHY

Independent of the mechanisms implicated in its pathogenesis, chronic chagasic cardiomyopathy is characterized by a focal, diffuse inflammatory process composed of lymphomononuclear cells that produce myocytolysis, severe reparative fibrosis encasing individual or groups of myocardial fibers, and dilated microvessels with thin and fibrotic walls, as shown in biopsy studies (**Fig. 3**). Endomyocardial biopsy studies have reported higher percentages of severe inflammation and fibrosis in patients with heart failure compared with indeterminate forms, suggesting a progressive character of the disease.[32]

This inflammatory process and subsequent reparative fibrosis affects multiple areas of the myocardium, explaining the segmental wall motion abnormalities most frequently reported in the posterior lateral and apical LV. This condition predisposes these patients to cardiac dilatation and heart failure as well as the formation of left ventricular aneurysms.[32,33] In addition, this process affects the parasympathetic cardiac nerves and all levels of the conduction system.[32,34] The sum of these

manifestations comprise the classic clinical features of chagasic cardiomyopathy, as described later.

## CLINICAL MANIFESTATIONS

As mentioned earlier, after the acute chagasic infection, most patients enter a chronic phase of an indeterminate form characterized by lifelong infection, with positive serologic tests and parasitemia but without clinical manifestations of the disease. However, 30% to 40% of patients with the initially chronic indeterminate form develop determinate forms with involvement of specific organs, including the heart, esophagus, colon, or mixed forms.

The cardiac electrical involvement in ChD is secondary to inflammatory and fibrotic changes at different levels of the electrical system and is manifested as sinus node dysfunction, bundle branch and fascicular block, and different grades of atrioventricular block.[31,32] The combination of right bundle branch block and left anterior fascicular block is one of the most prevalent ECG findings in patients with ChD.[31,32] However, left bundle branch block is also present in a minority of chagasic patients.

ChD is also associated with cardiac parasympathetic and sympathetic denervation secondary to inflammation and autoantibodies against cholinergic and adrenergic receptors.[25,32,35] Chagasic autonomic dysfunction produced by parasympathetic and sympathetic denervation can be detected in all the clinical phases of the disease, including the indeterminate form.[31,32,36,37] Parasympathetic denervation decreases vagal modulation of the sinus node causing reduced heart rate response to physiologic and pharmacologic stimuli.[31,32] Autopsy studies performed in chagasic patients without ventricular dilatation who died suddenly reported significant cardiac parasympathetic denervation.[17] In turn, sympathetic denervation detected by iodine-123 metaiodobenzylguanidine scintigraphic regional defects has been associated with the presence of sustained ventricular tachycardia (VT) in chagasic patients with preserved left ventricular ejection fraction (LVEF).[38] Detection of abnormal heart rate dynamics before the appearance of ventricular arrhythmias and the value of augmented T-wave variability as a marker of increased risk for sudden death suggest a role of cardiac dysautonomia in triggering malignant ventricular arrhythmias and secondary sudden death in ChD.[39,40] Although this hypothesis seems reasonable, there is only limited clinical evidence supporting this concept.[11,15]

Chagasic damage to the myocardium is considered a progressive process; in an adaptation of the international guidelines, it has been classified into

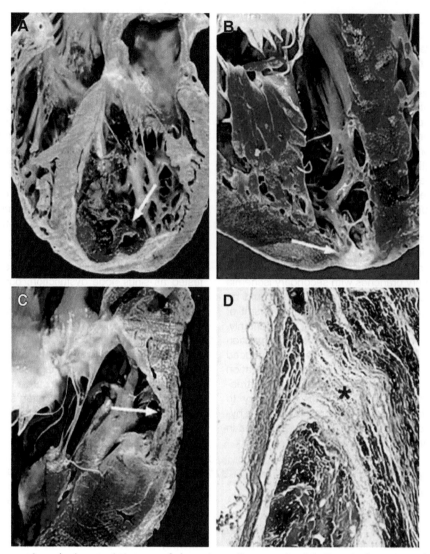

**Fig. 3.** Macroscopic and microscopic images of chagasic cardiomyopathy. (*A*) Chronic chagasic cardiomyopathy showing severe dilatation of both ventricles with thinning, fibrosis, and thrombosis of the left ventricular apex (*arrow*). (*B*) Moderately dilated and hypertrophic LV showing segmental fibrosis at the apex (*arrow*). (*C*) Fibrotic thinning of the myocardium adjacent to the mitral valve in the posterior wall of the LV (*arrow*). (*D*) Microscopic view of the bifurcation of the His bundle showing segmental fibrosis (*asterisk*) at the origin of the right bundle branch. (*From* Higuchi Mde L, Benvenuti LA, Martins Reis M, et al. Pathophysiology of the heart in Chagas' disease: current status and new developments. Cardiovasc Res 2003;60(1):96–107; with permission.)

clinical stages (**Table 1**).[11] Stage A includes those patients with the indeterminate form of the disease with positive serology but no evidence or symptoms of cardiac damage, and a normal ECG. Stage B1 refers to asymptomatic patients with appearance of ECG abnormalities (arrhythmias and conduction disorders that imply progression of the disease) and appearance of mild segmental echocardiographic contractile defects (posterior lateral and apical LV) with normal LVEF. Stage B2 includes patients with decreased LVEF who have never had signs or symptoms of heart failure.

Stages C and D include patients with decreased LVEF with prior or current symptoms of heart failure, and patients with refractory heart failure in New York Heart Association (NYHA) functional class IV, respectively. It is important to point out that sudden death can occur at any time during the evolution of the disease (even stage A or B) and can be related to ventricular arrhythmia, AV block, stroke, or refractory heart failure.[11,41]

As mentioned earlier, the myocardial damage in ChD can manifest as segmental contraction defects; LV dilatation with systolic dysfunction; and

| Table 1 | |
| --- | --- |
| **Clinical stages of chronic chagasic cardiomyopathy** | |
| **Stage** | **Definition** |
| Stage A | No present or previous symptoms of HF, no structural heart disease (normal ECG and chest radiograph). As long as the patient remains in this form of the disease, prognosis is not compromised |
| Stage B | Presence of structural heart disease but no signs or symptoms of HF |
| Stage B1 | Presence of ECG changes (arrhythmias or conduction disorders) with or without mild echocardiographic abnormalities (abnormalities of regional contractility) but normal global ventricular function |
| Stage B2 | Global ventricular dysfunction (decreased LV ejection fraction) |
| Stage C | LV dysfunction and prior or current symptoms of HF (NYHA I–IV) |
| Stage D | Symptoms of HF at rest, refractory to maximized medical therapy (NYHA IV) requiring specialized and intensive interventions |

*Abbreviations:* HF, heart failure; NYHA, New York Heart Association.
  *Data from* Andrade JP, Marin-Neto JA, Paola AA, et al. I Latin American Guidelines for the diagnosis and treatment of Chagas' heart disease: executive summary. Arq Bras Cardiol 2011;96:434–42.

LV aneurysms whose prevalence seems to increase with disease progression, varying from 8.5% among asymptomatic patients with mild cardiac damage to 45% of patients with heart failure.[42–44] The presence of LV aneurysms is a predictor of mural thrombus and stroke[44–47] and also can be the origin of VT.[48] In patients with ChD and normal coronary angiography, the presence of segmental myocardial damage (wall motion abnormalities on echocardiography or fixed myocardial perfusion defects) has been correlated with sustained VT induction and has prognostic value independent of systolic dysfunction.[43,46,47,49,50]

The myocardial damage in ChD is not exclusive to the LV and different grades of dysfunction can be seen in the right ventricle (RV).[36,51–54] It has been reported that RV involvement typically occurs in the setting of global cardiomyopathy with severe dilatation and dysfunction of both ventricles.[51,54] Similar to other cardiomyopathies, the association of RV with LV dysfunction portends a worse prognosis in dilated ChD.[52,54] There is some evidence that early RV involvement may occur in the absence of LV dysfunction. RV involvement has been observed in patients with the indeterminate form of the disease and no evidence of LV dysfunction.[53] There are also experimental and autopsy studies showing predominant RV dilatation in patients with overt ChD.[54] At the International Arrhythmia Center at the CardioInfantil Foundation (Bogota, Colombia), some patients with chagasic cardiomyopathy who underwent endoepicardial VT ablation guided by 3D mapping have shown larger scars in the RV than in the LV. In some of these cases the scar was completely confined to the RV (undetected by echocardiography) with normal LV voltage map and normal LVEF reported by echocardiography (Juan D. Ramírez, MD, unpublished data presented at the LATAM EP LIVE (Latin American Electrophysiology Live) meeting at July 2014, Bogota, Colombia). This finding suggests that, in some patients, RV involvement may precede LV involvement, which would present a significant challenge when attempting to stratify the risk of ventricular arrhythmias and sudden death in this population with normal or mildly impaired LVEF because significant RV scar may be undetected on echocardiography. In this regard, scar quantification by cardiac MRI may be the most valuable tool for defining arrhythmic risk in patients without LV dysfunction.

The involvement of the cardiac electrical system, the autonomic nervous system, and the myocardium in chagasic cardiomyopathy may present clinically as palpitations, dyspnea, chest pain, heart failure, thromboembolic events, syncope, and/or sudden death. In addition, the presence of the characteristic ECG changes mentioned earlier, atrial and ventricular arrhythmias, segmental contraction defects, LV aneurysms, and LV/RV dilatation and dysfunction constitute the clinical characteristics of chagasic cardiomyopathy (**Fig. 4**, **Table 2**). Moreover, the presence of any of these signs and symptoms with no evidence of another cardiac disorder to which the findings can be attributed, history of residence in an endemic area, and unequivocally positive serologic test for *T cruzi* confirm the diagnosis of ChD.[55]

## DIFFERENTIAL DIAGNOSIS

The previously described signs and symptoms are characteristics of ChD but are not pathognomonic of this disease. Chest pain, segmental perfusion

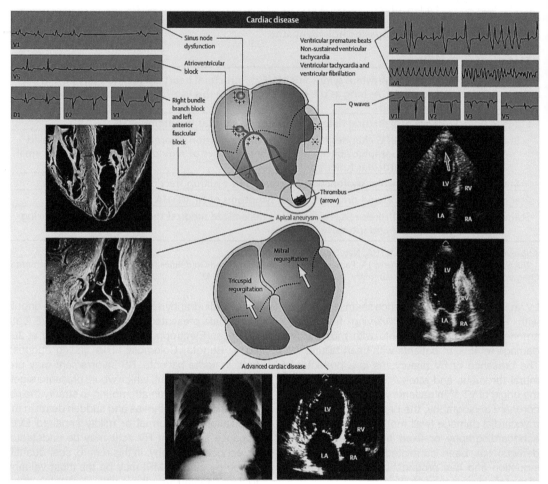

**Fig. 4.** Clinical characteristics of chagasic cardiomyopathy. LA, left atrium; RA, right atrium. (*From* Rassi A Jr, Rassi A, Marin-Neto JA. Chagas disease. Lancet 2010;375(9723):1388–402; with permission; and *Reproduced from* Rassi A, Rassi A Jr, Rassi SG, et al. Doença de Chagas. In: Lopes AC, editor. Tratado de clínica médica. 2nd edition. São Paulo (Brazil): Editora Roca; 2009. p. 4123–34; copyright 2009 Editora Roca.)

and contractile defects, and apical aneurysm can be seen in ischemic heart disease. Similarly, right bundle branch block, RV dilatation, and ventricular arrhythmias are part of the clinical presentation in RV dysplasia. Furthermore, most signs and symptoms present in ChD are also observed in patients with idiopathic dilated cardiomyopathy and explain why differentiation between the two can be challenging. The differential diagnosis between ChD and other cardiomyopathies is relevant because the worse prognosis seen in ChD may justify a more aggressive treatment approach. The differentiation is mainly based on residence in an endemic area and serologic confirmation for *T cruzi* (**Table 3**). Use of at least 2 serologic tests of different types (enzyme-linked immunosorbent assay, indirect immunofluorescence, or indirect hemagglutination) to confirm the existence of anti–*T cruzi* antibodies is required for serologic confirmation or exclusion of *T cruzi* infection.[11]

## IMAGING

The most useful initial imaging modality in suspected or confirmed ChD is echocardiography because of the wealth of data it can provide as well as the low cost and wide availability of the test. Abnormalities of structure and function on echocardiography may be observed in both symptomatic and asymptomatic patients with ChD. Early evidence of cardiac involvement may manifest as 1 or more areas of abnormal wall motion with preserved global systolic function. More severe forms of the disease are typically characterized by global dysfunction with or without the presence of ventricular aneurysms (see **Fig. 4**). Left ventricular apical aneurysm has been reported to occur in approximately half of patients with moderate to severe cardiac impairment but also may be present in up to 9% of asymptomatic patients.[56] Regional wall motion abnormalities may occur anywhere,

**Table 2**
Features of chagasic cardiomyopathy by stage

| | Cardiac Symptoms | NYHA Class | ECG Changes | Cardiomegaly on CXR | Echocardiogram | | Thromboembolism | Sustained VT | Sudden Death |
| --- | --- | --- | --- | --- | --- | --- | --- | --- | --- |
| | | | | | LV WMA | LV Apical Aneurysm | | | |
| Indeterminate | Absent | — | Absent | Absent | Absent | Absent | Absent | Absent | Absent |
| Digestive | Absent | — | Absent | Absent | Rare | Very rare | Absent | Absent | Absent |
| Cardiac | — | — | — | — | — | — | — | — | — |
| Stage I | Absent or minimal | — | Nonspecific | Absent | Rare | Very rare | Very rare | Rare | Rare |
| Stage II | Fairly common | I or II | RBBB ± LAFB, monomorphic PVCs, diffuse ST-T changes, first-degree or second-degree AVB | Absent or mild | Absent or segmental | Common | Fairly common | Common | Common |
| Stage III | Common | I, II, or III | As for stage II plus Q waves, polymorphic PVCs, high-degree AVB, severe bradycardia, low QRS voltage | Mild to moderate | Segmental or diffuse (mild to moderate) | Common | Fairly common | Common | Common |
| Stage IV | Common | II, III, or IV | As for stage III plus atrial flutter or fibrillation | Moderate to severe | Diffuse (severe) | Fairly common | Common | Fairly common | Fairly Common |

Dashes (—) indicate that data are not applicable.
*Abbreviations:* AVB, AV block; CXR, chest radiograph; LAFB, left anterior fascicular block; PVC, premature ventricular contraction; RBBB, right bundle branch block; WMA, wall motion abnormalities.
*Adapted from* Rassi A Jr, Rassi A, Marin-Neto JA. Chagas disease. Lancet 2010;375(9723):1388–402.

**Table 3**
**Comparison of clinical features in chagasic versus idiopathic cardiomyopathy**

| | Chagasic Cardiomyopathy | Idiopathic Cardiomyopathy |
|---|---|---|
| *T cruzi* serology | Positive | Negative |
| Demographic data | Male > female; age at diagnosis 30–50 y | 2.5-fold increased risk in black and male subjects, age at diagnosis 20–50 y |
| Epidemiology | Resident of rural endemic area in Latin America | Familial disease, alcohol consumption, recent viral illness |
| Clinical manifestation | Palpitations, syncope, chest pain, thromboembolic events, biventricular heart failure, predominantly right-sided failure in advanced disease | Left-sided heart failure predominates with progressive DOE. Palpitations and peripheral edema are less common. Thromboembolic events typically seen in advanced disease |
| ECG | RBBB, ± LAFB, PVCs, ST-T changes, abnormal Q waves, AV block, sick sinus syndrome, low-voltage QRS | Nonspecific repolarization abnormalities initially. Conduction abnormalities seen in 80% of cases (first-degree AVB, LBBB, and NSIVCD). RBBB is uncommon |
| Holter/exercise testing | Complex and frequent PVCs (usually asymptomatic); spontaneous or exercise-induced VT; bradyarrhythmias (AV block and sick sinus syndrome) | Ventricular arrhythmias are common but syncope and SCD are rarely the initial manifestation; bradyarrhythmias less frequent than in Chagas |
| Echocardiography | Apical LV aneurysm, mural thrombus, segmental LV WMA with akinesis or hypokinesis of inferolateral wall with preserved anteroseptal contraction, diastolic dysfunction in early stages, and RV involvement | LV dilatation with global hypokinesis, significant variability in extent of segmental WMA, mural thrombi frequently present in LV and in atria |
| Myocardial scintigraphy | Perfusion defects without obstructive coronary artery disease | Reversible and fixed perfusion abnormalities |
| Involvement of digestive system | Megaesophagus and/or megacolon | Absent |
| Outcome | High frequency of sudden unexpected death and poor prognosis compared with non-Chagas cardiomyopathy | Outcomes have improved with current treatment of heart failure |

*Abbreviations:* DOE, dyspnea on exertion; LBBB, left bundle branch block; NSIVCD, nonspecific interventricular conduction delay.

*Adapted from* Nunes MC, Dones W, Morillo CA, et al, Council on Chagas Disease of the Interamerican Society of Cardiology. Chagas disease: an overview of clinical and epidemiological aspects. J Am Coll Cardiol 2013;62(9):767–76.

but are frequently seen in the inferolateral wall, which is the most common source of macroreentrant VT.

Cardiac magnetic resonance (CMR), although more expensive and less readily available, provides significant advantages compared with echocardiography. CMR has the ability to identify the presence and extent of myocardial fibrosis detected by late gadolinium enhancement (**Fig. 5**), which correlates well with prognosis. In a series of 51 patients with ChD, myocardial fibrosis on CMR was present in 20% of patients without clinical cardiac involvement, 85% of those with clinical cardiac involvement, and 100% of those with VT. Furthermore, the extent of fibrosis increased across the

3 groups (0.9%, 16%, and 25% of LV mass, respectively).[57] In addition, CMR is well suited for precise evaluation of chamber dimensions, contractility, and tissue characterization. These qualities may make it the best approach to detect early right ventricular dysfunction.

## CHAGASIC VENTRICULAR ARRHYTHMIAS

Ventricular arrhythmias are common in ChD and may present as atypical chest pain, dyspnea, palpitations, syncope, or SCD. The prevalence and severity of chagasic ventricular arrhythmias correlates with the severity of the cardiomyopathy but can occur in patients with preserved LVEF.[58]

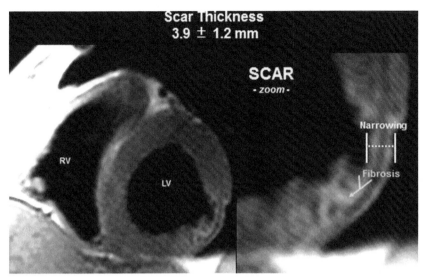

**Fig. 5.** CMR image showing an area of scar in the inferolateral left ventricular wall with associated narrowing and fibrosis.

Frequent monomorphic or polymorphic premature ventricular contractions (PVCs), couplets, and salvos of nonsustained VT (NSVT) are common on Holter monitoring in ChD.[59] NSVT is of higher prevalence compared with other cardiomyopathies and is present in 40% of chagasic patients with mild wall motion abnormalities and in 90% of those with heart failure.[60] Sustained VT is present in 2% of chagasic patients[58] and implies progression of cardiomyopathy when evident at early stages of the disease. Sustained VT is considered a hallmark of ChD, the main cause of SCD, and the most frequently observed life-threatening ventricular arrhythmia in chagasic patients with ICDs.[4]

## SUDDEN CARDIAC DEATH IN CHAGAS DISEASE

SCD is most common cause of death in ChD (55%–65%), followed by congestive heart failure in 25% to 30% and cerebral or pulmonary embolism in 10% to 15%.[61] The prevalence of SCD in chagasic populations varies from 29% to 37% in nonendemic and endemic regions, respectively.[62] Most SCD cases are in patients with manifest chagasic cardiomyopathy and mainly between 30 and 50 years of age, being rare after the sixth decade of life.[63] However, up to 20% of patients who die suddenly do not report previous symptoms.[63] SCD in chagasic patients is primarily an arrhythmic phenomenon but can be related to thromboembolic events (massive pulmonary or cerebral embolism) or rarely rupture of an LV aneurysm.[4] Accordingly, ventricular fibrillation (VF), either de novo or preceded by sustained VT, has

been reported as the main cause of SCD.[4] In a report of ambulatory Holter recordings of 10 chagasic patients who died suddenly, VF was the final event in 9 of them and bradyarrhythmia in 1. Of the 9 patients with VF, torsades de pointes was the precursor in 6 and sustained VT in the other 3.[64]

## IDENTIFICATION OF CHAGASIC POPULATIONS AT RISK

As mentioned previously, SCD in ChD is a catastrophic event that tends to occur in young and economically productive patients. SCD mostly occurs in patients with previous manifestations of cardiomyopathy but also can occur in asymptomatic patients without evidence LV dysfunction. This wide range of presentations implies that the risk of SCD is not similar for every patient and thus identifying factors that increase risk becomes extremely important. Previously proposed variables for the prediction of SCD in ChD include ventricular dysfunction and heart failure, nonsustained and sustained ventricular arrhythmias, severe bradyarrhythmias (sinus node dysfunction and advanced atrioventricular blocks), syncope, and previous cardiac arrest. The combined use of these predictors in this setting is difficult because most of the prediction models available in ChD have been designed to predict rick of death from all causes and not solely from SCD.

The presence of NSVT on Holter monitoring has a role in the identification of chagasic patients at risk for death. However, the highest value of NSVT as a predictor of mortality is in combination with LV dysfunction. Rassi and colleagues[65] developed and validated a risk score for predicting death in ChD based on a retrospective evaluation of 424 outpatients from a regional cohort who underwent routine noninvasive tests and were followed for a mean of 7.9 years. By using multivariable Cox proportional-hazard analysis, Rassi and colleagues[65] identified 6 independent prognostic factors: NYHA class III or IV (5 points), cardiomegaly on chest radiography (5 points), segmental or global wall motion abnormality on echocardiogram (3 points), NSVT on Holter monitoring (3 points), low QRS voltage (2 points), and male sex (2 points). Note that in this study NSVT on Holter monitoring was associated with an incremental increased mortality risk of 2.15-fold that increased to 15-fold when NSVT was combined with LV dysfunction. This score classifies chagasic patients into 3 groups: low (0–6 points), intermediate (7–11 points), and high risk (12–20 points), with 10-year mortalities of 10%, 44%, and 84%, respectively. The overall mortality was 3.9% per year, and the rate of sudden death was 2.4% per year. All of the variables included in this risk score were also strong predictors for increased risk of cardiovascular death and SCD, except for male sex and low QRS voltage, which had borderline value for predicting cardiovascular death and SCD, respectively. Conveniently, the score is based on noninvasive clinical variables that are easy to use and inexpensive. In addition, this score identifies chagasic patients with increased risk who could potentially benefit from a more aggressive therapeutic approach.

Spontaneous sustained VT has traditionally been associated with increased risk for SCD in ChD. At 8-year follow-up in chagasic patients with sustained VT, mortality has been reported at 93% with more than 70% of the deaths occurring in the first 2 years and 90% of the deaths occurring suddenly.[66] The value of sustained VT as a predictor of increased risk for SCD is also supported by results from analyses of the significance of sustained VT induced by programmed ventricular stimulation (PVS) during electrophysiologic study in patients with ChD. These studies have consistently shown that, in chagasic patients with spontaneous NSVT documented on Holter or syncope of unknown origin, the induction of sustained monomorphic VT by PVS is associated with a higher incidence of recurrent sustained VT, reappearance of syncope, and increased risk of death, driven mostly by SCD. As seen in other forms of cardiomyopathy, induction of polymorphic VT or VF by PVS has no prognostic significance in ChD.[67–69]

## INFORMATION DERIVED FROM SECONDARY PREVENTION IMPLANTABLE CARDIOVERTER-DEFIBRILLATOR OBSERVATIONAL STUDIES IN CHAGAS DISEASE

Cardinalli-Neto and colleagues[70] reported on 90 consecutive chagasic patients with aborted SCD or hemodynamically unstable VT who underwent ICD implantation. All patients were on amiodarone before the index event, and after device implantation they were followed for a mean of 25 months. The mean age was 59 ± 11 years at implantation and the mean LVEF was 47% ± 13%. Note that 28% of those included had no LV dysfunction. This study represents the largest observational series of patients with ChD at high risk for SCD (aborted SCD or hemodynamically unstable VT). Despite the high-risk nature of these patients, the LVEF was higher than that seen in historical secondary prevention ICD studies in other cardiomyopathies (34% ± 15% and 33% ± 14% for ICD and amiodarone groups, respectively, in a meta-analysis of ICD secondary prevention trials).[71] Moreover, a substantial number of the included patients had no LV dysfunction, further emphasizing the wide spectrum of clinical SCD risk in ChD. Those patients with normal LVEF who presented with SCD could not have been identified as being at increased arrhythmic risk by using LV function assessment alone. This finding is extremely important because it stresses the difference in arrhythmic risk for patients with ChD compared with ischemic and idiopathic dilated cardiomyopathy. Hypothetically, these limitations could be related to the complex interactions between the mechanisms triggering SCD, including chagasic dysautonomia, which can occur in the earliest stages of the disease even in the setting of preserved LVEF. In addition, the inflammatory and fibrotic process present in ChD affects both the LV and the RV. As described previously, patients with ICDs as secondary prevention have been seen who underwent endoepicardial bipolar voltage mapping and catheter ablation for frequent and appropriated ICD therapies in whom scar tissue was confined to the RV with preserved LVEF by echocardiography. The involvement of the RV can be difficult or impossible to identify by echocardiography, especially in early stages of ChD when significant symptoms and abnormalities in LVEF are not present.

In study by Cardinalli-Neto and colleagues,[70] despite amiodarone use in all patients and β-blocker use in 40%, life-threatening ventricular arrhythmias were detected in 64 of 90 patients (71%). Sustained VT was observed in 45 of 64 patients (70%) and VF not preceded by sustained

VT in 19 (30%) patients. The median number of ICD shocks per patient was 4.5. The investigators also reported that 31 of the 90 included patients (34%) died during follow-up. The total mortalities were also high (18% at 1 year, 27% at 2 years, 40% at 3 years, 50% at 4 years, and 73% at 5 years of follow-up) compared with historical secondary prevention ICD studies in other cardiomyopathies.[71] The calculated annual mortality was 16.6% and a cardiac origin for all of the reported deaths was also reported. The only independent predictor of increased risk for mortality was the number of ICD shocks per patient at 30 days.

In another secondary prevention ICD trial in ChD, Martinelli and colleagues[72] included 116 chagasic patients with aborted SCD (18%) or symptomatic sustained VT (82%), most of whom were taking amiodarone. The mean age and mean LVEF were 54 ± 10.7 years and 42% ± 16%, respectively. After a follow-up of 45 ± 32 months the study showed that 50% of the included patients experienced appropriate shocks, and the annual mortality was 7.1%. NYHA class III and LVEF were independent predictors of death. This study showed a lower annual mortality compared with the study published by Cardinalli-Neto and colleagues,[70] which is possibly attributable to more complete heart failure treatment and a higher rate of ablation procedures performed before and after ICD implantation to treat recurrent VT in the Martinelli and colleagues[72] study.

## INDICATIONS FOR IMPLANTABLE CARDIOVERTER-DEFIBRILLATOR IMPLANTATION IN CHAGAS DISEASE

As previously described, the available information about the results of ICD therapy in ChD consists of some observational studies following chagasic patients who underwent device implantation for secondary prevention and some registries comparing the results of ICD implantation in ChD versus patients without ChD. The available studies suggest that, in comparisons with historical cohorts and registries, patients with ChD implanted with an ICD for secondary prevention tend to have higher LVEF (even preserved in a substantial proportion of patients), higher burden of life-threatening ventricular arrhythmia, higher incidence of appropriate ICD therapies, lower survival free from device therapy or death, and higher all-cause mortalities.[71,72]

ICD therapy for secondary prevention has been associated with a significant reduction in the risk for SCD in ChD. However, the impact of ICD implantation on all-cause mortality in secondary prevention chagasic patients has shown contradictory results. As mentioned earlier, some studies have shown very high mortality in chagasic patients who underwent ICD implantation even though a significant portion of them had preserved LVEF and functional class. Pump failure has been reported as the main cause of death and the number of device shocks was the strongest predictor of all-cause death. The conflicting results of ICD therapy in this subset of chagasic patients has been for the subject of much debate and some investigators have proposed the urgent need for a randomized clinical trial comparing ICD therapy with amiodarone to elucidate the impact of device therapy for secondary prevention in patients with ChD.[73] This proposal has been questioned secondary to possible ethical issues. In addition, the positive results of ICD therapy in ischemic cardiomyopathy have been extended to other forms of cardiomyopathy, as proved in historical studies, which is an argument against starting secondary prevention trials in ChD.[72] Most groups working with ChD are extrapolating the secondary prevention ICD indications proposed by international guidelines to chagasic patients as reflected by the recommendations proposed by the I Latin American guidelines for the diagnosis and treatment of Chagas Heart Disease.[11]

The guidelines for diagnosis and treatment of ChD do not define recommendations about ICD implantation for primary prevention, reflecting the lack of clinical trials and observational studies in this area. Assuming that the benefits of ICD implantation have been proved independent of the type of cardiomyopathy, some groups have extrapolated the recommendation of primary prevention ICD implantation to chagasic cardiomyopathy. However, the cost-effectiveness of this approach is not known. The initiation of a randomized controlled trial in the subset of primary prevention patients with ChD is needed to clarify the role of ICD therapy in this specific population.

## PHARMACOLOGIC TREATMENT

Similar to ICD therapy, the evidence supporting the use of antiarrhythmic drugs to prevent SCD in ChD is scarce. The current guidelines in ChD establish that antiarrhythmic treatment is not required in asymptomatic chagasic patients with frequent isolated or repetitive PVCs when the LVEF is preserved. In patients with ChD with LV dysfunction and frequent PVCs/nonsustained VT, the guidelines recommend amiodarone as the only safe drug available. However, there are no clinical trials supporting a role for amiodarone to reduce the risk for SCD and total mortality in this context. Moreover, the use of amiodarone for the prevention of SCD in dilated cardiomyopathy has shown only a modest reduction in the risk of SCD, with no reduction in all-cause mortality and increased risk for pulmonary and thyroid side effects.[74] Amiodarone has also been used empirically to prevent the recurrence of sustained VT in patients with ChD. Scanavacca and colleagues[75] reported the results of amiodarone used in 35 chagasic patients with sustained VT and a mean LVEF of 56% ± 14%. After 27 ± 20 months of follow-up, the probability of suppressing sustained VT was 0.62 at 12 months, 0.56 at 24 months, and 0.44 at 36 months. Overall, survival probability was 96%, 89%, and 72% at 1-year, 2-year, and 3-year follow-up, respectively. Probability of freedom from SCD was 100%, 96%, and 89% at 1-year, 2-year, and 3-year follow-up, respectively. Importantly, all patients in functional class III or IV and with LVEF less than 30% had recurrence of sustained VT. Only 30% of patients in NYHA functional class I and II had recurrent VT (P<.05). Fifteen (43%) patients reported side effects. Thus, amiodarone seems to have limited efficacy to prevent sustained VT recurrence in patients with ChD, especially in patients with LV dysfunction and significantly reduced functional class.

As mentioned previously, parasite persistence likely contributes to the pathogenesis of chagasic cardiomyopathy, which suggests that trypanocidal therapy may have a positive impact on the clinical course of patients with ChD. However, the currently available experimental and clinical evidence is insufficient to support the routine use of treatment in these patients. The BENEFIT (Benznidazole Evaluation for Interrupting Trypanosomiasis) trial is an international, multicenter, double-blind, placebo-controlled trial designed to test whether antitrypanosomal therapy with benznidazole reduces mortality and other major cardiovascular clinical outcomes in patients with chronic Chagas heart disease.[76] Results of this trial are pending.

## CATHETER ABLATION OF SUSTAINED VENTRICULAR TACHYCARDIA IN CHAGASIC CARDIOMYOPATHY

The most common mechanism of sustained VT in chagasic cardiomyopathy is scar-related reentry. Scar is found in the inferolateral LV in more than 70% of these patients.[31] The reentrant circuit responsible for scar-related VT in these patients may be subendocardial, subepicardial, or intramyocardial. Occasionally, these circuits exist in

areas of the heart with thin walls and radiofrequency ablation may result in transmural injury effectively treating all portions of the myocardium involved in the arrhythmia circuit. However, scar commonly exists intramyocardially and/or subepicardially in an area with an associated thick layer of subendocardial myocardium. In these instances, endocardial radiofrequency ablation may not effectively treat all of the involved myocardium. For this reason, the transthoracic subxiphoid percutaneous approach may be necessary to explore the pericardial space in these patients.[77]

### Epicardial Ablation of Sustained Ventricular Tachycardia in Chagas Heart Disease

Transthoracic epicardial access for mapping and ablation of sustained VT in patients with chagasic cardiomyopathy was initially described in 1996.[78] Expert consensus documents report that epicardial access is necessary in greater than or equal to 20% of patients undergoing VT ablation in tertiary centers, and particularly in patients with nonischemic cardiomyopathies.[79,80]

Entering the pericardial space involves use of the Tuohy needle, which is curved at one end, making it ideal for penetrating pericardial membranes. The risk of pericardial bleeding is approximately 10% with this technique, although most of these bleeds are minor and transient. Severe bleeding requiring surgical repair occurs in only 1% to 2% of patients. Pericardial adhesions are frequently seen in patients with a history of prior ablation.[81] The electrograms obtained during epicardial mapping are similar to those seen during endocardial mapping both in patients with chagasic cardiomyopathy and in those with other forms of cardiomyopathy. Delayed potentials, mid-diastolic potentials, and continuous electrical activity are frequently seen in the area of interest. The critical isthmus of the reentrant circuit may be confirmed by entrainment maneuvers or interruption of VT with radiofrequency ablation during epicardial procedures, similar to techniques used with an endocardial approach. Previous reports have described a higher prevalence of epicardial VT in patients with chagasic cardiomyopathy (37%) compared with patients with ischemic or idiopathic dilated cardiomyopathy (28% and 24%, respectively).[82] The epicardial surface presents 3 major anatomic challenges that may affect the efficiency and safety of ablation: epicardial coronary arteries, thick epicardial fat, and potential injury to surrounding structures (phrenic nerve).[83] Because of these limitations as well as evolution of the disease, clinical recurrences are common even after endocardial and epicardial ablation.

Use of an irrigated-tip catheter may provide deeper injury, even in the presence of fat, resulting in more effective ablation. However, this may increase the risk of damage to the coronary arteries or extracardiac structures.[84,85] To understand the utility and risks of epicardial access for the ablation of sustained VT in chagasic cardiomyopathy, prospective randomized studies are needed. There is a subset of patient for whom catheter ablation can be useful: patients with recurrent ICD shocks despite antiarrhythmic therapy. In these patients, clinical outcomes are favorable at short-term and medium-term follow-up.[86]

## SURGERY

The use of surgical resection (aneurysmectomy) for the treatment of recurrent ventricular arrhythmias in ChD has been described.[87–89] In one report, electrophysiologic mapping was performed of the area adjacent to the aneurysm to identify abnormal potentials. These areas were excised along with the aneurysm. Pathologic examination revealed a chronic inflammatory reaction, myocytolysis, and fibrosis. In addition, interlaced fronts of healthy (normally conducting) and damaged (slowly conducting) myocytes were observed, resulting in an ideal configuration for reentry.[87] These case reports have noted positive results. However, the risks and benefits of this procedure remain poorly defined. The attendant morbidity and mortality of the procedure make its widespread use less desirable compared with catheter ablation.

## SUMMARY

ChD and chagasic cardiomyopathy represent an important and often underappreciated cause of heart failure and ventricular arrhythmias. Residence, even if remote, in an endemic area should prompt diagnostic evaluation for ChD in patients who present with appropriate signs or symptoms. The exact pathophysiologic processes at work that lead to ventricular remodeling and arrhythmias in ChD remain poorly defined and poorly understood. What is known is that the burden of ventricular arrhythmias is high in chagasic cardiomyopathy and may precede left ventricular dysfunction and signs of heart failure. Risk stratification for ventricular arrhythmias is also incompletely understood. LVEF is useful, but may not be as predictive in ChD as in other forms of cardiomyopathy. Ultimately, scar burden (as defined by MRI or other imaging modalities) may be a more useful way to assess arrhythmic risk. The use of ICDs and amiodarone has been studied but

remains to be understood with respect to the patients who will benefit most from these therapies. Catheter ablation has proved to be a useful tool in patients with ChD with recurrent ventricular arrhythmias, but epicardial access (a more challenging technique not used by all electrophysiologists) is required in a significant proportion of patients if optimal clinical results are to be achieved. If progress is to be made in the understanding and treatment of chagasic cardiomyopathy, large international registries and randomized clinical trials are required.

## REFERENCES

1. Botoni FA, Ribeiro AL, Marinho CC, et al. Treatment of Chagas cardiomyopathy. Biomed Res Int 2013; 2013:849504.
2. World Health Organization. First WHO report on neglected tropical diseases: working to overcome the global impact of neglected tropical diseases. Geneva (Switzerland): World Health Organization; 2010. p. 1–172.
3. World Health Organization. Chagas disease: control and elimination. World Health Organization. World Health Assembly report. Geneva (Switzerland): World Health Organization; 2010. p. 1–4.
4. Bestetti RB, Cardinalli-Neto A. Sudden cardiac death in Chagas' heart disease in the contemporary era. Int J Cardiol 2008;131:9–17.
5. Rassi A Jr, Rassi A, Rassi SG. Predictors of mortality in chronic Chagas disease: a systematic review of observational studies. Circulation 2007;115:1101–8.
6. Rassi A Jr, Rassi A, Little WC, et al. Development and validation of a risk score for predicting death in Chagas' heart disease. N Engl J Med 2006;355:799–808.
7. Rosa RF, Neto AS, Franken RA. Chagas' disease and the use of implantable cardioverter-defibrillators in Brazil. Am J Geriatr Cardiol 2006; 15(6):372–6.
8. Bern C, Montgomery SP. An estimate of the burden of Chagas disease in the United States. Clin Infect Dis 2009;49:e52–4.
9. Pereira Nunes MC, Dones W, Morillo C, et al. Chagas disease: an overview of clinical and epidemiological aspects. J Am Coll Cardiol 2013;62:767–76.
10. Lee BY, Bacon KM, Bottazzi ME, et al. Global economic burden of Chagas disease: a computational simulation model. Lancet Infect Dis 2013;13:342–8.
11. Andrade JP, Marin Neto JA, Paola AA, et al. I Latin American guidelines for the diagnosis and treatment of Chagas' heart disease: executive summary. Arq Bras Cardiol 2011;96:434–42.
12. Ribeiro AL, Rocha MO. Indeterminate form of Chagas disease: considerations about diagnosis and prognosis. Rev Soc Bras Med Trop 1998;31:301–14.

13. Pinto Dias JC. Natural history of Chagas disease. Arq Bras Cardiol 1995;65:359–66.

14. Rassi A Jr, Rassi A, Little WC. Chagas' heart disease. Clin Cardiol 2000;23:883–9.

15. Marin-Neto JA, Cunha-Neto E, Maciel BC, et al. Pathogenesis of chronic Chagas heart disease. Circulation 2007;115:1109–23.

16. Sterin-Borda E, Sterin Borda L. Antiadrenergic and muscarinic receptor antibodies in Chagas' cardiomyopathy. Int J Cardiol 1996;54:149–56.

17. Lopes ER, Tafuri WL. Involvement of the autonomic nervous system in Chagas' heart disease. Rev Soc Bras Med Trop 1983;16:206–11.

18. Andrade ZA, Andrade SG, Sadigursky M, et al. The indeterminate phase of Chagas disease: ultrastructural characterization of cardiac changes in the canine model. Am J Trop Med Hyg 1997;57(3):328–36.

19. Cunha-Neto E, Bilate AM, Hyland KV, et al. Induction of cardiac autoimmunity in Chagas heart disease: a case for molecular mimicry. Autoimmunity 2006;39: 41–54.

20. Cunha-Neto E, Iwai LK, Bilate AM, et al. Autoimmunity in Chagas' disease. In: Shoenfeld Y, Rose NR, editors. Infection and autoimmunity. Amsterdam (The Netherlands): Elsevier; 2004. p. 449–72.

21. Cunha-Neto E, Duranti M, Gruber A, et al. Autoimmunity in Chagas disease cardiopathy: biological relevance of a cardiac myosin-specific epitope crossreactive to an immunodominant *Trypanosoma cruzi* antigen. Proc Natl Acad Sci U S A 1995;92: 3541–5.

22. Franco MF. Experimental carditis induced by *Trypanosoma cruzi* (y strain) in guinea pigs: correlation between histopathology and the presence of *T cruzi* antigens identified by indirect immunofluorescence. Rev Soc Bras Med Trop 1990;23: 187–9.

23. Higuchi ML, Brito T, Reis MM, et al. Correlation between *T cruzi* parasitism and myocardial inflammation in human chronic chagasic myocarditis: light microscopy and immunohistochemical findings. Cardiovasc Pathol 1993;2:101–6.

24. Jones EM, Colley DG, Tostes S, et al. Amplification of *Trypanosoma cruzi* DNA sequence from inflammatory lesions in human chagasic cardiomyopathy. Am J Trop Med Hyg 1993;48:348–57.

25. Bellotti G, Bocchi E, de Moraes AV, et al. In vivo detection of *T cruzi* antigens in hearts of patients with chronic Chagas' heart disease. Am Heart J 1996;131:301–7.

26. Garcia S, Ramos CO, Senra JF, et al. Treatment with benznidazole during the chronic phase of experimental Chagas' disease decreases cardiac alterations. Antimicrob Agents Chemother 2005;49: 1521–8.

27. Silva JS, Rossi MA. Intensification of acute *Trypanosoma cruzi* myocarditis in BALB/c mice pretreated with low doses of cyclophosphamide or gamma irradiation. J Exp Pathol 1990;71:33–9.

28. Harms G, Feldmeier H. The impact of HIV infection on tropical diseases. Infect Dis Clin North Am 2005;19:121–35.

29. Higuchi ML, Fukasawa S, De Brito T, et al. Different microcirculatory and interstitial matrix patterns in idiopathic dilated cardiomyopathy and Chagas' disease: a three dimensional confocal microscopy study. Heart 1999;82(3):279–85.

30. Sambiase NV, Higuchi ML, Benvenuti LA. Narrowed lumen of the right coronary artery in chronic chagasic patients is associated with ischemic lesions of segmental thinnings of ventricles. Invest Clin 2010; 51(4):531–9.

31. Sarabanda AV, Sosa E, Simões MV, et al. Ventricular tachycardia in Chagas' disease: a comparison of clinical, angiographic, electrophysiologic and myocardial perfusion disturbances between patients presenting with either sustained or nonsustained forms. Int J Cardiol 2005;102(1):9–19.

32. Higuchi ML, Benvenuti LA, Martins Reis M, et al. Pathophysiology of the heart in Chagas' disease: current status and new developments. Cardiovasc Res 2003 15;60(1):96–107.

33. Regueiro A, García-Álvarez A, Sitges M, et al. Myocardial involvement in Chagas disease: insights from cardiac magnetic resonance. Int J Cardiol 2013;165(1):107–12.

34. Amorim DS, Marin-Neto JA. Functional alterations of the autonomic nervous system in Chagas' heart disease. Sao Paulo Med J 1995;113:772–84.

35. De Oliveira SF, Pedrosa RC, Nascimento JH, et al. Sera from chronic chagasic patients with complex cardiac arrhythmias depress electrogenesis and conduction in isolated rabbit hearts. Circulation 1996;96:2031–7.

36. Marin-Neto JA, Bromberg-Marin G, Pazin-Filho A, et al. Cardiac autonomic impairment and early myocardial damage involving the right ventricle are independent phenomena in Chagas' disease. Int J Cardiol 1998;65:261–9.

37. Ribeiro AL, Moraes RS, Ribeiro JP, et al. Parasympathetic dysautonomia precedes left ventricular systolic dysfunction in Chagas' disease. Am Heart J 2001;141:260–5.

38. Miranda CH, Figueiredo AB, Maciel BC, et al. Sustained ventricular tachycardia is associated with regional myocardial sympathetic denervation assessed with 123I-metaiodobenzylguanidine in chronic Chagas cardiomyopathy. J Nucl Med 2011;52:504–10.

39. Diaz JO, Makikallio TH, Huikuri HV, et al. Heart rate dynamics before the spontaneous onset of ventricular tachyarrhythmias in Chagas' heart disease. Am J Cardiol 2001;87:1123–5. A10.

40. Ribeiro AL, Rocha MO, Terranova P, et al. T-wave amplitude variability and the risk of death in

Chagas disease. J Cardiovasc Electrophysiol 2011;22:799–805.

41. Rassi A Jr, Rassi SG, Rassi AG, et al. Sudden death in Chagas disease. Arq Bras Cardiol 2001;76:75–96.

42. Rassi A Jr, Rassi A, Marin-Neto JA. Chagas disease. Lancet 2010;375(9723):1388–402.

43. Viotti RJ, Vigliano C, Laucella S, et al. Value of echocardiography for diagnosis and prognosis of chronic Chagas disease cardiomyopathy without heart failure. Heart 2004;90:655–60.

44. Nunes Mdo C, Barbosa MM, Rocha MO. Peculiar aspects of cardiogenic embolism in patients with Chagas' cardiomyopathy: a transthoracic and transesophageal echocardiographic study. J Am Soc Echocardiogr 2005;18:761–7.

45. Nunes MC, Barbosa MM, Ribeiro AL, et al. Ischemic cerebrovascular events in patients with Chagas cardiomyopathy: a prospective follow-up study. J Neurol Sci 2009;278:96–101.

46. Bestetti RB, Dalbo CM, Arruda CA, et al. Predictors of sudden cardiac death for patients with Chagas' disease: a hospital-derived cohort study. Cardiology 1996;87:481–7.

47. Pazin-Filho A, Romano MM, Almeida-Filho OC, et al. Minor segmental wall motion abnormalities detected in patients with Chagas' disease have adverse prognostic implications. Braz J Med Biol Res 2006;39:483–7.

48. Barros ML, Ribeiro A, Nunes Mdo C, et al. Association between left ventricular wall motion abnormalities and ventricular arrhythmia in the indeterminate form of Chagas disease. Rev Soc Bras Med Trop 2011;44:213–6.

49. Marin-Neto JA, Simões MV, Sarabanda AV. Chagas heart disease. Arq Bras Cardiol 1999;72:247–80.

50. Marin-Neto JA, Rassi A Jr, Maciel BC, et al. Chagas heart disease. In: Yusuf S, Cairns JA, Camm AJ, et al, editors. Evidence based cardiology. 3rd edition. London: BMJ Books; 2010. p. 823–41.

51. Nunes Mdo C, Barbosa Mde M, Brum VA, et al. Morphofunctional characteristics of the right ventricle in Chagas' dilated cardiomyopathy. Int J Cardiol 2004;94(1):79–85.

52. Nunes Mdo C, Rocha MO, Ribeiro AL, et al. Right ventricular dysfunction is an independent predictor of survival in patients with dilated chronic Chagas' cardiomyopathy. Int J Cardiol 2008;127(3):372–9.

53. Marin-Neto JA, Marzullo P, Sousa AC, et al. Radionuclide angiographic evidence for early predominant right ventricular. Can J Cardiol 1988;4:231–6.

54. Kumar R, Kline L, Abelman W. Experimental Trypanosoma cruzi myocarditis. Relative effects upon the right and left ventricles. Am J Pathol 1969;57:31–48.

55. Nunes MC, Dones W, Morillo CA, et al, Council on Chagas disease of the Interamerican Society of Cardiology. Chagas disease: an overview of clinical and epidemiological aspects. J Am Coll Cardiol 2013;62(9):767–76.

56. Acquatella H. Echocardiography in Chagas heart disease. Circulation 2007;115:1124–31.

57. Rochitte CE, Oliveira PF, Andrade JM, et al. Myocardial delayed enhancement by magnetic resonance imaging in patients with Chagas' disease: a marker of disease severity. J Am Coll Cardiol 2005;46(8):1553–8.

58. Carrasco HA, Guerrero L, Parada H, et al. Ventricular arrhythmias and left ventricular myocardial function in chronic chagasic patients. Int J Cardiol 1990;28:35–41.

59. Rassi Júnior A, Gabriel Rassi A, Gabriel Rassi S, et al. Ventricular arrhythmia in Chagas disease. Diagnostic, prognostic, and therapeutic features. Arq Bras Cardiol 1995;65:377–87 [in Portuguese].

60. Martinelli Filho M, De Siqueira SF, Moreira H, et al. Probability of occurrence of life-threatening ventricular arrhythmias in Chagas' disease versus non-Chagas' disease. Pacing Clin Electrophysiol 2000;23:1944–6.

61. Rassi A Jr, Rassi SG, Rassi AG, et al. Sudden death in Chagas' disease: review. Arq Bras Cardiol 2001;76:75–96.

62. Manzullo EC, Chuit R. Risk of death due to chronic chagasic cardiopathy. Mem Inst Oswaldo Cruz 1999;94(Suppl 1):317–20.

63. Bestetti RB, Freitas OC, Muccillo G, et al. Clinical and morphological characteristics associated with sudden cardiac death in patients with Chagas' disease. Eur Heart J 1993;14:1610–4.

64. Mendoza I, Moleiro F, Marques J. Morte súbita na doença de Chagas. Arq Bras Cardiol 1992;59:3–4.

65. Rassi A Jr, Rassi A, Little WC, et al. Development and validation of a risk score for predicting death in Chagas' heart disease. N Engl J Med 2006;355:799–808.

66. Rassi A. Curva atuarial da taquicardia ventricular sustentada na cardiopatia chagásica crônica. In: Anais do IV Simpósio Brasileiro de Arritmias Cardíacas. Recife (Brazil); 1987. p. 129.

67. Silva RM. Valor preditivo das variáveis clínicas e eletrofisiológicas nos pacientes com cardiopatia chagásica crônica e taquicardia ventricular não-sustentada? Análise terapêutica? (Tese). São Paulo (Brazil): Escola Paulista de Medicina da Universidade Federal de São Paulo; 1997. p. 147.

68. Rassi SG, Rassi A Jr, Rassi AG, et al. Avaliação da síncope e da pré-sincope na cardiopatía chagásica crônica através da estimulação elétrica programada. In: Anais do 2° Congresso da Sociedade Latino Americana de Estimulação Cardíaca. Porto Alegre (Brazil); 1989. p. 36.

69. Martinelli Filho M, Sosa E, Nishioka S, et al. Clinical and electrophysiologic features of syncope in chronic chagasic heart disease. J Cardiovasc Electrophysiol 1994;5:563–70.

70. Cardinalli-Neto A, Bestetti RB, Cordeiro JA, et al. Predictors of all-cause mortality for patients with chronic Chagas' heart disease receiving implantable cardioverter-defibrillator therapy. J Cardiovasc Electrophysiol 2007;18:1236–40.

71. Connolly SJ, Hallstrom AP, Cappato R, et al. Meta-analysis of the implantable cardioverter defibrillator secondary prevention trials. AVID, CASH and CIDS studies. Eur Heart J 2000;21:2071–8.

72. Martinelli M, Freitas de Siqueira S, Back Sternick E, et al. Long-term follow-up of implantable cardioverter-defibrillator for secondary prevention in Chagas' heart disease. Am J Cardiol 2012;110:1040–5.

73. Rassi A Jr. Implantable cardioverter-defibrillators in patients with Chagas heart disease: misperceptions, many questions and the urgent need for a randomized clinical trial. J Cardiovasc Electrophysiol 2007; 18:1241–3.

74. Piccini JP, Berger JS, O'Connor CM. Amiodarone for the prevention of sudden cardiac death: a meta-analysis of randomized controlled trials. Eur Heart J 2009;30(10):1245–53.

75. Scanavacca MI, Sosa EA, Lee JH, et al. Empiric therapy with amiodarone in patients with chronic Chagas cardiomyopathy and sustained ventricular tachycardia. Arq Bras Cardiol 1990;54:367–71 [in Portuguese].

76. Marin-Neto JA, Rassi A Jr, Avezum A Jr, et al, BENEFIT Investigators. The BENEFIT trial: testing the hypothesis that trypanocidal therapy is beneficial for patients with chronic Chagas heart disease. Mem Inst Oswaldo Cruz 2009;104(Suppl 1):319–24.

77. Scanavacca MI, de Brito FS, Maia I, et al, Sociedade Brasileira de Cardiologia. Guidelines for the evaluation and treatment of patients with cardiac arrhythmias. Arq Bras Cardiol 2002;79(Suppl 5):1–50.

78. Sosa E, Scanavacca M, d'Avila A, et al. A new technique to perform epicardial mapping in the electrophysiology laboratory. J Cardiovasc Electrophysiol 1996;7(6):531–6.

79. Natale A, Raviele A, Al-Ahmad A, et al, Venice Chart Members. Venice Chart International consensus document on ventricular tachycardia/ventricular fibrillation ablation. J Cardiovasc Electrophysiol 2010;21(3):339–79.

80. Aliot EM, Stevenson WG, Almendral-Garrote JM, et al. EHRA/HRS expert consensus on catheter ablation of ventricular arrhythmias: developed in a partnership with the European Heart Rhythm Association (EHRA), a registered branch of the European Society of Cardiology (ESC), and the Heart Rhythm Society (HRS); in collaboration with the American College of Cardiology (ACC) and the American Heart Association (AHA). Europace 2009;11:771–817.

81. Pisani CF, Lara S, Scanavacca M. Epicardial ablation for cardiac arrhythmias: techniques, indications and results. Curr Opin Cardiol 2014;29(1):59–67.

82. Scanavacca M, Sosa E. Epicardial ablation of ventricular tachycardia in Chagas heart disease. In: Shivkumar K, Boyle NG, editors. Cardiac electrophysiology clinics: epicardial interventions in electrophysiology, vol. 2. Philadelphia: Saunders; 2010. p. 55–67.

83. D'Avila A, Scanavacca M, Sosa E, et al. Pericardial anatomy for the interventional electrophysiologist. J Cardiovasc Electrophysiol 2003;14:422–30.

84. Viles-Gonzalez JF, de Castro Miranda R, Scanavacca M, et al. Acute and chronic effects of epicardial radiofrequency applications delivered on epicardial coronary arteries. Circ Arrhythm Electrophysiol 2011;4:526–31.

85. Koruth JS, Aryana A, Dukkipati SR, et al. Unusual complications of percutaneous epicardial access and epicardial mapping and ablation of cardiac arrhythmias. Circ Arrhythm Electrophysiol 2011;4:882–8.

86. Henz BD, do Nascimento TA, Dietrich Cde O, et al. Simultaneous epicardial and endocardial substrate mapping and radiofrequency catheter ablation as first-line treatment for ventricular tachycardia and frequent ICD shocks in chronic chagasic cardiomyopathy. J Interv Card Electrophysiol 2009; 26(3):195–205.

87. Milei J, Pesce R, Valero E, et al. Electrophysiologic-structural correlations in chagasic aneurysms causing malignant arrhythmias. Int J Cardiol 1991; 32(1):65–73.

88. Castagnino HE, Cicco JA, Coniglio J, et al. Chagasic ventricular aneurysm with ventricular tachycardia operated on with good results. Medicina (B Aires) 1975;35(2):166–79.

89. Iturralde P, Barragán R, Araya V, et al. Surgical resection of a focus of ventricular tachycardia guided by endocardial and epicardial mapping. Arch Inst Cardiol Mex 1992;62(1):69–75.

# Arrhythmias in Viral Myocarditis and Pericarditis

A. John Baksi, PhD, MRCP[a,b], G. Sunthar Kanaganayagam, PhD, MRCP[a,b],
Sanjay K. Prasad, MD, FRCP, FESC[a,b],*

## KEYWORDS

• Ventricular arrhythmia • Viral myocarditis • Acute pericarditis • CMR

## KEY POINTS

• Viral myocarditis is common and frequently unrecognized.
• Arrhythmia is common in acute viral myocarditis. The finding of ventricular arrhythmia (especially ventricular fibrillation [VF]) should prompt investigation to confirm the substrate.
• Cardiovascular magnetic resonance (CMR) is a powerful tool for the diagnosis and follow-up of acute myocarditis and also acute pericarditis; a normal CMR scan confers a good prognosis.
• Acute pericarditis in isolation does not seem to be frequently associated with ventricular arrhythmia but is often present as a perimyocarditis with an incumbent burden of arrhythmia related to the myocardial component.
• Management of arrhythmia in this setting is fundamentally usual management of the underlying arrhythmia and associated hemodynamic/clinical impact.

## INTRODUCTION

Acute viral myocarditis and acute pericarditis are typically self-limiting conditions that run a benign course and that may not even involve symptoms that lead to medical assessment. However, ventricular arrhythmia is a frequent occurrence in viral myocarditis; this may be in the form of premature ventricular contractions but may also be far more malignant as sustained ventricular tachycardia (VT) or unheralded VF. Myocarditis is thought to account for a large proportion of sudden cardiac deaths in young people without prior structural heart disease.[1–3] Identification of acute myocarditis either with or without pericarditis is therefore of importance. However, there are many potential hindrances to this. Furthermore, even when the diagnosis is made, therapeutic interventions remain limited and nonspecific. Identifying those at greatest risk of life-threatening arrhythmia is critical to reducing the mortality resulting from this condition.[4] This review summarizes current understanding of this challenging area.

## VIRAL MYOCARDITIS

Although there are many potential triggers, in economically developed countries, viruses are the most common cause of myocarditis (inflammation of the heart muscle).[5] The most frequently identified viruses in this setting are adenovirus,[6] parvovirus B19,[7] human herpes virus 6, and enterovirus.

The true incidence of viral myocarditis remains uncertain, largely as a result of its commonly asymptomatic course. Even when symptomatic, viral myocarditis frequently remains unrecognized

The authors have nothing to disclose.
[a] Cardiovascular Biomedical Research Unit, Royal Brompton Hospital & Harefield NHS Foundation Trust and Imperial College London, Sydney Street, London SW3 6NP, UK; [b] Cardiovascular Magnetic Resonance Unit, Royal Brompton Hospital, Sydney Street, London SW3 6NP, UK
* Corresponding author. Cardiovascular Magnetic Resonance Unit, Royal Brompton Hospital, Sydney Street, London SW3 6NP, UK.
E-mail address: s.prasad@rbht.nhs.uk

or unconfirmed. Myocarditis has been postulated in 1% to 40% of cases of sudden unexpected death, but the true incidence is poorly characterized. Myocarditis was identified as the cause of death in 40% of cases in a study of Air Force recruits who had sudden cardiac death.[8]

There are 3 phases to viral myocarditis.[9] The first phase consists of active viral replication within the myocardium causing direct lysis of cardiac myocytes and activation of the innate immune response. The consequent myocardial damage may be asymptomatic or may include symptoms anywhere along a spectrum to fulminant cardiogenic shock. Most patients recover fully from this initial acute phase. In some, persistent disease activity is thought to trigger an adaptive autoimmune response to viral and myocardial proteins. Again, in the majority, the pathogenic stimulus is cleared and the immune response diminished. But in some, as a consequence of the harmful inflammatory effect of this response on the myocardium, in this second phase of the disease process, often heart failure manifests. Furthermore, this autoimmune response seems to be the predominant driver of cellular injury, which may then lead to ventricular arrhythmia. The pivotal role of the autoimmune component is highlighted by experimental data that show that the severity of disease is modified by the major histocompatibility complex class 2 genes by modulation of the autoimmune element of myocarditis.[10]

Although left ventricular (LV) size and ejection fraction usually remain normal during acute viral myocarditis, a dilated cardiomyopathy phenotype may develop as a result of persistent myocarditis,[11,12] and this represents the third phase of the disease process. Diagnostic and therapeutic strategies are best directed according to the particular phase of the disease process. Arrhythmia in dilated cardiomyopathy is specifically considered elsewhere in this issue by John and colleagues.

The contribution of viral myocarditis to the development of dilated cardiomyopathy has been inferred by the common isolation of viral genomic material in the myocardium of affected individuals.[6,13] In addition, progressive myocardial dysfunction has been linked to viral persistence, in contrast to improvement of ventricular function wherein the virus is cleared.[14] The etiologic role of viruses is further supported by improvement in ventricular function after therapy with immunomodulators. However, with increased appreciation and understanding of the genetic basis of dilated cardiomyopathy,[15,16] the etiologic mechanisms may in cases be more complex. It is well recognized that the vast majority of the population is infected by cardiotropic viruses at one time or another, yet only a small minority of infected individuals (1%–5%) go on to develop histologically proven myocarditis.[17] It may be that in several cases, an episode of viral myocarditis is the trigger that unmasks a genetic predisposition to dilated cardiomyopathy. However, most of those who are infected with a virus that could cause myocarditis do not go on to develop clinically overt disease and of those who do, only a minority develop an overt cardiomyopathy. In a genome-wide association study, Bezzina and colleagues[18] identified a polymorphism adjacent to the gene encoding a viral receptor implicated in both dilated cardiomyopathy and modulation of the cardiac conduction system, which they found to be more frequently expressed in patients with VF than in controls.

## Investigations in Viral Myocarditis

Electrocardiographic (ECG) findings in acute myocarditis are most often nonspecific.[19] Sinus tachycardia is a typical finding. ST-segment elevation potentially mimicking acute myocardial infarction is frequently present. Arrhythmia or bundle branch block may be evident on the ECG. With regard to cardiac enzymes, the superior sensitivity of cardiac troponins over creatine kinase MB has been established,[20] and this is likely even more pronounced with high-sensitivity assays. Likewise, high-sensitivity C-reactive protein (CRP) assays also have good capability to detect acute viral myocarditis.[21]

Confirming a viral cause beyond a history of viral prodromal symptoms requires the detection of an appropriate virus, viral genome, or antibody on serology or in relevant tissue or fluid. Paired sera collected at least a fortnight apart may implicate a viral substrate, but more definitive evidence by direct identification of the virus from biopsy tissue by polymerase chain reaction (PCR) or in situ hybridization is desirable, but not routine.

## The Role of Imaging

Echocardiography remains the cornerstone of cardiac imaging. However, CMR has unique capability that makes it a powerful and an increasingly first-line investigation in the diagnosis and assessment of myocarditis. CMR uses the response of hydrogen protons to radiofrequency excitation and consequently is sensitive to regions of increased water content. Specific sequences, notably, short tau inversion recovery (STIR) T2 sequences, have been developed to identify regions of myocardial (**Fig. 1**) and pericardial inflammation or edema. In acute myocarditis, in which there is cell lysis and necrosis in addition to inflammation, regions of myocardial damage are further identified by the administration of gadolinium-based extracellular contrast agents,

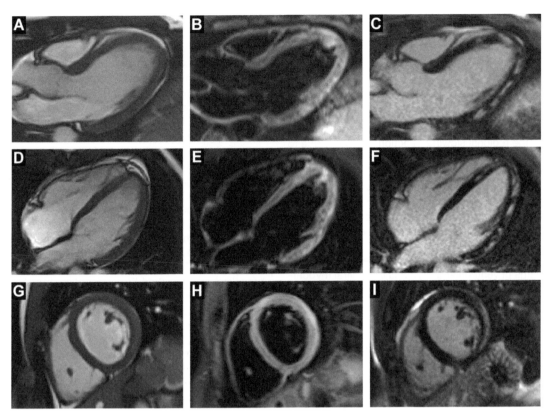

**Fig. 1.** Diagnostic CMR images of acute myocarditis. The upper row (A–C) is the LVOT (left ventricular outflow tract) view; the middle row (D–F), the HLA (horizontal long axis; 4-chamber equivalent) view; and the lower row (G–I) a basal short axis slice. In each series, the first column is SSFP (steady state free procession) imaging (for cine imaging). Even in these images, there is slightly higher signal in the myocardial regions, which are edematous. The middle column is STIR imaging for the detection of myocardial inflammation or edema. Regions of high signal are evident identifying myocardial inflammation or edema in regions similar to the late gadolinium enhancement (LGE) seen in the third column. This LGE is typically in a subepicardial/midwall distribution, in contrast to the subendocardial origin of LGE seen in myocardial infarction.

which in this setting are able to accumulate where the cell membrane has been compromised. In cases in which replacement fibrosis has occurred after acute myocarditis, the increased extracellular space is identified on late gadolinium imaging. These regions of scar highlighted by gadolinium-based contrast enhancement on delayed imaging are often considered to be the substrate for reentrant circuits that serve as the substrate for arrhythmia.[22] Typically the pattern of late gadolinium enhancement in myocarditis involves the subepicardium or midwall of the myocardium. Most often, this is predominantly in the lateral LV free wall.[23]

Of additional benefit is the ability of CMR to discriminate myocarditis from myocardial infarction based largely on the pattern of late gadolinium enhancement. Myocardial infarction typically has its origin in the subendocardium. Given the ability of CMR to readily identify regions of myocardial inflammation, endomyocardial biopsy is no longer necessary for the diagnosis of myocarditis in most

cases. Although this diagnosis may well be evident from a robust history, abnormal ECG result, and elevated levels of cardiac enzymes, CMR is able to confirm this definitively as well as assess the extent of myocardial inflammation and its impact on ventricular size and function. Extensive inflammation and/or late gadolinium enhancement may portend a higher likelihood of adverse remodeling and highlights the value of a follow-up study either by echocardiography or by CMR to assess for this. CMR is also useful in indicating the area to be targeted by endomyocardial biopsy.[23,24] Three-dimensional electroanatomical mapping has also been used successfully to guide biopsy and hence reduce sampling error and increase the sensitivity of biopsy by identifying ventricular segments with abnormal voltage.[22] However, clinically, endomyocardial biopsy is now generally reserved for those suspected of having giant cell myocarditis or those in whom there is progressive deterioration despite usual supportive treatment.

## Potential Mechanisms of Arrhythmia

Several molecular and immunopathogenetic mechanisms are likely involved in the disease process (**Box 1**). The precise mechanism or more likely mechanisms by which ventricular arrhythmia results from acute myocarditis are unclear, although several hypotheses have been postulated. The formation of reentry circuits consequent on the regional slowing of action potentials due to viral-induced myocardial fibrosis and secondary hypertrophy has been proposed.[22] The development of focal areas of inflammation in electrically sensitive regions of myocardium may also invoke ventricular arrhythmia. There is also the potential for myocardial ion channel dysfunction, as is seen in animal models,[25] as well as myocardial ischemia contributing to or underlying mechanisms of ventricular arrhythmia in my viral myocarditis. The inflammatory process itself seems proarrhythmic, and resolution of this may also lessen the proarrhythmic substrate.

There are animal data to support alteration in myocardial expression of connexins, important proteins involved in gap junction function and hence communication between myoctyes, during coxsackievirus B3 (CVB3)-induced myocarditis.[26]

Of interest, atorvastatin was able to modulate the downregulation of connexin expressivity, restoring gap junction channel function and outcome in viral myocarditis in mice after inoculation with CVB3. Altered calcium handling is also likely to be an important component of the perturbations of normal cardiomyocyte function during acute myocarditis.[27] Regions of myocardial infarction may result from prolonged vasospasm. Microvascular ischemia may also be a feature that promotes arrhythmia.

Some of the arrhythmic substrate of myocarditis seems to lie in the disease-unmasking cardiomyopathy or channelopathy. An inflammatory component is often identified in the myocardium of individuals with arrhythmogenic right ventricular cardiomyopathy (ARVC) at postmortem and likely promotes ventricular arrhythmia.[28] ARVC may be provoked or unmasked by myocarditis, but data suggest that myocarditis may frequently lead to structural changes that mimic ARVC.[29] In a group of 30 patients meeting noninvasive criteria for ARVC, half had histologic and immunohistochemical evidence of ARVC, whereas active myocarditis was identified in the other half. Endocmyocardial biopsy was required to determine which of them had ARVC and which had myocarditis. Individuals with ARVC had recurrent malignant arrhythmia, whereas those with myocarditis remained asymptomatic and free from arrhythmic events.

### Viral Myocarditis and Channelopathy

Several articles in the literature report the association of acute myocarditis and ventricular arrhythmia with myocardial channelopathies, notably Brugada syndrome, short QT syndrome and early repolarization.[30,31] Myocarditis of the right ventricle (RV) has frequently been identified in patients with a Brugada-like phenotype; in one study, it was identified in up to 77% of patients.[32]

### TREATMENT

In most cases, no therapy is required. As described, acute myocarditis may be asymptomatic or often just invoke self-limiting nonspecific viral symptoms for which affected individuals may at most seek over-the-counter medications. There is currently relatively little and weak evidence to substantiate the use of any specific disease-modifying therapy for acute viral myocarditis, although intravenous immunoglobulin, immunosuppression, interferon (IFN), and immune adsorption therapies have been used. These therapies are unsurprisingly most effective in phase 2 of the disease process, that is, the period of autoimmune response. Equally, there is a lack of

---

**Box 1**
**Mechanisms of arrhythmia in myocarditis**

*Mechanisms of myocardial injury*

- Direct viral-induced lysis of cardiac myocytes triggering innate immune responses
- Adaptive autoimmune response
- Viral persistence
- Apoptotic cell death

*Postulated and potential mechanisms of arrhythmia*

- Myocardial replacement fibrosis, favoring reentry mechanism
- Myocyte necrosis
- Proarrhythmic effects of cytokines
- Altered function at myocardial gap junctions
- Altered calcium handling
- Infarction, microvascular ischemic insult
- Protease release resulting in cleavage of dystrophin with consequent cytoskeletal abnormality
- Unmasking cardiomyopathy, dilated cardiomyopathy (DCM)/arrhythmogenic right ventricular cardiomyopathy (ARVC)
- Concomitant channelopathy

evidence to support the use of specific antiarrhythmic agents beyond the conventional strategies. Treatment of heart failure follows current guidelines.[33] The often self-limiting nature of myocarditis makes this an attractive condition for circulatory assistance as a bridge to recovery in patients in whom this is required. Longer-term strategies for influencing disease may well lie in prevention by either immunization or the development of molecules to block viral receptors. Fundamentally, treatment is supportive, where any is required. Traditionally, affected individuals are advised to avoid strenuous activity for several months.[34] The evidence to support the recommendation to avoid strenuous episode during viral illness per se is more equivocal.

## PROGNOSIS

There are limited data regarding the long-term prognosis after viral myocarditis. One study showed a 20% mortality at 5 years after viral myocarditis.[4] Many of the major studies in dilated cardiomyopathy specifically exclude cases considered to be due to overt myocarditis, although it is quite likely that even when this is an explicit exclusion criteria, the cause in several cases remains a viral myocarditis. In the absence of a dilated cardiomyopathy phenotype, the prognosis for individuals surviving cardiac arrest due to ventricular arrhythmia in the setting of acute myocarditis seems favorable if resuscitation was prompt and effective as such arrhythmias tend to be self-limiting.[35] However, further large long-term studies are required.

Risk stratification for patients with myocarditis has until recently been difficult because of a paucity of prognostic data and limited biomarkers of risk. One of the key limitations has been difficulty in establishing the diagnosis because of the broad spectrum of possible presentations and the frequently asymptomatic course of disease. Nevertheless, where there is diagnostic suspicion, CMR has emerged as a powerful diagnostic tool. Furthermore, there are increasing data that CMR appearances carry valuable prognostic information. Late gadolinium enhancement revealing replacement fibrosis has been shown to be an independent predictor of adverse outcome in dilated cardiomyopathy.[36] Schumm and colleagues[37] followed up 405 consecutive patients referred for CMR to assess for suspected myocarditis. In 55.6% of patients, initial CMR confirmed normal LV volumes and ejection fraction without late gadolinium enhancement. STIR T2 sequences were not performed. CMR was considered to confirm the diagnosis of myocarditis in 28.8% of patients.

The patients were followed up for a median duration of 1591 days. A normal result on CMR conferred a good prognosis regardless of symptoms or other findings. All 10 major adverse cardiac events (7 cardiac deaths, 1 aborted sudden cardiac death, and 2 appropriate implantable cardioverter-defibrillator [ICD] shocks) occurred in patients with abnormal results on CMR. However, exactly which patients should be offered primary prevention against ventricular arrhythmia with ICD remains somewhat inconclusive outside of the current recommendations for dilated cardiomyopathy; this is one key area where data are lacking.

## PERICARDITIS

Acute pericarditis is a clinical diagnosis made by the presence of at least 2 of the following 3 conditions: typical chest pain, pericardial friction rub, and widespread ST-segment elevation; it has an estimated incidence of 27.7 per 100,000 in Europe.[38] Elevated levels of inflammatory markers are found in the majority[39] accompanied by normal markers of myocardial damage. An exemplar case includes a recent viral prodrome; sharp chest pain worse on deep inspiration, coughing, or when lying flat; and an ECG with global saddle-shaped ST elevation as well as PR depression (a specific finding in pericarditis). The distinction from myopericarditis lies in the diagnosis of pericarditis together with the demonstration of myocardial damage using specific markers of myocardial injury without focally impaired LV function. In this case, inflammation of the pericardium is thought to lead to limited secondary involvement of the myocardium (found in approximately 15% in one observational cohort including 274 cases of idiopathic or viral pericarditis, and in 32% in a smaller cohort).[38,40] Myopericarditis is distinguished from perimyocarditis by the regional myocardial dysfunction in perimyocarditis as a dominantly myocarditic syndrome.[41]

### Etiology

Viral pericarditis is the commonest of many causes,[42] but unfortunately it can be a difficult diagnosis to make, with a lot of cases being placed in an idiopathic or viral category, including in the literature. One study used extensive serologic investigation in this group and found it to be not only diagnostically but also therapeutically futile.[43] A similar panel of cardiotropic viruses, notably coxsackieviruses, etiologic in myocarditis reappear as culprits in those cases of pericarditis identified; this includes the recently identified torque teno viruses and papilloma viruses via metagenome analysis of pericardial fluid from affected patients.[44] Recurrent postviral myocarditis is thought to have a largely autoimmune basis, via activation of both innate and adaptive immune systems and through subsequent cytokine release.[45] Increased levels of interleukin-6 and tumor necrosis factor (TNF)-$\alpha$ with low IFN-$\gamma$ concentrations in pericardial effusion fluid analysis in comparison to serum values were found in a study of patients with inflammatory pericardial processes. The cytokine pattern of high levels of TNF-$\alpha$ and low levels of transforming growth factor $\beta_1$ was signatory for patients with viral pericarditis indicating a unique mechanism of inflammation.[46]

## The Role of Imaging (Cardiovascular Magnetic Resonance and Computed Tomography)

Imaging in pericarditis can yield variable results, with no significant abnormality a possible finding regardless of the modality used; hence pericarditis remains a clinical diagnosis. However, echocardiography is a useful initial screen for effusions and associated physiology via assessment of RV diastole and transmitral and transtricuspid Doppler plus assessment of the rare complication of constriction. Pericardial brightness, however, remains subjective and an imprecise tool for defining pericardial inflammation, and accurate assessment of pericardial thickness is unreliable. Therefore in uncomplicated pericarditis with or without an effusion, echocardiography is appropriate. Dedicated imaging with CMR allows for pericardial characterization with inflammation sequences (such as STIR T2-weighted sequences) and late gadolinium imaging for pericardial enhancement (**Fig. 2**) as well as assessment of pericardial thickness and effusions (using basic sequences such as steady-state free precessions) and hemodynamic effects of possible pericardial constriction (free-breathing sequences). Cardiac

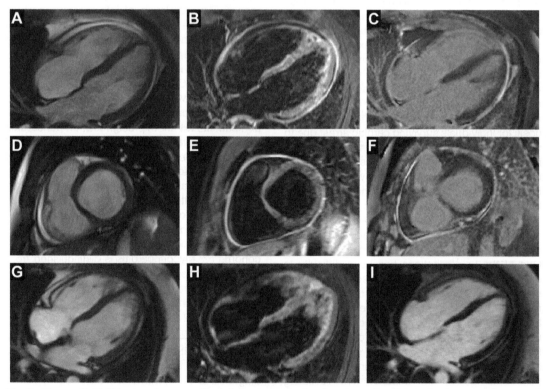

**Fig. 2.** Diagnostic CMR images from a patient during an episode of acute pericarditis and subsequent images after resolution of the episodes. The top 2 rows (A–F) show diagnostic CMR images of acute pericarditis (without myocardial involvement). The bottom row (G–I) shows CMR images from the same patient after resolution of the episode. The top and bottom rows present the HLA (4-chamber equivalent) view, and the middle row is a basal short axis slice. In each series, the first column is SSFP imaging (for cine imaging). The pericardium is dark and a small rim of bright pericardial fluid can be seen within it. The middle column is STIR imaging for the detection of inflammation or edema. The entire pericardium is bright in the images during the acute episode indicating inflammation. This signal has normalized in the lower images confirming resolution of the inflammation. Late gadolinium enhancement (LGE) of the pericardium is evident in the third column during the acute episode (top 2 images), but not after resolution of the inflammation (bottom image). The thickness of the pericardium seems slightly greater during the acute phase than on follow-up when the inflammation had resolved.

computed tomography (CT) is also a valuable imaging tool in the assessment of pericardial disease with accurate assessment of pericardial thickness, calcification, and effusions and the added benefit of possible preoperative planning plus delineation of coronary anatomy.[47] Retrospective cardiac CT can also be of use to an extent in the assessment of physiologic effects of adverse hemodynamics. The obvious disadvantages are ionizing radiation dose and lack of dedicated inflammation imaging.[48]

When there are acute or subacute symptoms of heart failure refractory to medical management, the development of compromising arrhythmias, heart failure with eosinophilia, suspicion of giant cell myocarditis, or a history of collagen vascular disease endomyocardial biopsy should be considered.[38]

## MANAGEMENT OF PERICARDITIS AND COMPLICATIONS

Briefly, the clinical management of pericarditis itself can be challenging with recurrent pericarditis a feature in almost one-third of patients.[49,50] Those with recurrent pericarditis tend to have a more benign course with little in the way of complications at recurrences.[51] Optimal treatment is with full-dose nonsteroidal antiinflammatory drugs for around 7 days (up to 6 weeks) or until symptom resolution with a subsequent tapering dose (**Box 2**). The addition of colchicine was found to significantly reduce the recurrence rate of pericarditis from 32.3% to 10.7% in a large prospective randomized trial, despite an 8% discontinuance because of diarrhea.[50] Steroids have been associated with recurrence[50] and are usually reserved for resistant and recurrent cases or in some tuberculous cases with associated effusions.[52,53] As with

---

**Box 2**
**Diagnosis and management of pericarditis**

- Diagnosis is based on the presence of 2 of the following: typical chest pain, pericardial friction rub, and widespread ST-segment elevation.

- Elucidating the underlying cause can be futile and unnecessary in uncomplicated cases.

- Pericarditis is a clinical diagnosis, but imaging can help and especially assess complications. CMR provides superior tissue characterization.

- Management is based on a combination of an antiinflammatory medications such as NSAIDs and colchicine.

*Abbreviation:* NSAID, nonsteroidal antiinflammatory drug.

---

myocarditis, cessation of physical activity is also advised for 6 months.[54]

The Colchicine for the Prevention of the Post-pericardiotomy Syndrome (COPPS) 2 trial by Imazio and colleagues[55] investigated the reduction of postoperative atrial fibrillation (AF) as well as postpericardiotomy syndrome and pericardial/pleural effusions upon administration of colchicine, started preoperatively. The investigators found no reduction in postoperative AF or effusions but a significant reduction in postpericardiotomy syndrome in an intention-to-treat analysis. Of note, there were significant gastrointestinal side effects in the treatment group (20% of patients), and when an on-treatment analysis was performed there was indeed a reduction in AF.[55]

Constrictive pericarditis is a rare complication of viral or idiopathic pericarditis. Other causes of pericarditis such as tuberculous, neoplastic, and purulent causes are associated with a significantly increased risk of constriction (found to be 0.76 cases per 1000 years for idiopathic/viral pericarditis vs 52.74 cases per 1000 years for purulent pericarditis in a median 72-month follow-up of 500 patients).[56]

### The Electrocardiographic in Pericarditis and Myopericarditis

ECG findings in patients with myopericarditis tend to be more pronounced than in patients with pericarditis only and evolve as the disease progresses. The stages of progression are described as follows: stage 1 involves ST elevation and upright T waves that usually resolve to normal (stage II) over several days or evolve further to T-wave inversion (stage III) and finally to normal or with potentially fixed T-wave inversion (stage IV).[57] There can also be PR-segment elevation in aVR that suggests an atrial current of injury.[58,59] Myopericarditis can lead to regional ST-segment change mimicking an acute infarction before normalization.[38] The initial presenting ECG of saddle-shaped ST elevation can be confused with early repolarization and LV hypertrophy with early repolarization. A ratio of the height of the ST-segment junction to the height of the apex of the T wave of more than 0.25 suggests pericarditis,[60] specifically in leads I, V4, V5, and V6, with lead I providing optimal predictive value in a series of 80 patients.[61]

### Pathologic and Postmortem Studies in Pericarditis and Myopericarditis

Pathologic data from the 1960s initially demonstrated involvement of the sinus node, because of its proximity to the visceral pericardium, in pericarditis specimens,[62] only for this to be later disproved in a larger series.[63]

In Croatia, over a 10-year period from 1998, there were 4 sudden unexpected deaths because of myopericarditis during or after physical exercise. The death rate in athletes was 0.15 per 100,000 versus 0.75 per 100,000 in all males practicing exercise and having myopericarditis ($P$ = .0014). Details on arrhythmias were limited, but 1 patient had ventricular premature beats while training.[44]

## ARRHYTHMIAS IN CASE REPORTS OF VIRAL PERICARDITIS

A PubMed search of case reports of pericarditis and arrhythmia from onset of electronic records to January 2015 yields very little in the way of documented arrhythmias in specifically viral pericarditis.[64–67] One case of myopericarditis from 1976 that documents a VF arrest in a 12-year-old child with confirmed coxsackievirus seems to be predominantly perimyocarditis, with nothing in the way of a pericardial rub on presentation but marked cardiomegaly on a chest radiograph shortly after resuscitation and a small effusion a month after presentation.[68] Another case is reported of a patient with sinus bradycardia at 35 beats per minute in whom an idiopathic, presumed viral, pericariditis was diagnosed based on chest pain, a pericardial rub, and concave ST segments.[69] Other investigations in this patient including coronary angiography yielded normal results, and the bradycardia resolved within a few hours and was put down to a vasovagal response to the chest pain. This observation is indeed converse to the predominant sinus tachycardia described at presentation, which at one point was managed solely with carotid sinus pressure.[70] More recently, the importance of heart-rate-lowering medication has been raised albeit with no clinical data in pericarditis, but with adverse outcomes in myocarditis managed without β-blockers.[71] Roubille and colleagues[72] theorize that a pharmacologically induced rest would likely reduce inflammation and therefore limit damage in pericarditis; however, clinical evidence remains limited with only a correlation between admission heart rate and discharge CRP levels.[73]

### Follow-up Studies on Arrhythmia Burden in Pericarditis

The 1984 Holter data in 49 patients with diagnosed pericarditis, via pericardial rub and typical ECG changes, and sinus rhythm at the time of diagnosis demonstrated a low incidence of arrhythmias outside of an acute infarct.[74] Isolated ectopics were the only ventricular arrhythmia recognized with only 4 cases of supraventricular arrhythmias in patients with no history of cardiac disease. In patients with a history (n = 29), including 21 with an acute infarction and Dressler type pericarditis, 3 had nonsustained VT, 3 had a junctional rhythm, 1 had paroxysmal atrial flutter, 1 had an ectopic atrial rhythm, 1 had a supraventricular tachycardia (SVT), and 1 had intermittent atrioventricular (AV) block.[74] A subsequent study in 1986 reported on 31 patients with pericarditis (24 of whom had idiopathic pericarditis) and found that 1 patient developed atrial fibrillation (AF) and 1 an SVT in follow-up of up to 19 years.[49]

Patients with myopericarditis have been found to have more arrhythmias than those with pericarditis alone.[38] In an observational study, among patients with acute pericarditis, 7.7% (n = 234) developed AF, 9% another supraventricular arrhythmia, and 0% undefined ventricular arrhythmias, whereas among patients with myopericarditis, 2.5% (n = 40) developed AF, 17.5% another supraventricular arrhythmia, 40% ventricular arrhythmia, and 5% AV block. Overall, 65% of patients with myopericarditis developed an arrhythmia.[38]

A retrospective 37-month follow-up of patients on the spectrum of pure pericarditis to pure myocarditis (with the majority having predominant pericarditis) found no mortality. Arrhythmias were not specifically reported.[75] Imazio and colleagues[76] studied 300 cases with a similar follow-up of 38 months and divided them into a low-risk group and a high-risk group that warranted in-hospital investigation and management. The high-risk group (of whom 22% had a presumed viral/idiopathic etiology) had subacute onset, immunodepression, trauma, anticoagulant therapy, a severe pericardial effusion, tamponade, or evidence of myopericarditis. The low-risk group (84.7%, of whom 91% had a presumed viral/idiopathic etiology) had a single day of basic investigations including an ECG and echocardiogram and then were discharged to clinic follow-up. Again, although arrhythmias were not specifically documented, there was no mortality in either group with the objective morbidity being constriction.[76]

Imazio and colleagues[77] in another cohort study of 486 patients over a median 36-month follow-up divided patients into those with myopericarditis (23%), perimyocarditis (5%), and pericarditis alone (71%). The investigators found a statistically significant difference in ventricular arrhythmias between the 4.4% and 7.7% of those with myopericarditis and perimyocarditis, respectively, and only 0.3% of those with a pure pericarditis. Supraventricular arrhythmias were found in 8.8% and 19.2% of those with myopericarditis and perimyocarditis, respectively, and only 5.8% of those with a pure pericarditis (not statistically significant). No AV block was demonstrated. Of the total cohort,

84.8% were deemed as having an idiopathic cause and only 4.5% were deemed to have infectious (including assessment of coxsackievirus, Epstein-Barr virus, parvovirus, adenovirus, cytomegalovirus, and influenza). Patients were advised against competitive, amateur, or leisure time sports for 3 months with pericarditis and 6 months otherwise. There were no deaths during total follow-up with a residual mild LV dysfunction in 8% of patients with myopericarditis and in 15% of those with perimyocarditis. Of note, CRP levels were higher in patients with simple pericarditis, and troponin elevation was related to the degree of myocardial involvement in myopericarditis and perimyocarditis, although it is known not to be a prognostic indicator.[40] Management of arrhythmias was not specified; however, most patients with myocardial involvement were treated with a β-blocker, possibly for LV impairment rather than for rhythm control per se.

## DEFINING ARRHYTHMIAS IN PERICARDITIS VERSUS MYOPERICARDITIS AND PERIMYOCARDITIS

A study that sought to define arrhythmias in acute pericarditis split patients into those with endomyocardial-biopsy-proven evidence of myocarditis (perimyocarditis and myopericarditis, n = 10) and those with no evidence (n = 40)[78]; 6 to 9 samples were taken from both ventricles to minimize sampling error, but this remains a possibility. The investigators found that supraventricular arrhythmias, VF, and AF occurred in 40%, 20%, and 0%, respectively, of patients with myocarditis and perimyocarditis compared with 5%, 0%, and 20%, respectively, of those with pericarditis alone. It was also found that 1 patient died of VF and 2 had ICD implantation in the myocarditis and perimyocarditis group. No difference was found in AV block between the groups, with both exhibiting low levels. Of the 40 patients with pericarditis only, 12.5% had confirmed viral pericarditis after pericardial biopsy and effusion analysis of viruses using PCR, but no specific data are presented in this group. In addition, limited data are presented on the group with biopsy-proven evidence of myocarditis with no further details of the patients with ICD implantation or VF.

A more recent study focused on the treatment of epicardial VT sought to address the difficulty in access in patients with prior pericarditis and non-coronary cardiac surgery with recurrent VT.[79]

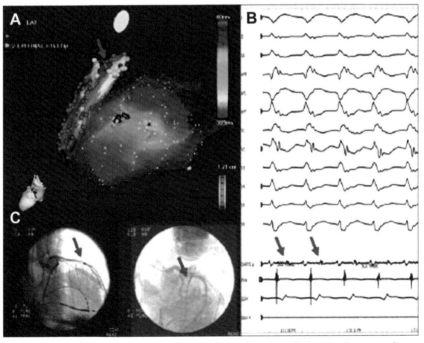

**Fig. 3.** Visualization of epicardial VT ablation. (*A*) Epicardial and endocardial activation maps from a 48-year-old man with pericarditis. The red arrow demonstrates earliest VT activation on the LV epicardium. (*B*) Middiastolic electrograms (*red arrows*) found at the location presented in panel A. Perfect entrainment response to pacing was demonstrated at this location (not shown). (*C*) Cineangiography confirmed catheter position away from coronary anatomy (*red arrows*) at the site showing middiastolic potentials. Ablation at this location successfully terminated the VT. (*From* Tschabrun CM, Haggani HM, Cooper JM, et al. Percutaneous epicardial ventricular tachycardia ablation after non-coronary cardiac surgery or pericarditis. Heart Rhythm 2013;10:168; with permission.)

Patients in whom an epicardial substrate was clear on imaging, those who had the epicardial VT morphology on their 12-lead ECG, and those with failed endocardial VT ablation were included for an attempt at epicardial access. Percutaneous puncture was then performed from the subxiphoid approach using a guidewire to circumscribe the heart, with contrast injection if this failed, in order to demonstrate adhesions. The catheter was then manipulated to disrupt these before electroanatomical mapping (**Fig. 3**). In this single-center study, over a 10-year period 10 patients with prior non-coronary cardiac surgery or pericarditis (n = 2) and recurrent VT with a need for epicardial access were recruited. Of the 2 patients with pericarditis, one had VT storm and the other had VT, and both had successful pericardial access but one had an RV perforation. Blunt catheter dissection allowed for disruption of adhesions and successful mapping in the target region in all but 1 patient, in whom adhesions proved too strong despite an eventual surgical pericardial window. Of the 10 patients 8 had noninducibility of target arrhythmia at the end of the ablation. In 1 patient in whom this was not achieved, there were 30 ablation lesions after mapping, but the arrhythmia remained inducible. Over a follow-up of 13 months 50% remained VT free.

There is clear evidence that myopericarditis and perimyocarditis carry a higher arrhythmic burden than pericarditis alone. Clinically, there remains a responsibility to determine the arrhythmias in this cohort,[80] especially if VF has been described in up to 20% in 1 small study,[78] although the number elsewhere seems much lower. AF and supraventricular arrhythmias seem to be the commonest findings in isolated pericarditis (**Box 3**), with rare cases of ventricular arrhythmias described in the literature. Owing to the infrequency of even supraventricular arrhythmias in this group, there are no trials on management in viral pericarditis, although extrapolations from other causes of pericarditis can be surmised.[81] In the few cases that have

been described in the literature, AV block and epicardial VT both feature.

## SUMMARY/DISCUSSION

The literature regarding the mechanism of arrhythmia in viral myocarditis and pericarditis remains limited with incomplete understanding of these conditions. Specifically, the precise mechanisms by which ventricular arrhythmias occur during myocarditis and pericarditis are unknown. It seems likely that several genetic factors influence and/or determine the sequelae of myocardial viral infection, including the development of arrhythmia. The broad principles of management remain centered around the particular rhythm perturbation and in particular its clinical impact and follow published guidelines.[82] The association with channelopathies supports exploration for arrhythmic substrate in patients with acute myocarditis complicated by VF. The power of CMR to identify myocardial inflammation and myocardial fibrosis and also provide accurate quantification of ventricular volumes and function supports increased utilization of this powerful and increasingly available technique in this setting. The combination of such imaging with biobanking and in particular genetic analysis will enhance the understanding of this condition and in particular the variable course of disease between individuals. In addition, much further basic scientific research and molecular biology is required to enhance the currently extremely limited understanding of the electrical basis of arrhythmia in this setting. The paramount importance of this is to better identify those individuals at risk of sudden cardiac death due to the acute viral myocarditis, as well as identifying those most likely to develop a dilated cardiomyopathy. Additional trials to assess the ability of pharmacologic intervention to abort or limit the development of both arrhythmia and dilated cardiomyopathy are much needed.

---

**Box 3**
**Arrhythmias in viral pericarditis**

- There are limited data on the subgroup of viral pericarditis
- Most data come from follow-up of large cohorts of mixed etiology pericarditis
- There is a low incidence of particularly ventricular arrhythmias in patients with pericarditis as a whole
- Supraventricular arrhythmias are the largest burden in patients with isolated pericarditis.

## REFERENCES

1. Sagar S, Liu PP, Cooper LT Jr. Myocarditis. Lancet 2012;379:738–47.
2. Fabre A, Sheppard MN. Sudden adult death syndrome and other non-ischaemic causes of sudden cardiac death. Heart 2006;92(3):316–20.
3. Doolan A, Semsarian C, Langlois N. Causes of sudden cardiac death in young Australians. Med J Aust 2004;180(3):110–2.
4. Grün S, Schumm J, Greulich S, et al. Long-term follow-up of biopsy-proven viral myocarditis: predictors of mortality and incomplete recovery. J Am Coll Cardiol 2012;59:1604–15.

5. Shauer A, Gotsman I, Keren A, et al. Acute viral myocarditis: current concepts in diagnosis and treatment. Isr Med Assoc J 2013;15:180–5.

6. Bowles NE, Ni J, Kearney DL, et al. Detection of viruses in myocardial tissues by polymerase chain reaction. Evidence of adenovirus as a common cause of myocarditis in children and adults. J Am Coll Cardiol 2003;42:466–72.

7. Bock CT, Klingel K, Kandolf R. Human parvovirus B19-associated myocarditis. N Engl J Med 2010; 362:1248–9.

8. Phillips MP, Robinowitz M, Higgins JR, et al. Sudden cardiac death in Air Force recruits. JAMA 1986;256: 2696–9.

9. Mason JW, Trehan S, Renlund DG. Myocarditis. In: Willerson JT, Cohn JN, Wellens HJ, et al, editors. Cardiovascular medicine. 3rd edition. London: Springer; 2007. p. 1314–47.

10. Li HS, Ligons DL, Rose NR. Genetic complexity of autoimmune myocarditis. Autoimmun Rev 2008; 7(3):168–73.

11. Kawai C. From myocarditis to cardiomyopathy: mechanisms of inflammation and cell death. Learning from the past for the future. Circulation 1999;99:1091–100.

12. D'Ambrosio A, Patti G, Manzoli A, et al. The fate of acute myocarditis between spontaneous improvement and evolution to dilated cardiomyopathy: a review. Heart 2001;85:499–504.

13. Kuhl U, Pauschinger M, Noutsias M, et al. High prevalence of viral genomes and multiple viral infections in the myocardium of adults with "idiopathic" left ventricular dysfunction. Circulation 2005;111:887–93.

14. Kühl U, Pauschinger M, Seeberg B, et al. Viral persistence in the myocardium is associated with progressive cardiac dysfunction. Circulation 2005; 112:1965–70.

15. Hershberger RE, Hedges DJ, Morales A. Dilated cardiomyopathy: the complexity of a diverse genetic architecture. Nat Rev Cardiol 2013;10(9):531–47.

16. Roberts AM, Ware JS, Herman DS, et al. Integrated allelic, transcriptional, and phenotypic dissection of the cardiac effects of titin truncations in health and disease. Sci Transl Med 2015;7(270):270.

17. Andreoletti L, Leveque N, Boulagnon C, et al. Viral causes of human myocarditis. Arch Cardiovasc Dis 2009;102(6–7):559–68.

18. Bezzina CR, Pazoki R, Bardai A, et al. Genome-wide association study identifies a susceptibility locus at 21q21 for ventricular fibrillation in acute myocardial infarction. Nat Genet 2010;42(8):688–91.

19. Punja M, Mark DG, McCoy JV, et al. Electrocardiographic manifestations of cardiac infectious-inflammatory disorders. Am J Emerg Med 2010;28: 364–77.

20. Smith SC, Ladenson JH, Mason JW, et al. Elevations of cardiac troponin I associated with myocarditis.

Experimental and clinical correlates. Circulation 1997;95:163–8.

21. Guo JG. Detection of cardiac troponin and high-sensitivity C reactive protein in children with viral myocarditis. Na Fang Yi ke Da Xue Xue Bao 2008; 28(6):1076–7.

22. Pieroni M, Smaldone C, Bellocci F. Myocarditis presenting with ventricular arrhythmias: role of electroanatomical mapping-guided endomyocardial biopsy in differential diagnosis. In: Cihakova D, editor. Myocarditis. InTech; 2011. p. 365–86. http://dx.doi.org/10.5772/22123. ISBN: 978-953-307-289-0. Available at: http://www.intechopen.com/books/myocarditis/myocarditis-presenting-with-ventricular-arrhythmias-role-of-electroanatomical-mapping-guided-endomyo. Accessed March 04, 2015.

23. Mahrholdt H, Goedecke C, Wagner A, et al. Cardiovascular magnetic resonance assessment of human myocarditis: a comparison to histology and molecular pathology. Circulation 2004;109:1250–8.

24. De Cobelli F, Pieroni M, Esposito A, et al. Delayed gadolinium-enhanced cardiac magnetic resonance in patients with chronic myocarditis presenting with heart failure or recurrent arrhythmias. J Am Coll Cardiol 2006;47:1649–54.

25. Saito J, Niwano S, Niwano H, et al. Electrical remodeling of the ventricular myocardium in myocarditis: studies of rat experimental autoimmune myocarditis. Circ J 2002;66:97–103.

26. Zhang A, Zhang H, Wu S. Immunomodulation by atorvastatin upregulates expression of gap junction proteins in coxsackievirus B3 (CVB3)-induced myocarditis. Inflamm Res 2010;59(4):255–62.

27. Li Y, Ge S, Peng Y, et al. Inflammation and cardiac dysfunction during sepsis, muscular dystrophy, and myocarditis. Burns Trauma 2013;1(3):109–21.

28. Thiene G, Basso C. Arrhythmogenic right ventricular cardiomyopathy: an update. Cardiovasc Pathol 2001;10:109–17.

29. Pieroni M, Dello Russo A, Marzo F, et al. High prevalence of myocarditis mimicking arrhythmogenic right ventricular cardiomyopathy differential diagnosis by electroanatomic mapping-guided endomyocardial biopsy. J Am Coll Cardiol 2009;53(8):681–9.

30. Salerno F, Girerd N, Chalabreysse L, et al. Myocarditis and cardiac channelopathies: a deadly association? Int J Cardiol 2011;147(3):468–70.

31. Buob A, Siaplaouras S, Janzen I, et al. Focal parvovirus B19 myocarditis in a patient with Brugada syndrome. Cardiol Rev 2003;11(1):45–9.

32. Frustaci A, Priori SG, Pieroni M, et al. Cardiac histological substrate in patients with clinical phenotype of Brugada syndrome. Circulation 2005;112:3680–7.

33. McMurray JJ, Adamopoulos S, Anker SD, et al. ESC Guidelines for the diagnosis and treatment of acute and chronic heart failure 2012. Eur Heart J 2012;33: 1787–847.

34. Pelliccia A, Corrado D, Bjornstad HH, et al. Recommendations for participation in competitive sport and leisure-time physical activity in individuals with cardiomyopathies, myocarditis and pericarditis. Eur J Cardiovasc Prev Rehabil 2006;13:876–85.

35. Chau EM, Chow WH, Chiu C, et al. Treatment and outcome in biopsy proven fulminant myocarditis in adults. Int J Cardiol 2006;110(3):405–6.

36. Gulati A, Jabbour A, Ismail TF, et al. Association of fibrosis with mortality and sudden cardiac death in patients with nonischemic dilated cardiomyopathy. JAMA 2013;309:896–908.

37. Schumm J, Greulich S, Wagner A, et al. Cardiovascular magnetic resonance risk stratification in patients with clinically suspected myocarditis. J Cardiovasc Magn Reson 2014;16:14.

38. Imazio M, Cecchi E, Demichelis B, et al. Myopericarditis versus viral or idiopathic acute pericarditis. Heart 2008;94:498–501.

39. Imazio M, Brucato A, Maestroni S, et al. Prevalence of C-reactive protein elevation and time course of normalisation in acute pericarditis: implications for the diagnosis, therapy, and prognosis of pericarditis. Circulation 2011;123:1092–7.

40. Imazio M, Demichelis B, Cecchi E, et al. Cardiac troponin I in acute pericarditis. J Am Coll Cardiol 2003;42:2144–8.

41. Imazio M, Cooper LT. Management of myopericarditis. Expert Rev Cardiovasc Ther 2013;11:193–201.

42. Oakley CM. Myocarditis, pericarditis and other pericardial diseases. Heart 2000;84:449–54.

43. Abu Fanne R, Banai S, Chorin U, et al. Diagnostic yield of extensive infectious panel testing in acute pericarditis. Cardiology 2011;119:134–9.

44. Fancello L, Monteil S, Popgeorgiev N, et al. Viral communities associated with human pericardial fluids in idiopathic pericarditis. PLoS One 2014;9:e93367.

45. Cantarini L, Lopalco G, Selmi C, et al. Autoimmunity and autoinflammation as the yin and yang of idiopathic recurrent acute pericarditis. Autoimmun Rev 2015;14:90–7.

46. Ristic AD, Pankuweit S, Maksimovic R, et al. Pericardial cytokines in neoplastic, autoreactive and viral pericarditis. Heart Fail Rev 2013;18:345–53.

47. Kanaganayagam GS, Ngo AT, Alsafi A, et al. CT coronary angiography in the investigation of chest pain—beyond coronary artery atherosclerosis: a pictorial review. Int J Cardiol 2014;176:618–29.

48. Verhaert D, Gabriel RS, Johnston D, et al. The role of multimodality imaging in the management of pericardial disease. Circ Cardiovasc Imaging 2010;3:333–43.

49. Fowler NO, Harbin AD 3rd. Recurrent acute pericarditis: follow-up study of 31 patients. J Am Coll Cardiol 1986;7:300–5.

50. Imazio M, Bobbio M, Cecchi E, et al. Colchicine in addition to conventional therapy for acute pericarditis: results of the Colchicine for Acute Pericarditis (COPE) trial. Circulation 2005;112:2012–6.

51. Soler-soler J, Sagrista-Sauleda J, Permanyer-Miralda G. Relapsing pericarditis. Heart 2004;90:1364–8.

52. Troughton RW, Asher CR, Klein AL. Pericarditis. Lancet 2004;363:717–27.

53. Hakim JG, Ternouth I, Mushangi E, et al. Double blind randomised placebo controlled trial of adjunctive prednisolone in the treatment of effusive tuberculous pericarditis in HIV seropositive patients. Heart 2000;84:183–8.

54. Durakovic Z, Misigoj Durakovic M, Skavic J, et al. Myopericarditis and sudden cardiac death due to physical exercise in male athletes. Coll Anthropol 2008;32:399–401.

55. Imazio M, Brucato A, Ferrazzi P, et al. Colchicine for prevention of postpericardiotomy syndrome and postoperative atrial fibrillation: the COPPS-2 randomised clinical trial. JAMA 2014;312:1016–23.

56. Imazio M, Brucato A, Mestroni S, et al. Risk of constrictive pericarditis after acute pericarditis. Circulation 2011;124:1270–5.

57. Braunwald E, Zipes DP, Libby P, et al. Pericardial diseases. In: Khan MG, editor. Heart disease: a textbook of cardiovascular medicine. 6th edition. Philadelphia: Saunders; 2001. p. 1823–76.

58. Spodick DH. Diagnostic electrocardiographic sequences in acute pericarditis. Significance of PR segment and PR vector changes. Circulation 1973;48:575–80.

59. Khandaker MH, Espinosa RE, Nishimura RA, et al. Pericardial disease: diagnosis and management. Mayo Clin Proc 2010;85:572–93.

60. Ginzton LE, Laks MM. The differential diagnosis of acute pericarditis from the normal variant: new electrocardiographic criteria. Circulation 1982;65:1004–9.

61. Bhardwaj R, Berzingi C, Miller C, et al. Differential diagnosis of acute pericarditis from normal variant early repolarisation and left ventricular hypertrophy with early repolarisation: an electrocardiographic study. Am J Med Sci 2013;345:28–32.

62. James TN. Pericarditis and the sinus node. Arch Intern Med 1962;110:305–11.

63. Le Kieffre J, Medvedowsky JL, Thery C. Le node sinusale normale et pathologie. Rueil-Malmaison (France): Sandoz ed; 1979. p. 162.

64. Lee WS, Lee KJ, Kwon JE, et al. Acute viral myopericarditis presenting as a transient effusive constrictive pericarditis caused by coinfection with coxsackieviruses A4 and B3. Korean J Intern Med 2012;27:216–20.

65. De A, Myridakis D, Kerrigan M, et al. Varicella myopericaeditis mimicking myocardial infarction in a 17 year old boy. Tex Heart Inst J 2011;38:288–90.

66. Morita H, Kitaura Y, Deguchi H, et al. Coxsackie B5 myopericarditis in a young adult—clinical course and endomyocardial biopsy findings. Jpn Circ J 1983;47:1077–83.
67. Biton A, Herman J. Perimyocarditis. Report on an unusual case. Postgrad Med 1989;85:77–80.
68. Ward C. Severe arrhythmias in coxsackievirus B3 myopericarditis. Arch Dis Child 1978;53:174–6.
69. Gosselink AT, Van den Berg MP, Crijns HJ. Acute pericarditis presenting with sinus bradycardia. Int J Cardiol 1997;60:307–10.
70. Dressler W. Sinus tachycardia complicating and outlasting pericarditis. Am Heart J 1966;72:422–3.
71. Kindermann I, Kindermann M, Kandolf R, et al. Predictors of outcome in patients with suspected myocarditis. Circulation 2008;118:639–48.
72. Roubille F, Tournoux F, Roubille C, et al. Management of pericarditis and myocarditis: could heart rate reducing drugs hold a promise? Arch Cardiovasc Dis 2013;106:672–9.
73. Khoueiry Z, Roubille C, Nagot N, et al. Could heart rate play a role in pericardial inflammation? Med Hypotheses 2012;79:512–5.
74. Spodick DH. Frequency of arrhythmias in acute pericarditis determined by Holter monitoring. Am J Cardiol 1984;53:842–5.
75. Leitman M, Tyomkin V, Peleg E, et al. Left ventricular function in acute inflammatory peri-myocardial diseases – new insights and long term follow up. Cardiovasc Ultrasound 2012;10:42.
76. Imazio M, Demichelis B, Parrini I, et al. Day hospital treatment of acute pericarditis: a management program for outpatient therapy. J Am Coll Cardiol 2004;43:1042–6.
77. Imazio M, Brucato A, Barbieri A, et al. Good prognosis for pericarditis with and without myocardial involvement: results from a multicentre, prospective cohort study. Circulation 2013;128:42–9.
78. Ristic AD, Maisch B, Hufnagel G, et al. Arrhythmias in acute pericarditis. An endomyocardial biopsy study. Herz 2000;25:729–33.
79. Tschabrun CM, Haggani HM, Cooper JM, et al. Percutaneous epicardial ventricular tachycardia ablation after non-coronary cardiac surgery or pericarditis. Heart Rhythm 2013;10:165–9.
80. Chevalier P, Scridon A. Ventricular arrhythmias complicating acute myocarditis. E-Journal of the ESC Council for Cardiology Practice 2011;9(26). Available at. http://www.escardio.org/communities/councils/ccp/e-journal/volume9/Pages/Ventricular-arrhythmias-complicating-acute-myocarditis-Chevalier-Scridon.aspx#.VQ8lnOFvLr4. Accessed March 04, 2015.
81. Imazio M, Brucato A, Ferrazzi P, et al. Colchicine reduced postoperative atrial fibrillation: results of the Colchicine for the Prevention of the Postpericardiotomy Syndrome (COPPS) atrial fibrillation substudy. Circulation 2011;124:2290–5.
82. Caforio AL, Pankuweit S, Arbustini E, et al. Current state of knowledge on aetiology, diagnosis, management, and therapy of myocarditis: a position statement of the European Society of Cardiology Working Group on Myocardial and Pericardial Diseases. Eur Heart J 2013;34:2636–48.

# Arrhythmias in Fabry Cardiomyopathy

Deepak Acharya, MD[a],*, Harish Doppalapudi, MD[b], José A. Tallaj, MD[a]

## KEYWORDS

- Fabry disease • Cardiomyopathy • Bradycardia • Tachycardia • Arrhythmia • Pacemaker
- Defibrillator

## KEY POINTS

- Fabry cardiomyopathy is a multisystem disorder with important cardiovascular involvement.
- Arrhythmias can cause significant morbidity and mortality in Fabry disease.
- Fabry disease can be diagnosed by measurement of plasma α-galactosidase A or mutation analysis.
- Specific treatment consists of enzyme replacement with agalsidase alfa or agalsidase beta.
- Arrhythmias in Fabry disease can be treated with device or pharmacologic therapy.

## INTRODUCTION

Anderson-Fabry disease (FD) is a multisystem disorder caused by the deficiency of α-galactosidase A, which leads to abnormal lysosomal accumulation of glycolipids. It is the second most common lysosomal storage disease, after Gaucher's disease. It is an X-linked disorder, but females can also be affected because of random X chromosome inactivation. Clinical findings include angiokeratomas, neuropathy, gastrointestinal symptoms, renal failure, stroke, and cardiovascular disease. Women typically have later onset, fewer symptoms, and slower progression than men. Life expectancy is decreased by 20 years in men and 10 to 15 years in women, and the principal cause of death is renal failure followed by cardiac and cerebrovascular causes.[1,2] Treatment involves enzyme replacement therapy (ERT) with agalsidase alfa or agalsidase beta. Early treatment leads to improved clinical outcomes.

## CARDIOVASCULAR MANIFESTATIONS

Left ventricular hypertrophy is the most common cardiac manifestation (**Figs. 1–3**).[3] The hypertrophy can be related to abnormal lysosomal storage and myocyte hypertrophy and fibrosis.[4] The hypertrophy can be so severe that it resembles hypertrophic cardiomyopathy. In fact, 1% to 6% of patients presenting with hypertrophic cardiomyopathy may have FD by genetic analysis.[5,6] Coronary and cerebrovascular disease and microvascular dysfunction may be present. Valvular regurgitation is frequently observed by echocardiogram but typically not clinically significant.[5] Patients can present with angina, myocardial infarction, palpitations, syncope, and heart failure.[6] Hypertrophy is usually the primary cardiac presentation in women. However, women in particular can have fibrosis without hypertrophy.[7] Arrhythmias are important causes of morbidity and mortality in FD and are the focus of this article.

## ELECTROCARDIOGRAPHIC FINDINGS

The first electrocardiographic descriptions in FD were those of abbreviated PR intervals.[8,9] Subsequent series described short PR intervals and atrioventricular (AV) block, sinus node dysfunction,

The authors have nothing to disclose.
[a] Section of Advanced Heart Failure and Transplant Cardiology, Division of Cardiovascular Diseases, University of Alabama at Birmingham, 1900 University Boulevard, THT 321, Birmingham, AL 35294, USA; [b] Section of Electrophysiology, Division of Cardiovascular Diseases, University of Alabama at Birmingham, Faculty Office Tower, Room 930, 1530 3rd Avenue South, Birmingham, AL 35294-3400, USA
* Corresponding author.
E-mail address: dacharya@uab.edu

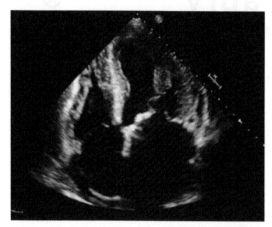

**Fig. 1.** Apical 4-chamber view of a patient with FD shows hypertrophied right and left ventricles and biatrial enlargement.

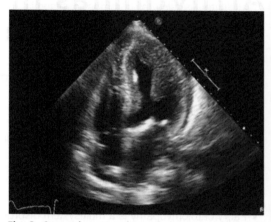

**Fig. 3.** Severe hypertrophy and narrowing of the LV outflow tract in a man with FD.

intraventricular conduction delay, right bundle branch block, atrial enlargement, left ventricular (LV) hypertrophy, and ST-T changes (**Fig. 4**).[10–13] Short PR intervals and ST-T changes can be restored to normal with enzyme replacement therapy.[14,15] In a study of 207 patients with FD, PR interval shortening was found in 14% and AV block in 1.4%.[16] In another study of 30 patients with FD compared with controls, P wave duration, PR interval, and QRS width are shorter in patients with FD.[17] In a cross-sectional study of 150 patients with FD, there was a positive correlation between LV mass on cardiovascular magnetic resonance and QRS duration and the Sokolow index for left ventricular hypertrophy (LVH) on electrocardiogram, and the absence of ST or T alterations on electrocardiogram excluded late enhancement on cardiovascular magnetic resonance.[18]

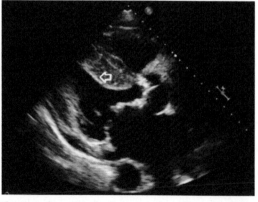

**Fig. 2.** Left ventricular hypertrophy with a characteristic endocardial stripe (*arrow*) and thinning of the basal posterolateral wall in an FD patient.

## BRADYCARDIA

Patients with FD can have sinus node dysfunction, AV nodal disease, or His-Purkinje system disease. Sinus bradycardia may be poorly responsive to atropine.[19] AV conduction abnormalities can occur without other cardiovascular manifestations and may be related to infiltration of the conduction system.[19,20] A longitudinal study of 204 patients with FD showed that QRS duration and PR interval duration increased with age and were independent future predictors of need for pacemaker.[21] Patients who have pacemakers and defibrillators have high utilization of pacing in atria and ventricles.[22]

## TACHYCARDIA

A longitudinal study of arrhythmias in FD followed up with 78 patients for 1.9 years. There was 1 sudden death, 4 patients received pacemakers, and 1 patient received a biventricular implantable cardioverter defibrillator (ICD). Of the 60 patients in this cohort who underwent Holter monitoring, 3.9% had persistent atrial fibrillation, 13.3% had paroxysmal atrial fibrillation, and 8.3% had nonsustained ventricular tachycardia. Age was an independent predictor of atrial fibrillation.[23] A review of the 1448 untreated patients with FD showed a 13% incidence of ventricular arrhythmias in men and 20% in women, highlighting the significant arrhythmic risk in women.[24] Clinically significant ventricular tachycardia, ventricular fibrillation, atrial tachycardia, atrial flutter, and supraventricular tachycardia have all been described in individual cases and series.[25–28] In a long-term study of 40 patients, 6 patients had sudden cardiac death (SCD), and these patients all had previously documented ventricular tachycardia and fibrosis.[29] We follow more than 30 patients in our FD Clinic, most of who are on enzyme replacement therapy. The incidence of ventricular arrhythmias in these patients is low, but the incidence of bradycardia and AV block and need for pacemaker are high. This observation suggests that enzyme replacement may decrease the risk of ventricular arrhythmias.

## ELECTROPHYSIOLOGIC FINDINGS AND PATHOPHYSIOLOGY

Little has been published on electrophysiologic study (EPS) findings in FD. EPS findings in patients with short PR intervals have shown short AH and HV intervals in the absence of accessory pathways (bypass tracts).[9,30,31] Although there is at least 1 case report of a patient with multiple bypass tracts,[32] most studies find no evidence of bypass tracts by mapping or para-Hisian pacing.[31,33] This finding suggests that enhanced AV conduction (through the AV node or His-Purkinje system) rather than ventricular pre-excitation is the most likely cause of the short PR intervals. Enhanced conduction could be caused by deposition of glycosphingolipids in the AV node (resulting in a short AH interval) or in the distal conduction system (resulting in a short HV interval). The normalization of PR intervals with enzyme replacement therapy is also consistent with this hypothesis.[34]

Progressive infiltration of the conduction system and fibrosis seems to be responsible for the conduction abnormalities seen in later stages of the disease, such as sinus node dysfunction, AV block, and bundle branch block.[20]

Various mechanisms have been proposed for atrial fibrillation including infiltration and fibrosis of the atrial myocardium and diastolic dysfunction caused by hypertrophy and fibrosis of the ventricular myocardium.[23]

Abnormalities demonstrated in FD patients with ventricular ectopy and nonsustained and sustained VT include infiltration of the cardiac conduction tissue, myocardial hypertrophy, localized fibrosis, and, in the later stages, severe LV dysfunction with diffuse fibrosis. The major mechanism of sustained VT in FD appears to be reentry related to myocardial fibrosis. Although diffuse myocardial hypertrophy is the characteristic finding in FD, localized thinning and fibrosis, typically of the basal posterior or lateral wall, has been described.[35] Voltage mapping in one patient with recurrent VT found fractionated electrograms in the epicardial lateral wall, and activation mapping found a re-entrant circuit in the lateral wall (**Fig. 5**).[36] Another patient with asymptomatic nonsustained ventricular tachycardia had abnormal fractionation of the ventricular electrograms but no inducible arrhythmia or conduction abnormality.[37] The utility of programmed ventricular stimulation in predicting risk of SCD in FD is unknown.

## DIAGNOSIS

A high index of suspicion is necessary for the diagnosis of FD. An electrophysiologist may encounter undiagnosed FD when evaluating a patient for a pacemaker, ICD, or ablation. Left ventricular hypertrophy without risk factors, such as hypertension, particularly in a patient with significant renal, neurologic, or gastrointestinal symptoms, should raise concern for FD. Echocardiogram can show LVH, sometimes with thinning of the base of the LV posterior wall or a prominent endocardial stripe (see **Figs. 1–3**).[38] Electrocardiographic findings are not specific, but the combination of a short PR interval with LVH should raise suspicion for FD and other storage disorders. Cardiovascular MRI can show hypertrophy, fibrosis, and reduced noncontrast myocardial T1 values. Basal inferolateral hyperenhancement sparing the subendocardium and reduced myocardial noncontrast T1 values may be specific to FD and assist in differentiation from other hypertrophic cardiomyopathies.[39] Endomyocardial biopsy is seldom necessary, but it has a role in the decision to institute ERT in women who do not otherwise have indications (eg, renal involvement) for ERT. The myocardial biopsy can show osmiophilic bodies on electron microscopy and dense cytoplasmic inclusion bodies by light microscopy (**Fig. 6**).[40,41] Diagnosis of FD is made by measurement of α-galactosidase A in leukocytes or plasma in men and by mutation analysis of the α-galactosidase A in women. **Table 1** outlines the cardiac follow-up that we use in our patients with documented FD.

## TREATMENT

The cornerstone of treatment for FD is ERT with agalsidase alfa or beta. ERT has been found to clear globotriaosylceramide from tissues, improve renal function, relieve neuropathic pain, improve cardiovascular conduction, reduce LV mass, decrease diastolic dysfunction, and improve systolic function.[6,34,42–47] Response to ERT can be dramatic, and patients with New York Heart Association (NYHA) IV listed for heart transplant have improved to NYHA I with normal LV ejection fraction with 2 years of treatment.[34] In general, early treatment leads to the best responses to ERT, and patients treated late in the course of disease may progress

**A**

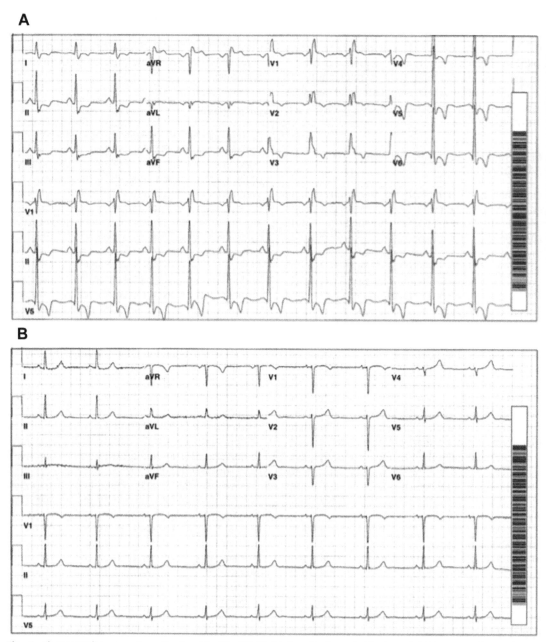

**B**

**Fig. 4.** Electrocardiograms in patients with FD. (*A*) Right bundle branch block and LV hypertrophy with ST-T changes. (*B*) Sinus bradycardia in an asymptomatic patient.

toward organ failure and death, underscoring the need for timely diagnosis.[29] Given the utility of ERT, it is crucial to consider FD in otherwise unexplained LV hypertrophy, as the efficacy of electrophysiologic treatments will be limited if the underlying disease process remains untreated.

There are no large-scale trials of other medical therapies, and recommendations for treatment are derived from individual experiences, published case reports, case series, and consensus recommendations. There may be significant practice variations across centers and countries. Patients with heart failure are treated with angiotensin-converting enzyme inhibitors and diuretics. Beta-blockers may be useful for heart failure and tachyarrhythmias, but caution is advised in patients who do not have pacemakers, as it may precipitate further conduction abnormalities.

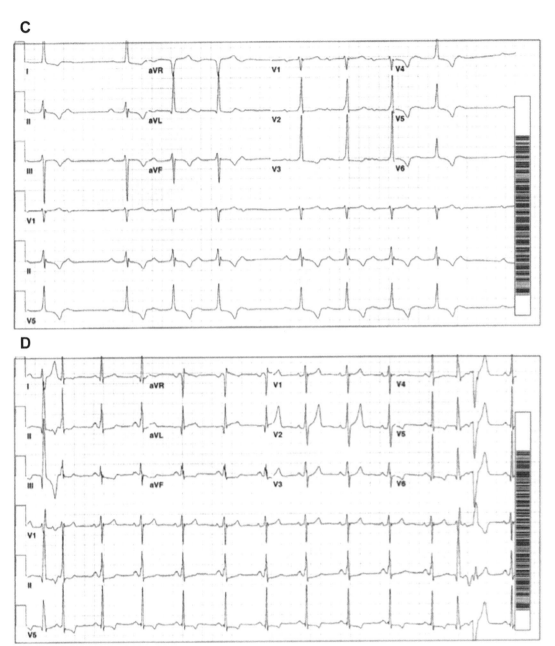

**Fig. 4.** (*continued*). (*C*) Mobitz I AV block in an asymptomatic patient. (*D*) ST-T wave changes and premature ventricular complexes.

Coronary artery disease is treated along standard guidelines. LV outflow tract obstruction, if severe and refractory to medications and pacing, can be treated with alcohol ablation or myomectomy. Patients with advanced disease may be considered for transplantation in selected cases.

Bradycardia and heart block are important sources of morbidity and may contribute to sudden death. Symptomatic bradycardia or asymptomatic patients with progressive conduction system abnormalities, intermittent AV block, or significant bradycardia should be treated with a pacemaker. Holter monitoring can provide some guidance in detecting high-risk asymptomatic patients (**Fig. 7**). If significant LV systolic dysfunction is present and pacing requirements are expected to be significant, biventricular pacing should be considered. It has been the practice of the authors

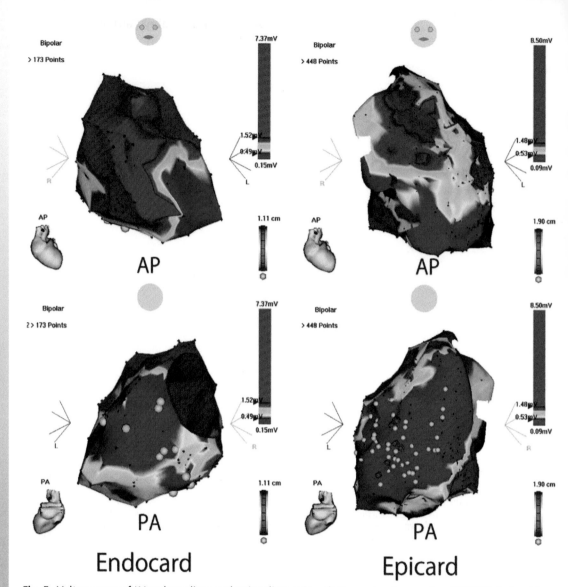

Bipolar

> 173 Points

7.37mV

1.52mV
0.49mV
0.15mV

1.11 cm

AP

Bipolar

> 448 Points

8.50mV

1.48mV
0.53mV
0.09mV

1.90 cm

AP

Bipolar

?> 173 Points

7.37mV

1.52mV
0.49mV
0.15mV

1.11 cm

PA

Bipolar

> 448 Points

8.50mV

1.48mV
0.53mV
0.09mV

1.90 cm

PA

Endocard

Epicard

**Fig. 5.** Voltage map of LV endocardium and epicardium using electroanatomic mapping (CARTO) during biventricular pacing. A low-amplitude area was seen on the lateral wall during endocardial and epicardial mapping. Fractionated electrograms, late potentials (*pink dots*), and dense scar (*gray dots*) were predominantly recorded at the epicardial site. AP, anteroposterior; PA, posteroanterior. (*From* Higashi H, Yamagata K, Noda T, et al. Endocardial and epicardial substrates of ventricular tachycardia in a patient with Fabry disease. Heart Rhythm 2011;8(1):134; with permission.)

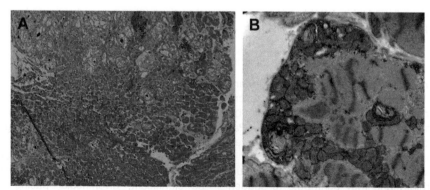

**Fig. 6.** (*A*) Endomyocardial biopsy specimen shows vacuolated myocytes. (*B*) Electron microscopy shows lamellar bodies typical of FD.

**Table 1**
**Example of routine follow-up testing in patients with Fabry cardiomyopathy**

| Recommended Test(s) | Frequency | Reason |
|---|---|---|
| Electrocardiogram | Yearly | Evaluation of the conduction system, bradycardia |
| Holter | Yearly | Evaluation of asymptomatic bradycardia, chronotropic incompetence, and asymptomatic ventricular tachycardia |
| Echocardiogram | Yearly | Evaluation of LVH, valvular heart disease, LV function |
| Myocardial perfusion imaging | At diagnosis and based on symptoms | Evaluation of coronary artery disease |

to implant defibrillators in FD patients who have an indication for pacing.

Atrial fibrillation and flutter can be treated with antiarrhythmics or ablation in conjunction with anticoagulation. Short PR intervals typically seem to be related to enhanced conduction through the AV node or His-Purkinje system and can normalize with enzyme replacement therapy, but an EPS may be considered if there is a high suspicion for an accessory pathway.

There are no international guidelines for device therapy specific to FD. The European Society of Cardiology Guidelines for Hypertrophic Cardiomyopathy include FD, with the explicitly stated caveat

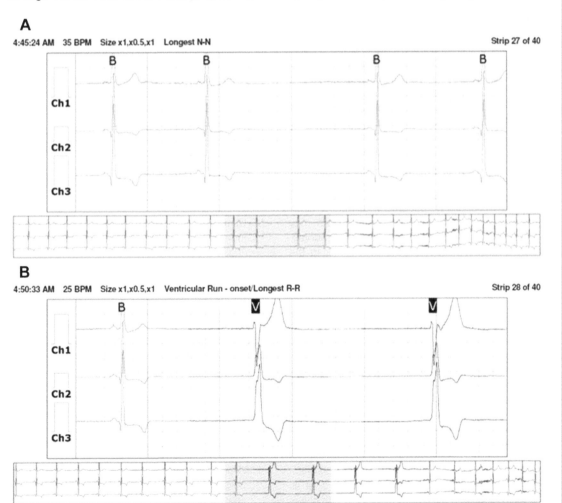

**Fig. 7.** (A) Holter monitor tracing in a patient with FD with sinus node dysfunction. (B) Holter monitor tracing in the same patient as in 7A shows sinus arrest and ventricular escape rhythm.

that there are no randomized trials or validated prediction models to guide ICD implantation.[48] FD patients with documented sustained ventricular tachyarrhythmias or cardiac arrest should receive ICDs for secondary prevention of SCD. Antiarrhythmic drugs or catheter ablation are useful adjuncts for patients with recurrent VT or ICD therapies. Patients with FD with LVEF less than 35% (like all such patients with any nonischemic cardiomyopathy) should be offered ICDs for primary prophylaxis against SCD. Patients with unexplained syncope, especially those who have any LV dysfunction or significant LVH, may have had ventricular arrhythmias or bradycardia and are most appropriately managed with a defibrillator. In the absence of clinical symptoms, identification of patients who would benefit from ICDs for primary prevention is challenging, with little guidance from published reports or guidelines. The ESC guidelines for hypertrophic cardiomyopathy have developed an SCD risk score to guide ICD implantation but specifically state that this score should not be used for infiltrative diseases such as FD.[48] Patients who have significant fibrosis on MRI and those who have nonsustained ventricular tachycardia on Holter monitoring are at higher risk for arrhythmic complications and may be considered for defibrillators.[49] EPS can be considered for risk stratification in such patients with high-risk features (syncope, fibrosis on imaging, nonsustained ventricular tachycardia) and mild to moderate LV dysfunction. The role of EPS to detect inducible arrhythmias, and how this relates to subsequent clinically significant arrhythmias, is not well known. Similarly, patients with family members who have had sudden cardiac death may be at higher risk for arrhythmias, and close surveillance is required, but their individual risk in the setting of ERT has not been well established.

# REFERENCES

1. MacDermot KD, Holmes A, Miners AH. Anderson-Fabry disease: clinical manifestations and impact of disease in a cohort of 60 obligate carrier females. J Med Genet 2001;38(11):769–75.
2. MacDermot KD, Holmes A, Miners AH. Anderson-Fabry disease: clinical manifestations and impact of disease in a cohort of 98 hemizygous males. J Med Genet 2001;38(11):750–60.
3. O'Mahony C, Elliott P. Anderson-Fabry disease and the heart. Prog Cardiovasc Dis 2010;52(4):326–35.
4. Weidemann F, Sanchez-Niño MD, Politei J, et al. Fibrosis: a key feature of Fabry disease with potential therapeutic implications. Orphanet J Rare Dis 2013;8:116.
5. Weidemann F, Strotmann JM, Niemann M, et al. Heart valve involvement in Fabry cardiomyopathy. Ultrasound Med Biol 2009;35(5):730–5.
6. Pierre-Louis B, Kumar A, Frishman WH. Fabry disease: cardiac manifestations and therapeutic options. Cardiol Rev 2009;17(1):31–5.
7. Niemann M, Herrmann S, Hu K, et al. Differences in Fabry cardiomyopathy between female and male patients: consequences for diagnostic assessment. JACC Cardiovasc Imaging 2011;4(6):592–601.
8. Roudebush CP, Foerster JM, Bing OH. The abbreviated PR interval of Fabry's disease. N Engl J Med 1973;289(7):357–8.
9. Rowe JW, Caralis DG. Accelerated atrioventricular conduction in Fabry's disease: a case report. Angiology 1978;29(7):562–8.
10. Mehta J, Tuna N, Moller JH, et al. Electrocardiographic and vectorcardiographic observations in Fabry's disease. Adv Cardiol 1978;21:220–2.
11. Sheth KJ, Thomas JP Jr. Electrocardiograms in Fabry's disease. J Electrocardiol 1982;15(2):153–6.
12. Suzuki M, Goto T, Kato R, et al. Combined atrioventricular block and sinus node dysfunction in Fabry's disease. Am Heart J 1990;120(2):438–40.
13. Doi Y, Toda G, Yano K. Sisters with atypical Fabry's disease with complete atrioventricular block. Heart 2003;89(1):e2.
14. Waldek S. PR interval and the response to enzyme-replacement therapy for Fabry's disease. N Engl J Med 2003;348(12):1186–7.
15. Prinz C, Farr M, Hering D, et al. Reduction in ECG abnormalities and improvement of regional left ventricular function in a patient with Fabry's disease during enzyme-replacement therapy. Clin Res Cardiol 2010;99(1):53–5.
16. Namdar M, Kampmann C, Steffel J, et al. PQ interval in patients with Fabry disease. Am J Cardiol 2010; 105(5):753–6.
17. Namdar M, Steffel J, Vidovic M, et al. Electrocardiographic changes in early recognition of Fabry disease. Heart 2011;97(6):485–90.
18. Niemann M, Hartmann T, Namdar M, et al. Cross-sectional baseline analysis of electrocardiography in a large cohort of patients with untreated Fabry disease. J Inherit Metab Dis 2013;36(5):873–9.
19. Kouris NT, Kontogianni DD, Pavlou MT, et al. Atrioventricular conduction disturbances in a young patient with Fabry's disease without other signs of cardiac involvement. Int J Cardiol 2005;99(2):327–8.
20. Ikari Y, Kuwako K, Yamaguchi T. Fabry's disease with complete atrioventricular block: histological evidence of involvement of the conduction system. Br Heart J 1992;68(3):323–5.
21. O'Mahony C, Coats C, Cardona M, et al. Incidence and predictors of anti-bradycardia pacing in patients with Anderson-Fabry disease. Europace 2011;13(12):1781–8.

22. Acharya D, Robertson P, Kay GN, et al. Arrhythmias in Fabry cardiomyopathy. Clin Cardiol 2012;35(12): 738–40.

23. Shah JS, Hughes DA, Sachdev B, et al. Prevalence and clinical significance of cardiac arrhythmia in Anderson-Fabry disease. Am J Cardiol 2005;96(6): 842–6.

24. Pinderski LJ, Strotmann J. Congestive heart failure in Fabry cardiomyopathy: natural history experience in an international cohort of 1,448 patients. J Heart Lung Transpl 2006;25(2):S70.

25. Efthimiou J, McLelland J, Betteridge DJ. Short PR intervals and tachyarrhythmias in Fabry's disease. Postgrad Med J 1986;62(726):285–7.

26. Chimenti C, Russo MA, Frustaci A. Atrial biopsy evidence of Fabry disease causing lone atrial fibrillation. Heart 2010;96(21):1782–3.

27. Frustaci A, Chimenti C. Images in cardiovascular medicine. Cryptogenic ventricular arrhythmias and sudden death by Fabry disease: prominent infiltration of cardiac conduction tissue. Circulation 2007; 116(12):e350–1.

28. Fukuzawa K, Yoshida A, Onishi T, et al. Dilated phase of hypertrophic cardiomyopathy caused by Fabry disease with atrial flutter and ventricular tachycardia. J Cardiol 2009;54(1):139–43.

29. Weidemann F, Niemann M, Störk S, et al. Long-term outcome of enzyme-replacement therapy in advanced Fabry disease: evidence for disease progression towards serious complications. J Intern Med 2013; 274(4):331–41.

30. Pochis WT, Litzow JT, King BG, et al. Electrophysiologic findings in Fabry's disease with a short PR interval. Am J Cardiol 1994;74(2):203–4.

31. Jastrzebski M, Bacior B, Dimitrow PP, et al. Electrophysiological study in a patient with Fabry disease and a short PQ interval. Europace 2006;8(12): 1045–7.

32. Omar AR, Harris L, Cameron DA, et al. WPW and Fabry's disease: evidence foratrioventricular and atriohisian accessory pathway conduction. Heart Rhythm 2006;3:5S.

33. Aryana A, Fifer MA, Ruskin JN, et al. Short PR interval in the absence of preexcitation: a characteristic finding in a patient with Fabry disease. Pacing Clin Electrophysiol 2008;31(6):782–3.

34. Frustaci A, Chimenti C, Ricci R, et al. Improvement in cardiac function in the cardiac variant of Fabry's disease with galactose-infusion therapy. N Engl J Med 2001;345(1):25–32.

35. Moon JC, Sachdev B, Elkington AG, et al. Gadolinium enhanced cardiovascular magnetic resonance in Anderson-Fabry disease. Evidence for a disease specific abnormality of the myocardial interstitium. Eur Heart J 2003;24(23):2151–5.

36. Higashi H, Yamagata K, Noda T, et al. Endocardial and epicardial substrates of ventricular tachycardia in a patient with Fabry disease. Heart Rhythm 2011; 8(1):133–6.

37. Li J, Warth A, Schnabel P, et al. Electrophysiological findings in Fabry cardiomyopathy: mapping the maze of risk stratification. Acta Cardiol 2012;67(4): 481–5.

38. Takenaka T, Teraguchi H, Yoshida A, et al. Terminal stage cardiac findings in patients with cardiac Fabry disease: an electrocardiographic, echocardiographic, and autopsy study. J Cardiol 2008;51(1):50–9.

39. Thompson RB, Chow K, Khan A, et al. T(1) mapping with cardiovascular MRI is highly sensitive for Fabry disease independent of hypertrophy and sex. Circ Cardiovasc Imaging 2013;6(5):637–45.

40. Gambarin FI, Disabella E, Narula J, et al. When should cardiologists suspect Anderson-Fabry disease? Am J Cardiol 2010;106(10):1492–9.

41. Thurberg BL, Fallon JT, Mitchell R, et al. Cardiac microvascular pathology in Fabry disease: evaluation of endomyocardial biopsies before and after enzyme replacement therapy. Circulation 2009; 119(19):2561–7.

42. Schiffmann R, Kopp JB, Austin HA 3rd, et al. Enzyme replacement therapy in Fabry disease: a randomized controlled trial. JAMA 2001;285(21):2743–9.

43. Eng CM, Guffon N, Wilcox WR, et al. Safety and efficacy of recombinant human alpha-galactosidase A–replacement therapy in Fabry's disease. N Engl J Med 2001;345(1):9–16.

44. Spinelli L, Pisani A, Sabbatini M, et al. Enzyme replacement therapy with agalsidase beta improves cardiac involvement in Fabry's disease. Clin Genet 2004;66(2):158–65.

45. Hughes DA, Elliott PM, Shah J, et al. Effects of enzyme replacement therapy on the cardiomyopathy of Anderson-Fabry disease: a randomised, double-blind, placebo-controlled clinical trial of agalsidase alfa. Heart 2008;94(2):153–8.

46. Germain DP, Weidemann F, Abiose A, et al. Analysis of left ventricular mass in untreated men and in men treated with agalsidase-beta: data from the Fabry Registry. Genet Med 2013;15(12):958–65.

47. Weidemann F, Breunig F, Beer M, et al. Improvement of cardiac function during enzyme replacement therapy in patients with Fabry disease: a prospective strain rate imaging study. Circulation 2003;108(11):1299–301.

48. Authors/Task Force Members, Elliott PM, Anastasakis A, et al. 2014 ESC Guidelines on diagnosis and management of hypertrophic cardiomyopathy: the Task Force for the Diagnosis and Management of Hypertrophic Cardiomyopathy of the European Society of Cardiology (ESC). Eur Heart J 2014;35(39):2733–79.

49. Kramer J, Niemann M, Störk S, et al. Relation of burden of myocardial fibrosis to malignant ventricular arrhythmias and outcomes in Fabry disease. Am J Cardiol 2014;114(6):895–900.

# Mitochondrial Cardiomyopathy and Related Arrhythmias

David Montaigne, MD, PhD[a,b,c],*, Anju Duva Pentiah, MD[c,d]

## KEYWORDS

- Mitochondrial cardiomyopathy • Mitochondrial syndrome • Mitochondrial DNA mutation
- Diabetic cardiomyopathy • Arrhythmia mechanisms • Arrhythmia management

## KEY POINTS

- Inherited mitochondrial cardiomyopathy results from a mutation of the mitochondrial DNA, most often on a maternal inheritance pattern, and commonly shows multisystemic dysfunction, that is, mitochondrial syndromes.
- Mitochondrial cardiomyopathy commonly presents as nonobstructive symmetric left ventricular (LV) hypertrophy and more rarely as dilated cardiomyopathy with systolic dysfunction, the latter most often being a complication of the former phenotype called the burn-out form.
- Atrioventricular (AV) block and supraventricular arrhythmias associated with pre-excitation syndrome are the most common rhythmic issues in mitochondrial disease, irrespective of the phenotype.
- Progressive and unpredictable hallmarks of AV block prompt prophylactic cardiac pacing device implantation even on early occurrence of conduction disorders in asymptomatic patients.
- Incidence of ventricular arrhythmia depends on the cardiomyopathy phenotype rather than on its mitochondrial origin.

## INTRODUCTION

Mitochondria have emerged as a key actor in arrhythmogenesis, apart from their core role in cardiomyocyte energetic homeostasis and life/death pathways. Basic laboratory studies pointed out mitochondria-related modulations of electrophysiological and calcium cycling properties of cardiomyocyte in both physiologic and pathologic situations.

After being first reported 30 years ago in encephalomyopathy,[1,2] mutations in mitochondrial DNA responsible for mitochondrial respiratory chain disorders have been proved a rare but classic cause of inherited cardiomyopathy, presenting with associated multisystem disorders in mitochondrial syndrome and a specific mode of inheritance. Mitochondrial dysfunction has been involved in acquired cardiomyopathy, such as ischemic or diabetic cardiomyopathies, and their related arrhythmias, opening a new area for promising mitochondria-targeted drugs.

This article briefly discusses the basics of mitochondrial physiology and details the mechanisms underlying mitochondrial function and arrhythmia. The clinical spectrum of inherited and acquired cardiomyopathies associated with mitochondrial dysfunction is discussed, followed by the general

The authors have nothing to disclose.
[a] Lille University, Inserm U1011, European Genomic Institute for Diabetes, Place de Verdun-amphi J&K, Lille F-59045, France; [b] Institut Pasteur de Lille, Boulevard Louis XV, Lille F-59019, France; [c] Cardiovascular Explorations Department, University Hospital of Lille, Lille F-59000, France; [d] Division of Cardiomyopathy, Department of Cardiology, University Hospital of Lille, Rue du Pr Laguesse, Lille F-59000, France
* Corresponding author. Cardiovascular Explorations Depatment, Hôpital Cardiologique-CHRU Lille, Rue du Pr Laguesse, Lille F-59000, France. Lille F-59000, France.
E-mail address: david.montaigne@chru-lille.fr

aspects of the management of mitochondrial cardiomyopathy and related arrhythmia.

## MITOCHONDRIAL PHYSIOLOGY

Mitochondria are subcellular organelles that play an important role in most cellular biological processes. The following are the most critical functions (**Fig. 1**):

- Providing the cell with a constant and adaptive amount of energy in synthesizing ATP through oxidative phosphorylation by the respiratory chain complexes
- Dealing with cellular reactive oxygen species (ROS), which are mainly by-products of mitochondrial respiration that can lead to cell death signaling activation
- Participating in calcium homeostasis through sarcoplasmic reticulum-mitochondria calcium

cross talk, energized mitochondria being able to accumulate calcium

The heart is a tissue with one of the highest rates of energy conversion in the body, critically depending on mitochondrial oxidative phosphorylation as a major source of ATP.[3] Thus, cardiac mitochondria represent a key actor of the biological systems addressed to prevent any mismatch between ATP production and utilization. Therefore, mitochondrial respiratory chain disorders often present with cardiac features.

## MECHANISMS BY WHICH MITOCHONDRIAL DYSFUNCTION CAUSES ARRHYTHMIA

As detailed further, mitochondrial disorders are responsible for contractile cardiac dysfunction and can thus indirectly lead to arrhythmias,

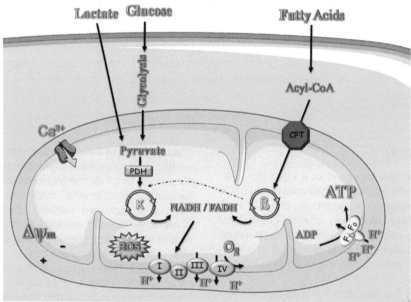

**Fig. 1.** Mitochondrial phosphorylative oxidation. Mitochondrial phosphorylative oxidation takes place along the mitochondrial inner membrane and corresponds to the oxidation of reduced form of nicotinamide adenine dinucleotide (NADH) and flavin adenine dinucleotide (FADH) by oxygen, allowing the synthesis of adenosine triphosphate (ATP). The oxidative process is catalyzed by the 4 respiratory chain complexes (complex I, II, III, and IV), with oxygen as the final electron acceptor at complex IV. Along the oxidoreduction reactions, part of the high redox energy of the electrons from NADH and FADH is turned into an electrochemical gradient of proton across the mitochondrial inner membrane, protons being pumped from the matrix to the intermembrane space by complexes I, III, and IV. Mitochondrial respiration creates a mitochondrial membrane potential ($\Delta\Psi$m), which is the driving force allowing mitochondria to participate to cardiomyocyte calcium homeostasis. The proton gradient is used by the ATP synthase (F1-F0 ATPase) to synthesize the energy-enriched ATP from ADP, a process called phosphorylation. In physiology, oxidation and phosphorylation are coupled. Reactive oxygen species (ROS) are highly reactive compounds harmful when produced in large amounts. Minute amounts of ROS are by-products of normal mitochondrial respiration and are involved in physiologic signaling of cardiomyocyte. Yet, produced in large amounts during mitochondrial dysfunction, ROS activate cardiomyocyte cell death signaling. ß, fatty acid ß-oxidation; CPT, carnitine palmitoyltransferase complex; κ, Krebs cycle; PDH, pyruvate dehydrogenase.

complicating this myocardial remodeling in an unspecific manner.

Evidence for direct involvement of mitochondria in cardiac electrical function has emerged from in vitro studies showing that modulation of the mitochondrial respiration, membrane potential, and ion channels alter action potential genesis and myocardial conduction properties.[4,5]

Almost half of cardiomyocyte ATP consumption is used for ion channels homeostasis, that is, sarcolemmal and sarcoplasmic reticulum pumps and transporters, which is mandatory for proper electrical activity. In conditions of mitochondrial dysfunction or increased metabolic stress such as myocardial ischemia, the resulting loss in mitochondrial membrane potential diminishes ATP synthesis, which readily disrupts the electrical stability by reducing the energy supply to these channels and transporters (**Fig. 2**). Moreover, a decrease in the ATP/ADP ratio results in the opening of the sarcolemmal $K_{ATP}$ channels, which slows electrical propagation by creating current sinks in the myocardium and shortens refractory periods, both promoting arrhythmias.[6–8]

ROS are by-products of mitochondrial respiration, and mitochondria harbor major cellular anti-ROS systems (eg, manganese superoxide dismutase, glutathione peroxidase, glutathione). Mitochondria are thus a master regulator of redox status and signaling in cardiomyocyte. Mitochondrial dysfunction leads to increased ROS production, which has been shown to directly alter cardiomyocyte excitability and cell-to-cell coupling (see **Fig. 2**).[9–11]

The authors' group has demonstrated that preoperative mitochondrial dysfunction of the atrial myocardium is associated with atrial fibrillation occurrence after cardiac surgery, identifying for the first time the mitochondrion as a potential key player in clinically relevant arrhythmia.[12] Along the same line, in a small study, remote ischemic preconditioning has been reported to preserve atrial mitochondrial function during cardiac surgery and decrease postoperative atrial fibrillation incidence in patients.[13] These promising translational data warrant further investigation to explore mitochondria as potential therapeutic target in clinical arrhythmias.

## INHERITED MITOCHONDRIAL CARDIOMYOPATHY
### Mitochondrial Genetics

Mitochondria contain small circular DNAs (mtDNA) that encode for 13 proteins of the respiratory chain complexes, 22 transfer RNAs and 2 ribosomal RNAs, the last 2 being involved in mitochondrial RNA and protein synthesis.[14] The other mitochondrial proteins, nearly a thousand, are encoded by the nuclear DNA and imported into the mitochondria. This bigenomic dependence of mitochondrial proteins gives rise to several noteworthy characteristics of the mitochondrial genetic disorders and related cardiomyopathies.

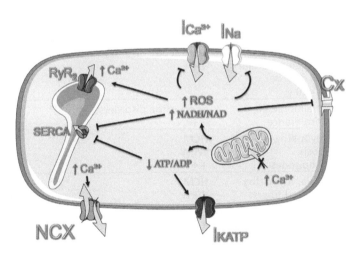

Fig. 2. Mechanisms linking mitochondrial dysfunction and arrhythmia. Mitochondrial dysfunction is responsible for shortening of the action potential as a result of the opening of the sarcolemmal $K_{ATP}$ channel, mediated by a low ATP/ADP ratio and inhibition of the calcium ($ICa^{++}$) and sodium ($INa^{+}$) depolarizing current by redox modifications of their related sarcolemmal channel. Weak $INa^{+}$ current and ROS-induced connexin (Cx) modifications lead to poor cell-to-cell coupling and decreased conduction velocities in the myocardium. Both increased NADH/NAD ratio and ROS production associated with mitochondrial dysfunction modify the ryanodine receptor ($RyR_2$) and sarcoplasmic calcium ATPase (SERCA), responsible for sarcoplasmic calcium leak for the former and incomplete removal of calcium from cytosol during diastole for the latter. In the absence of proper respiratory chain complex function, mitochondrial membrane potential is low and mitochondria unable to participate in cardiomyocyte calcium homeostasis. The resulting elevated diastolic calcium concentration in the cytosol activates the sarcolemmal Na-Ca exchanger (NCX), which is responsible for delayed after-depolarizations (DAD). Shortened action potential, low conduction velocities, and DAD make the myocardium with mitochondrial dysfunction more prone to arrhythmias.

Mitochondria in the embryo derive only from the ovule, as such mtDNA mutations are only transmitted on a maternal inheritance pattern, which is the most frequent inheritance pattern encountered in mitochondrial cardiomyopathy. However, when the mutation concerns a mitochondrial protein encoded by the nuclear DNA, a classic mendelian inheritance pattern is observed.

Each cell contains hundreds of mitochondria and a thousand copies of mtDNA. Mutation in some of these copies is responsible for mitochondrial dysfunction when the proportion of abnormal over normal mitochondria (heteroplasmy) exceeds a threshold beyond which oxidative phosphorylation performance is hampered. Thus, mitochondrial genetic disorders usually present as multisystemic syndromes involving the most energy-demanding organs, that is, the brain, fast-twitch extraocular muscles, heart, retina, auditory cells, and endocrine systems.

Mitochondria are randomly distributed during cell division, and daughter cells can present different degrees of heteroplasmy. This mitotic segregation can explain changes in tissue phenotype during life. Moreover, as mtDNA is continuously replicated, the proportion of mutant mtDNA can increase within the cell, even in postmitotic cells such as cardiomyocytes, underlying clinical progression.

## Clinical Features

As a result of heteroplasmy and mitotic segregation, mutation carriers within a family may be asymptomatic or oligosymptomatic or suffer from severe multisystemic disorders. Cardiac disorders related to inherited mitochondrial deficiency may be isolated, presenting primarily as an isolated cardiomyopathy, or associated with distant organ dysfunction, for example, neuromuscular, endocrine, and neurosensorial disorders. The most common mitochondrial syndromes are described in **Table 1**.[15–27] Poor correlation exists between clinical phenotypes and the mutation variant, even with single gene defects.

The cardiac phenotype associated with genetic mitochondrial dysfunction is unspecific, being hypertrophic or dilated. Conduction disorders and ventricular pre-excitation syndrome are encountered.

### Cardiomyopathy

Few data exist on the incidence of cardiomyopathy in patients displaying mitochondrial respiratory chain disorder. Yet, echocardiographic evidence for cardiomyopathy has been reported

**Table 1**
**Common mitochondrial syndromes**

| Syndrome | Characteristic Disorders | Type & Prevalence of Cardiac Disorders | Reference |
|---|---|---|---|
| Kearns-Sayre syndrome | Retinitis pigmentosa, external ophthalmoplegia, cardiac conduction disorder, onset age <20 y | Conduction disorders +++ | 15,16 |
| Chronic progressive external ophthalmoplegia | Ptosis, ophthalmoplegia, exercise intolerance | Conduction disorders ++ | 17,18 |
| Myopathy, encephalopathy, lactic acidosis, and strokelike episodes | Encephalomyopathy, lactic acidosis, strokelike episodes | HCM WPW ++ | 19,20 |
| Myoclonic epilepsy and ragged red fibers | Seizures, ataxia, myopathy with ragged red fibers | HCM WPW ++ | 21,22 |
| Pearson syndrome | Sideroblastic anemia, exocrine pancreatic dysfunction | + | 23,24 |
| Leigh syndrome | Psychomotor retardation, seizures, ataxia | + | 25,26 |
| Barth syndrome | Myopathy, cardiomyopathy, growth retardation, leucopenia | Dilated cardiomyopathy +++ | 27 |

(+++), high; (++), medium; (+), low prevalence.
*Abbreviations:* HCM, hypertrophic cardiomyopathy; WPW, Wolff-Parkinson-White syndrome.

in at least 25% of those patients in a small study.[28] Cardiomyopathy is thus most probably underdiagnosed rather than truly being rare, and a systematic screening for cardiomyopathy should be done in patients diagnosed for mitochondrial disorders.

Mitochondrial cardiomyopathy commonly presents as hypertrophic cardiomyopathy (HCM), described in up to 40% of patients with myopathy, encephalopathy, lactic acidosis, and strokelike episodes (MELAS) and myoclonic epilepsy and ragged red fibers (MERRF).[28–31] If the echocardiographic aspect may completely mimic the sarcomeric form of HCM, the hypertrophic phenotype observed in mitochondrial diseases is classically concentric without LV outflow tract obstruction and can also involve the right ventricle. Mitochondrial cardiomyopathy presenting as a hypertrophic phenotype is more prone to evolve to the dilated phenotype (dilated cardiomyopathy [DCM]) with associated LV systolic dysfunction than to sarcomeric HCM.[30,32] As such, DCM associated with heart failure in the context of mitochondrial disorders is much more of a poor evolution of the HCM phenotype rather than that of an initial presentation.[22,31,33]

Inherited mitochondrial disorder is also described in LV myocardial noncompaction, which is a rare presentation characterized by persistence of fetal features in the LV responsible for hypertrabeculation of the LV walls; heart failure with systolic dysfunction; arrhythmia, including sudden cardiac death; and systemic embolic events.[34–36]

Finally, few cases of restrictive and histiocytoid cardiomyopathies have been reported in patients with mtDNA mutations.[37,38]

Even if the precise incidence of life-threatening ventricular arrhythmias and end-stage heart failure in patients with mitochondrial cardiomyopathy is unknown, cardiac presentation is associated with a significant deleterious survival rate. In pediatric populations, patients presenting with cardiomyopathy show a survival rate divided by 3 to 5 compared with those presenting neuromuscular features solely.[31,34]

### Cardiac conduction disorders

Conduction disorders are the main cardiac signs encountered in KKS (Kearns-Sayre Syndrome) and chronic progressive external ophthalmoplegia syndromes.[28,29] They extend from simple PR-interval prolongation to infranodal high-degree AV block. Progression in intraventricular conduction defect is unpredictable and responsible for sudden cardiac death.[39,40] Prophylactic cardiac pacing device implantation is thus generally proposed to prevent cardiac death.[41] In the absence of consistent data regarding the incidence of ventricular arrhythmia in patients with mitochondrial cardiomyopathy, implantable cardiac defibrillator should be proposed according to current guidelines.

### Ventricular pre-excitation syndrome

Prevalence of Wolff-Parkinson-White syndrome among patients with mtDNA mutations is high (up to 15%), specifically in patients with MELAS and MERRF.[22,42]

## Diagnosis Strategy

In cardiac presentations that suggest mitochondriopathy (**Box 1**), both genetic testing and histochemical analysis of biopsied tissue are useful to confirm diagnosis.

Screening mtDNA can be done for the most common mutations, such as those most frequently encountered in Kearns-Sayre syndrome, MERRF, and MELAS. Given the lack of robust association between genotype and phenotype, the impact of genetic testing on clinical management is weak. Yet, identification of causative mutations facilitates presymptomatic diagnosis of family members, allows accurate follow-up, and helps preconception genetic counseling.

Because major challenges remain on making a reliable distinction between pathogenic mutations and benign variants, analysis of muscle biopsy specimen remains the gold standard for mitochondrial disease diagnosis, even if the specificity and sensitivity is not 100% and the technique is performed in few specialized centers. The pathologic hallmark of mtDNA disease in muscle fiber is the subsarcolemmal accumulation of abnormal mitochondria, which stains red with a Gomori trichrome stain (ragged red fibers), and cytochrome c oxidase–deficient fibers.

---

**Box 1**
**Cardiac presentations that suggest mitochondrial cardiomyopathy**

Conduction disorder, pre-excitation syndrome, cardiomyopathy associated with either

- Familial history with maternal inheritance pattern
- Classic mitochondrial syndrome
- Echocardiographic specific features, that is, biventricular hypertrophy and/or nonobstructive left ventricular hypertrophy
- Involvement of many organs, that is, neurosensorial and neurologic symptoms, diabetes
- Lactic acidosis at rest

## ACQUIRED MITOCHONDRIAL CARDIOMYOPATHY

Mitochondrial dysfunction plays a key role in the pathogenesis of ischemia-reperfusion injury. In addition, regardless of the cause, altered mitochondrial bioenergetics seem to play a substantial role in acquired cardiomyopathies as detailed further.

### Mitochondrial Dysfunction in the Failing Human Heart

Studies in rodent models of cardiotoxic agents such as anthracyclines,[43,44] alcohol,[45,46] and heart failure[47,48] have identified intrinsic cardiomyocyte dysfunction secondary to alteration in energy substrate utilization, mitochondrial dysfunction, increased oxidative stress, and mitochondrial-dependant cardiomyocyte death.

In the same line, studies in humans have shown mitochondrial network disorganization[49] and dysfunction as major characteristics of the failing heart of subjects regardless of the cause. Exploration of human failing myocardium clearly showed reduced mitochondrial respiration and increased oxidative stress.[50,51]

Poor mitochondrial function in the failing heart has been consistently described using technetium Tc 99m sestamibi cardiac imaging in patients with dilated and hypertrophic cardiomyopathy.[52–55]

### Diabetic Cardiomyopathy as an Acquired Mitochondrial Cardiomyopathy

Type 2 diabetes mellitus (DM) is an independent risk factor for the development of heart failure.[56,57] Epidemiologic and clinical studies strongly support the existence of obesity and diabetic-related cardiomyopathies irrespective of coronary artery disease, hypertension, or other comorbidities.[58]

Preclinical models of DM have identified mitochondrial dysfunction as responsible for the poor performance of cardiomyocytes and as a potent target to prevent cardiomyopathy in this metabolic disease.[58,59]

Dysregulation of the energy conversion process is a hallmark in the heart of patients with diabetes.[60] Exploration of human diabetic myocardium samples demonstrated reduced mitochondrial respiration, identifying a role for mitochondrial dysfunction in the pathophysiology of heart failure in patients with DM[61]: worsening of intrinsic myocardial contraction in the transition from the prediabetic state to DM has been related to worsening of cardiac mitochondrial function, because impaired mitochondrial function and structure and contractile dysfunction have been observed in diabetic patients but not in patients with early-stage insulin resistance. Besides, hyperglycemia has been hypothesized as a major driver of both mitochondrial dysfunction and mitochondrial fragmentation in the human diabetic heart.

Knowing the link between mitochondria and arrhythmia, mitochondrial dysfunction as described in DM can be responsible for the propensity of the diabetic myocardium to arrhythmia such as atrial fibrillation.

## MANAGEMENT OF MITOCHONDRIAL CARDIOMYOPATHY AND RELATED ARRHYTHMIA

- There is currently no established systemic treatment of mitochondrial disorders, and the clinical management of individuals is largely supportive, the aim being to provide prognostic information and genetic counseling. The common use of antioxidants and respiratory chain substrates and cofactors, such as coenzyme Q10, L-arginine, vitamins, carnitine, and creatinine, has failed to show consistent beneficial effects.[62]
- Conditions responsible for a high metabolic demand (ie, fever, stress) and drugs that potentially interfere with enzymes involved in energetic metabolism (ie, metformin, statins, valproic acid, propofol, erythromycine) should be avoided to prevent acute multiorgan failure secondary to enhanced mitochondrial dysfunction.
- AV block and supraventricular and ventricular arrhythmias are the most common cardiac presentations in patients with mitochondrial disease in association with HCM or not. As a result of lack of data, little evidence exists for a specific treatment of arrhythmia encountered in mitochondrial cardiomyopathy. Therefore, conventional drugs, pacing, and implantable cardioverter defibrillator indications should be applied in most cases.[63–66] Yet, as detailed earlier, knowing the progressive and unpredictable hallmarks of AV block in mitochondrial disorders, prophylactic cardiac pacing implantation is generally proposed on early PR-interval prolongation or bundle branch block even in asymptomatic patients.[41]
- Standard heart failure therapy, including β-blockers, angiotensin-converting enzyme inhibitors, aldosterone blockers, and loop diuretics, is used with success in patients with heart failure.[33] Implantable cardioverter defibrillator should be considered regarding the

standard guidelines for DCM associated with heart failure and for HCM, keeping in mind that life expectancy should be taken in account for these multiorgan disorders. In the same line, cardiac transplantation is controversial in multisystemic diseases but has been performed successfully in patients with mtDNA disease.[67,68]

- A regular cardiac evaluation (clinical examination, electrocardiography, and echocardiography) should be performed in patients diagnosed with mitochondrial syndrome, even in the absence of initial cardiac involvement knowing the progressive nature of mitochondrial disorders.

## SUMMARY

Mitochondrial dysfunction is present in arrhythmogenic cardiac diseases, including inherited and acquired cardiomyopathies. Reduced ATP synthesis and increased ROS production secondary to mitochondrial dysfunction can lead to malfunction of cellular mechanisms involved in maintaining normal electrical functioning and intracellular ionic homeostasis in cardiomyocytes. Because no targeted treatment has been proved useful in the management of mitochondrial cardiomyopathy, conventional treatment of arrhythmia is still the rule.

## REFERENCES

1. Holt IJ, Harding AE, Morgan-Hughes JA. Deletions of muscle mitochondrial DNA in patients with mitochondrial myopathies. Nature 1988;331:717–9.
2. Wallace DC, Singh G, Lott MT, et al. Mitochondrial DNA mutation associated with Leber's hereditary optic neuropathy. Science 1988;242:1427–30.
3. Balaban RS. Perspectives on: SGP symposium on mitochondrial physiology and medicine: metabolic homeostasis of the heart. J Gen Physiol 2012;139:407–14.
4. Brown DA, O'Rourke B. Cardiac mitochondria and arrhythmias. Cardiovasc Res 2010;88:241–9.
5. Jeong EM, Liu M, Sturdy M, et al. Metabolic stress, reactive oxygen species, and arrhythmia. J Mol Cell Cardiol 2012;52:454–63.
6. O'Rourke B, Ramza BM, Marban E. Oscillations of membrane current and excitability driven by metabolic oscillations in heart cells. Science 1994;265:962–6.
7. Zhou L, Solhjoo S, Millare B, et al. Effects of regional mitochondrial depolarization on electrical propagation: implications for arrhythmogenesis. Circ Arrhythm Electrophysiol 2014;7:143–51.
8. Smith RM, Visweswaran R, Talkachova I, et al. Uncoupling the mitochondria facilitates alternans formation in the isolated rabbit heart. Am J Physiol Heart Circ Physiol 2013;305:H9–18.
9. Sovari AA, Rutledge CA, Jeong EM, et al. Mitochondria oxidative stress, connexin 43 remodeling, and sudden arrhythmic death. Circ Arrhythm Electrophysiol 2013;6(3):623–31.
10. Zima AV, Kockskämper J, Mejia-Alvarez R, et al. Pyruvate modulates cardiac sarcoplasmic reticulum Ca2+ release in rats via mitochondria-dependent and -independent mechanisms. J Physiol 2003;550:765–83.
11. Liu M, Liu H, Dudley SC Jr. Reactive oxygen species originating from mitochondria regulate the cardiac sodium channel. Circ Res 2010;107:967–74.
12. Montaigne D, Marechal X, Lefebvre P, et al. Mitochondrial dysfunction as an arrhythmogenic substrate: a translational proof-of-concept study in patients with metabolic syndrome in whom postoperative atrial fibrillation develops. J Am Coll Cardiol 2013;62:1466–73.
13. Slagsvold KH, Rognmo O, Høydal M, et al. Remote ischemic preconditioning preserves mitochondrial function and influences myocardial microRNA expression in atrial myocardium during coronary bypass surgery. Circ Res 2014;114:851–9.
14. DiMauro S, Schon EA. Mitochondrial respiratory-chain diseases. N Engl J Med 2003;348:2656–68.
15. Kearns TP, Sayre GP. Retinitis pigmentosa, external ophthalmophegia, and complete heart block: unusual syndrome with histologic study in one of two cases. AMA Arch Ophthalmol 1958;60:280–9.
16. Polak PE, Zijlstra F, Roelandt JR. Indications for pacemaker implantation in the Kearns-Sayre syndrome. Eur Heart J 1989;10:281–2.
17. Danta G, Hilton RC, Lynch PG. Chronic progressive external ophthalmoplegia. Brain 1975;98:473–92.
18. Galetta F, Franzoni F, Mancuso M, et al. Cardiac involvement in chronic progressive external ophthalmoplegia. J Neurol Sci 2014;345:189–92.
19. Finsterer J. MELAS in the heart. Int J Cardiol 2009;137:e65–6.
20. Fayssoil A. Heart diseases in mitochondrial encephalomyopathy, lactic acidosis, and stroke syndrome. Congest Heart Fail 2009;15:284–7.
21. Mancuso M, Orsucci D, Angelini C, et al. Phenotypic heterogeneity of the 8344A>G mtDNA "MERRF" mutation. Neurology 2013;80:2049–54.
22. Wahbi K, Larue S, Jardel C, et al. Cardiac involvement is frequent in patients with the m.8344A>G mutation of mitochondrial DNA. Neurology 2010;74:674–7.
23. Pearson HA, Lobel JS, Kocoshis SA, et al. A new syndrome of refractory sideroblastic anemia with vacuolization of marrow precursors and exocrine pancreatic dysfunction. J Pediatr 1979;95:976–84.

24. Krauch G, Wilichowski E, Schmidt KG, et al. Pearson marrow-pancreas syndrome with worsening cardiac function caused by pleiotropic rearrangement of mitochondrial DNA. Am J Med Genet 2002;110:57–61.

25. Taylor RW, Turnbull DM. Mitochondrial DNA mutations in human disease. Nat Rev Genet 2005;6: 389–402.

26. Bugiani M, Invernizzi F, Alberio S, et al. Clinical and molecular findings in children with complex I deficiency. Biochim Biophys Acta 2004;1659:136–47.

27. Barth PG, Wanders RJ, Vreken P, et al. X-linked cardioskeletal myopathy and neutropenia (Barth syndrome) (MIM 302060). J Inherit Metab Dis 1999;22: 555–67.

28. Limongelli G, Tome-Esteban M, Dejthevaporn C, et al. Prevalence and natural history of heart disease in adults with primary mitochondrial respiratory chain disease. Eur J Heart Fail 2010;12:114–21.

29. Lev D, Nissenkorn A, Leshinsky-Silver E, et al. Clinical presentations of mitochondrial cardiomyopathies. Pediatr Cardiol 2004;25:443–50.

30. Vydt TC, de Coo RF, Soliman OI, et al. Cardiac involvement in adults with m.3243A>G MELAS gene mutation. Am J Cardiol 2007;99:264–9.

31. Holmgren D, Wåhlander H, Eriksson BO, et al. Cardiomyopathy in children with mitochondrial disease; clinical course and cardiological findings. Eur Heart J 2003;24:280–8.

32. Okajima Y, Tanabe Y, Takayanagi M, et al. A follow-up study of myocardial involvement in patients with mitochondrial encephalomyopathy, lactic acidosis, and stroke-like episodes (MELAS). Heart 1998;80:292–5.

33. Stalder N, Yarol N, Tozzi P, et al. Mitochondrial A3243G mutation with manifestation of acute dilated cardiomyopathy. Circ Heart Fail 2012;5:e1–3.

34. Scaglia F, Towbin JA, Craigen WJ, et al. Clinical spectrum, morbidity, and mortality in 113 pediatric patients with mitochondrial disease. Pediatrics 2004;114:925–31.

35. Stollberger C, Finsterer J, Blazek G. Left ventricular hypertrabeculation/noncompaction and association with additional cardiac abnormalities and neuromuscular disorders. Am J Cardiol 2002;90:899–902.

36. Tang S, Batra A, Zhang Y, et al. Left ventricular noncompaction is associated with mutations in the mitochondrial genome. Mitochondrion 2010;10:350–7.

37. Thebault C, Ollivier R, Leurent G, et al. Mitochondriopathy: a rare aetiology of restrictive cardiomyopathy. Eur J Echocardiogr 2008;9:840–5.

38. Vallance HD, Jeven G, Wallace DC, et al. A case of sporadic infantile histiocytoid cardiomyopathy caused by the A8344G (MERRF) mitochondrial DNA mutation. Pediatr Cardiol 2004;25:538–40.

39. Charles R, Holt S, Kay JM, et al. Myocardial ultrastructure and the development of atrioventricular block in Kearns-Sayre syndrome. Circulation 1981; 63:214–9.

40. Subbiah RN, Kuchar D, Baron D. Torsades de pointes in a patient with Kearns-Sayre syndrome: a fortunate finding. Pacing Clin Electrophysiol 2007; 30:137–9.

41. Young TJ, Shah AK, Lee MH, et al. Kearns-Sayre syndrome: a case report and review of cardiovascular complications. Pacing Clin Electrophysiol 2005; 28:454–7.

42. Sproule DM, Kaufmann P, Engelstad K, et al. Wolff-Parkinson-White syndrome in patients with MELAS. Arch Neurol 2007;64:1625–7.

43. Marechal X, Montaigne D, Marciniak C, et al. Doxorubicin-induced cardiac dysfunction is attenuated by ciclosporin treatment in mice through improvements in mitochondrial bioenergetics. Clin Sci (Lond) 2011;121:405–13.

44. Montaigne D, Hurt C, Neviere R. Mitochondria death/survival signaling pathways in cardiotoxicity induced by anthracyclines and anticancer-targeted therapies. Biochem Res Int 2012;2012:951539.

45. Laurent D, Mathew JE, Mitry M, et al. Chronic ethanol consumption increases myocardial mitochondrial DNA mutations: a potential contribution by mitochondrial topoisomerases. Alcohol Alcohol 2014;49:381–9.

46. Das AM, Harris DA. Regulation of the mitochondrial ATP synthase is defective in rat heart during alcohol-induced cardiomyopathy. Biochim Biophys Acta 1993;1181:295–9.

47. Nakayama H, Chen X, Baines CP, et al. Ca2+- and mitochondrial-dependent cardiomyocyte necrosis as a primary mediator of heart failure. J Clin Invest 2007;117:2431–44.

48. Elrod JW, Wong R, Mishra S, et al. Cyclophilin D controls mitochondrial pore-dependent Ca(2+) exchange, metabolic flexibility, and propensity for heart failure in mice. J Clin Invest 2010;120: 3680–7.

49. Schaper J, Froede R, Hein S, et al. Impairment of the myocardial ultrastructure and changes of the cytoskeleton in dilated cardiomyopathy. Circulation 1991;83:504–14.

50. Lemieux H, Semsroth S, Antretter H, et al. Mitochondrial respiratory control and early defects of oxidative phosphorylation in the failing human heart. Int J Biochem Cell Biol 2011;43:1729–38.

51. Sharov VG, Todor AV, Silverman N, et al. Abnormal mitochondrial respiration in failed human myocardium. J Mol Cell Cardiol 2000;32:2361–7.

52. Matsuo S, Nakae I, Tsutamoto T, et al. A novel clinical indicator using Tc-99m sestamibi for evaluating cardiac mitochondrial function in patients with cardiomyopathies. J Nucl Cardiol 2007;14:215–20.

53. Isobe S, Ohshima S, Unno K, et al. Relation of 99mTc-sestamibi washout with myocardial properties in patients with hypertrophic cardiomyopathy. J Nucl Cardiol 2010;17:1082–90.

54. Shiroodi MK, Shafiei B, Baharfard N, et al. 99mTc-MIBI washout as a complementary factor in the evaluation of idiopathic dilated cardiomyopathy (IDCM) using myocardial perfusion imaging. Int J Cardiovasc Imaging 2012;28:211–7.
55. Hayashi D, Ohshima S, Isobe S, et al. Increased 99mTc-sestamibi washout reflects impaired myocardial contractile and relaxation reserve during dobutamine stress due to mitochondrial dysfunction in dilated cardiomyopathy patients. J Am Coll Cardiol 2013;61:2007–17.
56. Kannel WB, Hjortland M, Castelli WP. Role of DM in congestive heart failure: the Framingham study. Am J Cardiol 1974;34:29–34.
57. Bertoni AG, Tsai A, Kasper EK, et al. DM and idiopathic cardiomyopathy: a nationwide case-control study. Diabetes Care 2003;26:2791–5.
58. Boudina S, Abel ED. Diabetic cardiomyopathy revisited. Circulation 2007;115:3213–23.
59. Lancel S, Montaigne D, Marechal X, et al. Carbon monoxide improves cardiac function and mitochondrial population quality in a mouse model of metabolic syndrome. PLoS One 2012;7:e41836.
60. Scheuermann-Freestone M, Madsen PL, Manners D, et al. Abnormal cardiac and skeletal muscle energy metabolism in patients with type 2 DM. Circulation 2003;107:3040–6.
61. Montaigne D, Marechal X, Coisne A, et al. Myocardial contractile dysfunction is associated with impaired mitochondrial function and dynamics in type 2 diabetic but not in obese patients. Circulation 2014;130:554–64.
62. Pfeffer G, Majamaa K, Turnbull DM, et al. Treatment for mitochondrial disorders. Cochrane Database Syst Rev 2012;(4):CD004426.
63. Elliott PM, Anastasakis A, Borger MA, et al. Authors/Task Force members. 2014 ESC Guidelines on diagnosis and management of hypertrophic cardiomyopathy: The Task Force for the Diagnosis and Management of Hypertrophic Cardiomyopathy of the European Society of Cardiology (ESC). Eur Heart J 2014;35:2733–79.
64. Gersh BJ, Maron BJ, Bonow RO, et al. 2011 ACCF/AHA guideline for the diagnosis and treatment of hypertrophic cardiomyopathy: a report of the American College of Cardiology Foundation/American Heart Association Task Force on Practice Guidelines. Developed in collaboration with the American Association for Thoracic Surgery, American Society of Echocardiography, American Society of Nuclear Cardiology, Heart Failure Society of America, Heart Rhythm Society, Society for Cardiovascular Angiography and Interventions, and Society of Thoracic Surgeons. American College of Cardiology Foundation/American Heart Association Task Force on Practice Guidelines. J Am Coll Cardiol 2011;58:e212–60.
65. Epstein AE, DiMarco JP, Ellenbogen KA, et al. 2012 ACCF/AHA/HRS focused update incorporated into the ACCF/AHA/HRS 2008 guidelines for device-based therapy of cardiac rhythm abnormalities: a report of the American College of Cardiology Foundation/American Heart Association Task Force on Practice Guidelines and the Heart Rhythm Society. J Am Coll Cardiol 2013;61:e6–75.
66. Brignole M, Auricchio A, Baron-Esquivias G, et al. 2013 ESC Guidelines on cardiac pacing and cardiac resynchronization therapy: the Task Force on Cardiac Pacing and Resynchronization Therapy of the European Society of Cardiology (ESC). Developed in collaboration with the European Heart Rhythm Association (EHRA). Eur Heart J 2013;34:2281–329.
67. Bonnet D, Rustin P, Rötig A, et al. Heart transplantation in children with mitochondrial cardiomyopathy. Heart 2001;86:570–3.
68. Schmauss D, Sodian R, Klopstock T, et al. Cardiac transplantation in a 14-yr-old patient with mitochondrial encephalomyopathy. Pediatr Transplant 2007;11:560–2.

# Arrhythmias in the Muscular Dystrophies

Archana Rajdev, MD[a], William J. Groh, MD, MPH[b],*

## KEYWORDS

- Muscular dystrophy • Arrhythmia • Sudden cardiac death • Genetics • Pacemaker
- Implantable cardioverter-defibrillator

## KEY POINTS

- Duchenne, Becker, and limb-girdle 2C-2F and 2I muscular dystrophies frequently develop a dilated cardiomyopathy, which precedes arrhythmia and conduction disturbance. Decision for prophylactic device implant is based on current guidelines for nonischemic cardiomyopathy.
- Myotonic dystrophy, Emery-Dreifuss, and limb-girdle type 1B muscular dystrophies are variably associated with cardiomyopathy and frequently develop conduction disturbances requiring pacing. Recent studies support use of cardioverter-defibrillator rather than pacemakers.
- Fascioscapulohumeral is a common muscular dystrophy, only variably associated with cardiac involvement and arrhythmias.

## INTRODUCTION

The muscular dystrophies are a group of inherited disorders affecting skeletal muscle diseases and to variable degree, cardiac muscle, with manifestations including heart failure, conduction disease and heart block, atrial and ventricular arrhythmias, and sudden death. With improved multidisciplinary care and increase in the life span, the prevalence of later-onset cardiac involvement is increasingly being recognized. Electrophysiologists are typically part of the care team involved in the management of patients with muscular dystrophies due to associated atrial and ventricular arrhythmias and the risk of sudden cardiac death. The aim of this article is to familiarize the reader with the nature, prevalence, treatment, and outcome of arrhythmias in muscular dystrophies and present the recent advances in this arena.

Classification of the muscular dystrophies is shown in **Box 1**.

## DUCHENNE AND BECKER MUSCULAR DYSTROPHIES
### Genetics and Cardiac Pathology

Duchenne and Becker muscular dystrophy are X-linked recessive disorders caused by mutations in the dystrophin gene. Abnormalities in dystrophin and in dystrophin-associated glycoproteins underlie the degeneration of cardiac and skeletal muscle in several inherited myopathies, including X-linked dilated cardiomyopathy. In Duchenne muscular dystrophy (DMD), dystrophin is nearly absent, whereas in Becker muscular dystrophy (BMD), dystrophin is present but reduced in size or amount. This leads to the characteristic rapidly progressive skeletal muscle disease in DMD and the more benign course in BMD. Cardiac involvement is seen in both disorders, and the severity is not correlated with the severity of skeletal muscle involvement. Mutations in specific domains of the large dystrophin gene are

Disclosure: Dr Archana Rajdev has nothing to disclose. Dr William J. Groh is Consultant at Isis Pharmaceuticals Inc., and receives Research Grant from Biogen.
[a] Krannert Institute of Cardiology, Indiana University School of Medicine, Indianapolis, IN 46202, USA;
[b] William Jennings Bryan Dorn Veterans Affairs Medical Center, University of South Carolina, 6439 Garners Ferry Road, Columbia, SC 29209-1639, USA
* Corresponding author.
E-mail address: wgroh@iu.edu

associated with a higher risk for cardiomyopathy.[1] Most patients with DMD develop a cardiomyopathy with a predilection for involvement in the inferobasal and lateral left ventricle. In BMD, cardiac disease can be even more pronounced than skeletal muscle weakness.[2]

## Electrocardiography

Most patients with DMD have an abnormal electrocardiogram (ECG) with the classically described electrocardiographic pattern of distinctive tall R waves and increased R/S amplitude in V1[3] and deep narrow Q waves in the left precordial leads, possibly related to the posterolateral left ventricular involvement.[4] Other common findings include short PR interval and right ventricular hypertrophy. No association between the presence of a dilated cardiomyopathy and ECG abnormalities has been established.[5] Left bundle branch block may be seen in patients with a dilated cardiomyopathy.

## Arrhythmias

In patients with DMD, persistent or labile sinus tachycardia is the most common arrhythmia recognized. Atrial arrhythmias, including atrial fibrillation and atrial flutter, can occur, often in the setting of respiratory dysfunction with cor pulmonale and in those with a dilated cardiomyopathy. Abnormalities in atrioventricular conduction have been observed with both short and prolonged PR intervals recognized. Ventricular arrhythmias occur on monitoring in 30%, primarily as ventricular premature beats. Complex ventricular arrhythmias have been reported, more commonly in patients with severe skeletal muscle disease. The presence of systolic dysfunction was a powerful predictor of mortality but ECG abnormalities, late potentials, or ventricular arrhythmias were not predictive.[6] In a cohort of patients with DMD, QT dispersion was an independent risk factor for the occurrence of ventricular tachycardia.[7] Sudden death occurs in DMD, typically in patients with end-stage muscular disease. Whether the sudden death is caused by

arrhythmias is unclear. Several follow-up studies have shown a correlation between sudden death and the presence of complex ventricular arrhythmias.[8] The presence of ventricular arrhythmias was not a predictor for all-cause mortality. Arrhythmia manifestations in BMD typically relate to the severity of the associated structural cardiomyopathy. Distal conduction system diseases with complete heart block and bundle branch reentry ventricular tachycardia have been observed.

## Screening, Treatment, and Prognosis

Clinical care guidelines recommend screening echocardiography at diagnosis or by the age of 6 years and subsequently every 2 years; until the age of 10 and annually thereafter in boys with DMD.[9] In patients with DMD, with improvement in respiratory support, age at death has increased so that most patients survive into their 30s.[10] Decision of implantation of an implantable cardioverter-defibrillator (ICD) should be considered individually based on patient status and wishes. Advanced heart failure therapy, including primary prevention ICDs, is appropriately considered in patients with cardiomyopathy. Patients with BMD often develop cardiac complications and death from congestive heart failure and arrhythmias are estimated to occur in up to 50% of cases.[9] BMD has a high heart transplantation rate in the first year after diagnosis of cardiomyopathy.[11] Female carriers of DMD and BMD do not develop a cardiomyopathy during childhood, but it can occur later in life. Screening echocardiography should be done in adults or with symptoms.

# MYOTONIC DYSTROPHIES
## Genetics and Cardiac Pathology

The myotonic dystrophies are autosomal dominant disorders characterized by myotonia (delayed muscle relaxation after contraction), weakness and atrophy of skeletal muscles, and systemic manifestations. Two distinct mutations are responsible for the myotonic dystrophies. In myotonic dystrophy type 1 (DM1), the mutation is an amplified trinucleotide cytosine-thymine-guanine (CTG) repeat found on chromosome 19.[12] It is typical for the CTG repeat to expand as it is passed from parents to offspring, resulting in the characteristic worsening clinical manifestations in subsequent generations, termed anticipation.[13] Myotonic dystrophy type 2 (DM2), also called proximal myotonic myopathy, has generally less severe skeletal muscle and cardiac involvement than in DM1 and is a tetranucleotide, CCTG repeat expansion occurs on chromosome 3. A recent study suggests that cardiac pathology in both DM1 and DM2 is related to gap junction (GJA1) and calcium channel (CAC-NA1C) protein overexpression.[14] Cardiac pathology involves degeneration, fibrosis, and fatty infiltration, preferentially targeting the specialized conduction tissue, including the sinus node, atrioventricular node, and His-Purkinje system. Degenerative changes are observed in working atrial and ventricular tissue but only rarely progress to a symptomatic dilated cardiomyopathy. The primary cardiac manifestations of the myotonic dystrophies are arrhythmias and are age-dependent and although the pathology appears similar in types 1 and 2, DM1 typically has earlier and more severe cardiac involvement. No correlation has been established between spontaneous ventricular arrhythmia and the severity of muscular weakness,[15] the size of CTG repetition,[16] premature ventricular contractions on 24-hour ambulatory ECG,[15] the presence of late ventricular potentials,[17] or ventricular arrhythmia induced by programmed ventricular stimulation.[15]

## Electrocardiography

Most adult patients with DM1 exhibit ECG abnormalities. In a large, unselected, middle-aged US myotonic population, abnormal ECG patterns were seen in 65% of the patients.[18] Abnormalities included first-degree atrioventricular block in 42%, right bundle branch block in 3%, left bundle branch block in 4%, and nonspecific intraventricular conduction delay in 12%. Q waves not associated with a known myocardial infarction are common. Conduction disease worsens with advancing age. ECG abnormalities are less common in DM2, occurring in approximately 20% of middle-aged patients.

## Arrhythmias

Patients with DM1 demonstrate a wide range of arrhythmias. At cardiac electrophysiological study, the most common abnormality found is a prolonged His-ventricular interval. Conduction system disease can progress to symptomatic atrioventricular block and necessitate pacemaker implantation. The prevalence of permanent cardiac pacing in patients with DM1 varies widely between studies. Updated practice guidelines have recognized that asymptomatic conduction abnormalities in neuromuscular diseases such as myotonic dystrophy may warrant special consideration for pacing.[19]

Atrial arrhythmias, primarily fibrillation and flutter, are common. Patients with atrial arrhythmias are often asymptomatic, possibly because of a controlled ventricular response from concomitant conduction disease.

Up to one-third of individuals with DM1 die suddenly. The mechanisms leading to sudden death are not clear, but are believed to be related primarily to arrhythmia. Asystole, owing to complete heart block without an appropriate escape rhythm, has been considered a probable cause. Sudden death can occur despite pacemakers, implicating ventricular arrhythmias.

Patients with DM1 are at risk for bundle branch reentry tachycardia because of associated conduction disease. Arrhythmias are observed in patients with DM2, but are less frequent and occur later in life. Patients with DM1 are at a higher risk of sudden death if they have significant ECG conduction disease.[18] Up to 18% of patients with DM1 and minor depolarization/repolarization at baseline present with Brugada ECG pattern after drug challenge.[20] This was not related to the occurrence of significant conduction disturbances or ventricular arrhythmias during follow-up. It may be useful to rule out Brugada ECG pattern in myotonic patients with the idea of avoiding some medications (ie, use of Class 1 drugs for decreasing myotonia in myotonic dystrophy) or in cases of unexplained syncope/palpitations. However, the role of drug challenge to unmask Brugada for purpose of risk stratification in these patients is uncertain. The prospective long-term multicenter RAMYD study is a large-scale clinical trial designed to investigate the course of cardiac disease in patients with DM1 and to explore the value of noninvasive and invasive findings to predict the occurrence of sudden death, resuscitated cardiac arrest, ventricular fibrillation, sustained ventricular tachycardia, severe sinus node dysfunction, or grade II or III atrioventricular block.[21]

## EMERY-DREIFUSS MUSCULAR DYSTROPHIES
### Genetics and Cardiac Pathology

The X-linked recessive Emery-Dreifuss muscular dystrophy (EDMD) disorder (EDMD1) is characterized by mild skeletal involvement, but life-threatening cardiac and arrhythmia manifestations. Mutations in the genes coding for the nuclear membrane protein Emerin[22] result in fibrotic replacement of cardiac muscle and conduction tissue and is thought to be responsible for the abnormalities in impulse generation and conduction that are commonly encountered in this group. The autosomal dominant EDMD (EDMD2) and a rare autosomal-recessive form of EDMD are caused by a mutation in the lamin A/C gene. Lamin A/C mutations can cause several other phenotypes, including limb-girdle muscular dystrophy type 1B (LGMD1B). Because of the different implications of laminopathy and emerinopathy both from the point of view of management and genetic counseling, a precise diagnosis should be sought in all patients.

## Arrhythmias

First-degree atrioventricular block and atrial arrhythmias are among the early manifestations. Classically, atrial standstill with junctional bradycardia may be seen. Pacing support is recommended once conduction disease is evident. Heart failure and ventricular arrhythmias seem to occur in only a minority of patients, but the risk may increase as patients with a pacemaker may survive longer.[23] In both XLEDMD (X-linked Emery-Dreifuss Muscular Dystrophy) and ADEDMD (autosomal dominant Emery-Dreifuss Muscular Dystrophy), atrial fibrillation/flutter and atrial standstill occur frequently, even after pacemaker implantation, and this carries a substantial risk of thromboembolic events, including ischemic stroke and initiation of therapeutic anticoagulation should be strongly considered.

## Screening, Treatment, and Prognosis

Sudden death is the most common cause of death and can be highly unpredictable.[24] Risk factors for sudden death and appropriate ICD therapy include nonsustained ventricular tachycardia, left ventricular ejection fraction less than 45%, male sex, and lamin A or C non-missense mutations.[25] Female carriers of X-linked EDMD are at risk of cardiac conduction disease and sudden death, typically occurring late in life. Affected patients should be monitored carefully for ECG conduction abnormalities and left ventricular dysfunction. Ambulatory monitoring can reveal asymptomatic ventricular arrhythmias that have prognostic significance. An ICD rather than bradycardia protection alone is the preferred prophylactic therapy.

## LIMB-GIRDLE MUSCULAR DYSTROPHIES
### Genetics and Cardiac Pathology

The muscular dystrophies with a limb–shoulder and pelvic girdle distribution of weakness and heterogeneous inheritance are called limb-girdle muscular dystrophies (LGMD, autosomal recessive, subtypes 2A to 2P; dominant, subtypes 1A to 1H, sporadic inheritance). Genes involved include those encoding dystrophin-associated glycoproteins, sarcomeric proteins, sarcolemma proteins, nuclear membrane proteins, and cellular enzymes.

## Arrhythmias

Occurrence of arrhythmias related to specific genetic subtypes with high incidence seen in subtype 1B (mutation in the gene coding lamin A/C akin to EDMD).

## Screening, Treatment, and Prognosis

The recommendations for cardiac surveillance in this group depend very much on the particular type of LGMD. Patients with LGMD2I are at risk of cardiomyopathy and should be assessed as for DMD/BMD. The severity of cardiomyopathy may be out of proportion to that of skeletal muscle involvement. Present perception is that the incidence of tachyarrhythmias or bradyarrhythmias in sarcoglycanopathies (LGMD 2C, 2D, 2E, and 2F) is low, but this issue is not fully resolved. Some arrhythmia surveillance with Holter ECG or similar recordings is still justified. In LGMD1B, risk factors for sudden death and appropriate ICD therapy include nonsustained ventricular tachycardia, left ventricular ejection fraction less than 45%, male sex, and lamin A or C non-missense mutations.[26] Prophylactic implantation of an ICD rather than pacemaker is recommended in patients with LGMD1B when cardiac conduction disease is present.[27]

## FACIOSCAPULOHUMERAL MUSCULAR DYSTROPHY

Facioscapulohumeral muscular dystrophy is the third most common muscular dystrophy after the Duchenne and myotonic types inherited in an autosomal dominant fashion characterized by slowly progressive muscle weakness. Because significant clinical cardiac involvement is rather rare in this form of muscular dystrophy, specific monitoring or treatment recommendations are not well defined. Discussion of arrhythmia-related symptoms and yearly electrocardiograms has been recommended.

## SUMMARY

With progress in the respiratory management of patients and prolonged survival of patients with muscular dystrophy, heart failure and arrhythmias contribute to a larger extent to premature death. Recognition of cardiac involvement requires active investigation and remains challenging because typical signs and symptoms of cardiac dysfunction may not be present and progression is unpredictable. On initial evaluation, the diagnostic workup for arrhythmias would depend on the type of muscular dystrophy, age of the patient, disease stage, symptoms attributable to cardiac involvement and previous cardiac events. Careful monitoring of cardiac symptoms, and surveillance using electrocardiogram, Holter and event monitoring, and/or implantable loop recorder as dictated by clinical situation would allow timely management of bradycardia and tachycardia rhythm disturbances with device implantation and can potentially improve prognosis. Because this clinical need frequently arises late in the life of many patients with muscular dystrophy, kyphoscoliosis, and muscle wasting might complicate device implantation. Experimental therapy for muscular dystrophies, including cell-based therapies, are also being explored for the regeneration of skeletal and cardiac muscle; skeletal muscle stem cells, when delivered systemically, might also home to cardiac muscle and result in muscle regeneration, which would alter electrical properties and cardiac function.

## REFERENCES

1. Spurney CF. Cardiomyopathy of Duchenne muscular dystrophy: current understanding and future directions. Muscle Nerve 2011;44:8.
2. Melacini P, Fanin M, Miorin M, et al. Myocardial involvement is very frequent among patients affected with subclinical Becker's muscular dystrophy. Circulation 1996;94:3168–75.
3. D'Orsogna L, O'Shea JP, Miller G. Cardiomyopathy of Duchenne muscular dystrophy. Pediatr Cardiol 1988;9:205–13.
4. Perloff JK, Roberts WC, Leon AC Jr, et al. The distinctive electrocardiogram of Duchenne's progressive muscular dystrophy. An electrocardiographic–pathologic correlative study. Am J Med 1967;42:179–88.
5. Thrush PT, Allen HD, Viollet L, et al. Re-examination of the electrocardiogram in boys with Duchenne muscular dystrophy and correlation with its dilated cardiomyopathy. Am J Cardiol 2009;103:262.
6. Corrado G, Lissoni A, Beretta S, et al. Prognostic value of electrocardiograms, ventricular late potentials, ventricular arrhythmias and left ventricular systolic dysfunction in patients with Duchenne muscular dystrophy. Am J Cardiol 2002;89:838.
7. Yotsukura M, Yamamoto A, Kajiwara T. QT dispersion in patients with Duchennes muscular dystrophy. Am Heart J 1999;137:62.
8. Chenard AA, Becane HM, Tertrain F, et al. Ventricular arrhythmia in Duchenne muscular dystrophy: prevalence, significance and prognosis. Neuromuscul Disord 1993;3:201–6.
9. Bushby K, Finkel R, Birnkrant DJ, et al. Diagnosis and management of Duchenne muscular dystrophy, part 1: diagnosis, and pharmacological and psychosocial management. Lancet Neurol 2010;9:77.
10. Eagle M, Baudouin SV, Chandler C, et al. Survival in Duchenne muscular dystrophy: improvements in life expectancy since 1967 and the impact of home nocturnal ventilation. Neuromuscul Disord 2002;12: 926–9.
11. Connuck DM, Sleeper LA, Colan SD, et al. Characteristics and outcomes of cardiomyopathy in children with Duchenne or Becker muscular dystrophy: a comparative study from the Pediatric Cardiomyopathy Registry. Am Heart J 2008;155: 998–1005.
12. Brook JD, McCurrach ME, Aburatani H, et al. Molecular basis of myotonic dystrophy: expansion of a trinucleotide (CTG) repeat at the 3′ end of a transcript encoding a protein kinase family member. Cell 1992;69:385.
13. Höweler CJ, Busch HF, Geraedts JP, et al. Anticipation in myotonic dystrophy: fact or fiction? Brain 1989;112:779–97.
14. Rau F, Freyermuth F, Fugier C, et al. Misregulation of miR-1 processing is associated with heart defects in myotonic dystrophy. Nat Struct Mol Biol 2011;18: 840.
15. Lazarus A, Varin J, Babuty D, et al. Long-term follow-up of arrhythmias in patients with myotonic dystrophy treated by pacing: a multicenter diagnostic pacemaker study. J Am Coll Cardiol 2002;40:1645–52.
16. Nishioka S, Filho M, Marie S, et al. Myotonic dystrophy and heart disease: behavior of arrhythmic events and conduction disturbances. Arq Bras Cardiol 2005;84:330–6.
17. Babuty D, Fauchier L, Tena-Carbi D, et al. Significance of late ventricular potentials in myotonic dystrophy. Am J Cardiol 1999;84:1099–101.
18. Groh WJ, Groh MR, Chandan S, et al. Electrocardiographic abnormalities and risk of sudden death in myotonic dystrophy type 1. N Engl J Med 2008; 358:2688.
19. Epstein A, Dimarco J, Ellenbogen K, et al. ACC/AHA/HRS 2008 guidelines for device-based therapy of cardiac rhythm abnormalities. Circulation 2008; 117:e350.
20. Maury P, Audoubert M, Razcka F, et al. Prevalence of type 1 Brugada ECG pattern after administration of Class 1C drugs in patients with type 1 myotonic dystrophy: myotonic dystrophy as a part of the Brugada syndrome. Heart Rhythm 2014;11(10):1721–7.
21. Russo A, Mangiola F, Bella P, et al. Risk of arrhythmias in myotonic dystrophy: trial design of the RA-MYD study. J Cardiovasc Med (Hagerstown) 2009; 10:51–8.
22. Manilal S, Nguyen TM, Sewry CA, et al. The Emery–Dreifuss muscular dystrophy protein, emerin, is a nuclear membrane protein. Hum Mol Genet 1996; 5:801–8.
23. Boriani G, Gallina M, Merlini L, et al. Clinical relevance of atrial fibrillation/flutter, stroke, pacemaker implant, and heart failure in Emery–Dreifuss muscular dystrophy: a long-term longitudinal study. Stroke 2003;34:901–8.

24. Merlini L, Granata C, Bonfiglioli S, et al. Emery–Drei-
    fuss muscular dystrophy: report of five cases in a
    family and review of the literature. Muscle Nerve
    1986;9:481–5.
25. Fanselme G, Moubarak A, Savouré A, et al. Implant-
    able cardioverter-defibrillators in lamin A/C mutation
    carriers with cardiac conduction disorders. Heart
    Rhythm 2013;10(10):1492–8.

26. Berlo JH, Voogt WG, Kooi AJ, et al. Meta-analysis of
    clinical characteristics of 299 carriers of LMNA gene
    mutations: do lamin A/C mutations portend a high
    risk of sudden death? J Mol Med 2005;83:79–83.
27. Meune C, Van Berlo JH, Anselme F, et al. Primary
    prevention of sudden death in patients with lamin
    A/C gene mutations. N Engl J Med 2006;354:
    209–10.

# Arrhythmias in Peripartum Cardiomyopathy

Michael C. Honigberg, MD, MPP[a],
Michael M. Givertz, MD[b],*

## KEYWORDS

• Peripartum cardiomyopathy • Pregnancy • Maternal-fetal health • Sudden cardiac death
• Antiarrhythmic medications • Implantable cardioverter-defibrillator • Arrhythmias

## KEY POINTS

• Peripartum cardiomyopathy (PPCM) is a complication of late pregnancy and the early postpartum period characterized by dilated cardiomyopathy and heart failure with reduced ejection fraction.
• Although the prevalence of specific arrhythmias in PPCM is unknown, an estimated 1 in 4 deaths in women with this condition is sudden and presumed secondary to ventricular tachyarrhythmia.
• Management of PPCM entails standard treatment of heart failure with reduced ejection fraction and prevention of sudden cardiac death (SCD) in patients at increased risk, with special considerations for women who are predelivery or breastfeeding.

## INTRODUCTION

PPCM is a rare, dilated cardiomyopathy of unknown cause characterized by heart failure with reduced ejection fraction.[1] According to the US National Heart, Lung, and Blood Institute, PPCM is diagnosed when a woman develops heart failure in the last month of pregnancy or up to 5 months postpartum, with a left ventricular (LV) ejection fraction less than 45% and no other identifiable cause of heart failure.[2] Alternative criteria allowing for earlier and later diagnosis have also been proposed.[3] Pregnancy-associated heart failure is a term used to describe women who develop signs and symptoms of heart failure at any time during pregnancy.[4]

### Clinical Presentation

In the United States, a majority of women with PPCM are diagnosed in the early postpartum period (**Fig. 1**).[5,6] Patients typically present with heart failure symptoms, although rarely they may present with symptomatic or even unstable arrhythmias.[1,7,8] More common electrocardiographic findings include nonspecific ST-T wave changes, occasionally with conduction abnormalities, such as bundle branch block. Echocardiography shows varying degrees of depressed ventricular systolic function and ventricular dilatation, often with biatrial enlargement as a consequence of valvular regurgitation.[5] Chest radiography may show cardiomegaly, pulmonary edema, and/or pleural effusions. Natriuretic peptide levels (eg, B-type natriuretic peptide (BNP) and N-terminal pro-BNP) may be markedly elevated, in contrast with normal pregnancies.[9] Low-level troponin elevations also may be seen and predict adverse remodeling.[4]

### Epidemiology

Well-established risk factors for PPCM include African American race,[10] older maternal age (with increased risk above age 30), chronic hypertension,

The authors report no conflicts of interest.
[a] Department of Medicine, Brigham and Women's Hospital, Harvard Medical School, 75 Francis Street, Boston, MA 02115, USA; [b] Cardiovascular Division, Department of Medicine, Brigham and Women's Hospital, Harvard Medical School, 75 Francis Street, Boston, MA 02115, USA
* Corresponding author.
E-mail address: mgivertz@partners.org

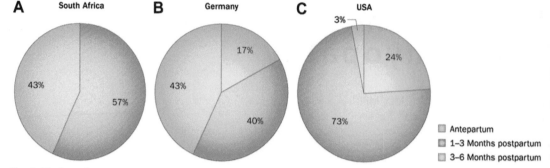

**Fig. 1.** Timing of presentation in patients with PPCM in (*A*) South Africa, (*B*) Germany, and (*C*) USA. (*From* Hilfiker-Kleiner D, Sliwa K. Pathophysiology and epidemiology of peripartum cardiomyopathy. Nat Rev Cardiol 2014;11(6):365; with permission.)

pregnancy-associated hypertensive conditions (eg, preeclampsia and eclampsia), and multifetal gestation as well as prolonged use of tocolytics in labor.[11–13] Hispanic women seem to have the lowest incidence.[12]

The incidence of PPCM in the United States seems to be increasing (**Fig. 2**),[14] with an average rate of 1 in 968 live births between 2004 and 2011.[15] During this period, incidence rose from 8.5 to 11.8 per 10,000 live births.[15] Proposed explanations for this trend include climbing rates of advanced maternal age and preeclampsia (secondary to increasing rates of obesity, diabetes, and chronic hypertension), more multifetal gestations due to increased use of assisted reproductive technologies, and growing recognition of PPCM as a disease entity.[5,6,15]

### Approach to Management

Standard medical therapies for heart failure are used to manage PPCM, with some exceptions for women who have not yet delivered. For example, diuresis in pregnant women should be undertaken cautiously to avoid maternal hypotension and uterine hypoperfusion. With respect to afterload reduction, angiotensin-converting enzyme inhibitors and angiotensin-receptor blockers are teratogenic and are contraindicated in pregnancy. The combination of hydralazine and isosorbide dinitrate may be used instead. $\beta_1$-Selective blockers are preferred to nonselective $\beta$-blockers due to risk of uterine stimulation via $\beta_2$-sympathetic innervation. For pregnant women with severely depressed LV ejection fraction at high risk of thrombus formation, unfractionated heparin and low-molecular-weight heparin are preferred, because warfarin crosses the placenta and may cause fetal hemorrhage.[5]

For women with acute decompensated heart failure refractory to medical management, mechanical support with an intra-aortic balloon pump, ventricular assist device, or extracorporeal membrane oxygenation may be necessary as a bridge to recovery or transplant.[16]

### Prognosis

Recovery of LV function occurs in approximately half of women, although there is considerable variation reported across studies likely due to selection bias. African American race seems to be associated with decreased likelihood of LV recovery.[17] A wide range of mortality rates, as high as 20%, has been reported in US series, with most mortality occurring within 6 months of diagnosis.[5] A recently published study reported that in-hospital mortality secondary to PPCM in the United States was 1.3%.[15] Other major adverse events associated with PPCM are the need for mechanical circulatory support (1.5%), heart transplant (0.5%), and cardiac arrest (2.1%).[15] Among women requiring mechanical circulatory support for PPCM, approximately half ultimately require cardiac transplantation; 2-year survival in this group is reported to be 83%.[16]

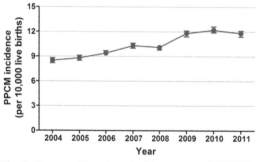

**Fig. 2.** Temporal trends in incidence rate of PPCM in the United States. (*From* Kolte D, Khera S, Aronow WS, et al. Temporal trends in incidence and outcomes of peripartum cardiomyopathy in the United States: a nationwide population-based study. J Am Heart Assoc 2014;3(3):e001056; with permission.)

## Risk of Subsequent Pregnancy

Data suggest that 20% to 50% of women with a history of PPCM experience PPCM recurrence with a subsequent pregnancy.[18,19] The risk seems increased among women whose LV ejection fraction failed to normalize after their first episode of PPCM.[18,20] Even in women with recovery of resting LV function, there is a small excess risk of recurrent heart failure, although patients demonstrating normal contractile reserve appear to do well.[20]

## ARRHYTHMIAS IN PERIPARTUM CARDIOMYOPATHY

Atrial and ventricular arrhythmias are common in patients with heart failure and cardiomyopathy.[21] Data on arrhythmia associated specifically with PPCM are sparse, and underlying mechanisms are unclear (Fig. 3). Available data are limited to case reports and small case series, which are summarized in Table 1. In a series of 19 patients in Senegal with PPCM who underwent 24-hour continuous electrocardiographic monitoring, 89% had sinus tachycardia, 37% had premature ventricular contractions, 21% had nonsustained ventricular tachycardia (VT), and 1 patient had first-degree atrioventricular block.[22] The exact prevalence of VT and other ventricular arrhythmias in PPCM is unknown.[23] In patients presenting with VT, other causes of cardiomyopathy should be considered, including arrhythmogenic right ventricular cardiomyopathy, sarcoidosis, and ischemia/infarction from coronary artery dissection or spasm.

## Sudden Cardiac Death

A recent study reported that 2.1% of women with PPCM in the United States suffered cardiac arrest in the period 2004 to 2011 (Fig. 4).[15] In the same study, the in-hospital mortality rate in women with PPCM was 1.3%. Based on limited data, an estimated 1 in 4 deaths in PPCM is caused by ventricular tachyarrhythmia leading to SCD.[24] Some women are only diagnosed with PPCM after presenting with SCD.[25] In an American cohort of 100 women with PPCM, 11 subjects died at a mean follow-up of 98 months. Among these patients, 1 had an implantable cardioverter-defibrillator (ICD) but died of heart failure; 2 patients without ICDs died from arrhythmias; and the cause of death was unknown for the other 8 women.[17]

## MANAGEMENT OF ARRHYTHMIA IN PERIPARTUM CARDIOMYOPATHY

### Medical Management

Some women who develop arrhythmias secondary to PPCM may require intravenous antiarrhythmic drugs (AADs) in the acute setting or oral AADs for chronic management. In women requiring AADs prior to delivery, consideration must be given to the effects of AADs on fetal heart rhythm, fetal growth, and uterine activity.[23]

There is a dearth of data on the risk of AADs to the fetus in pregnancy. As a result, most AADs are Food and Drug Administration (FDA) pregnancy category C (risk cannot be ruled out). Notable exceptions include lidocaine and sotalol, which are FDA category B (no evidence of risk in studies); amiodarone, which is FDA category D (positive evidence of risk, specifically fetal hypothyroidism and prematurity); and dronedarone, which is FDA category X (contraindicated in pregnancy).[23,26] Risk categories of AADs are summarized in Table 2. For women requiring treatment of PPCM-associated arrhythmia after delivery, many AADs are compatible with breastfeeding (see Table 2).

### External Cardioversion

Direct current cardioversion (DCCV) should be performed for patients with unstable arrhythmias

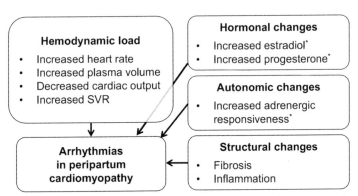

Fig. 3. Potential mechanisms of arrhythmias in PPCM. The asterisk indicates changes occurring during pregnancy. SVR, systemic vascular resistance.

**Table 1**
Summary of case series and reports documenting specific arrhythmias in peripartum cardiomyopathy

**Atrial arrhythmias**

| Case Series | Study Subjects | Major Finding(s) | Comments |
|---|---|---|---|
| Biteker et al,[35] 2012 | 42 women in Turkey | 5 (11.9%) developed AF | No apparent effect of AF on survival or recovery of LV function |
| Kane et al,[36] 2010 | 33 women in Senegal | 1 (3%) with AF; 1 (3%) with MAT | |
| Isezuo and Abubakar,[37] 2007 | 65 women in Nigeria | 2 (3.1%) developed AF | |

**Ventricular tachycardia**

| Case Series | Study Subjects | Major Finding(s) | Comments |
|---|---|---|---|
| Laghari et al,[38] 2013 | 45 women in Pakistan | 3 (6.6%) had VT at presentation | No further description of arrhythmias provided |
| Diao et al,[22] 2004 | 19 women in Senegal | 4 (21%) had NSVT | |

| Case reports | Patient | | Comments |
|---|---|---|---|
| Tokuda et al,[30] 2013 | 38-year-old woman with PPCM presented with sustained VT | | Patient with known PPCM and LV ejection fraction 20%; ICD placed 1 y before presentation for monomorphic VT. Mapping revealed low-voltage epicardial scar that was ablated with resolution of VT. |
| Puri et al,[7] 2009 | 25-year-old woman at 36 wk gestation found to have VT | | Echocardiography revealed depressed LV ejection fraction leading to diagnosis of PPCM. |
| Gemici et al,[8] 2004 | 30-year-old woman at 38 wk gestation (asymptomatic) found to have VT | | Echocardiography revealed depressed LV ejection fraction leading to diagnosis of PPCM. |

| | Study Subjects | Major Finding(s) | Comments |
|---|---|---|---|
| Palma et al,[39] 2001 | 33-year-old woman with PPCM presenting with incessant VT | | Patient underwent VT ablation that was transiently successful before VT recurred, leading to hemodynamic collapse and death. |
| **Ventricular fibrillation** | | | |
| **Case Series** | | | |
| Duncker et al,[33] 2014 | 12 women in Germany with PPCM: 9 with LV ejection fraction <35%, of whom 7 received a WCD | 4 appropriate shocks for VF in 3 women with WCDs (median follow-up 81 d) | |
| **Case report** | | **Patient** | **Comments** |
| Nelson et al,[40] 2012 | 35-year-old woman at 36 wk gestation suffered VF arrest at home | | Patient was defibrillated 5 times with return of spontaneous circulation. After emergent cesarean delivery, started on amiodarone and later received an ICD. |
| Colombo et al,[41] 2002 | 30-year-old woman with PPCM status post–ventricular assist device developed sustained VF | | Patient was defibrillated to sinus rhythm with 360 J after 13 d in VF. LV assist device was subsequently converted to biventricular assist devices. |
| Hetey et al,[42] 1996 | 26-year-old woman presented 9 wk postpartum with heart failure and VF | | |
| Pearl,[43] 1995 | 24-year-old woman developed postpartum CMP and died of refractory VF | | Patient's mother and sister also died from PPCM, suggesting a genetic predisposition. |

*Abbreviations*: AF, atrial fibrillation; ICD, implantable cardioverter-defibrillator; LV, left ventricular; MAT, multifocal atrial tachycardia; NSVT, nonsustained VT; PPCM, peripartum cardiomyopathy; VF, ventricular fibrillation; VT, ventricular tachycardia; WCD, wearable cardioverter-defibrillator.

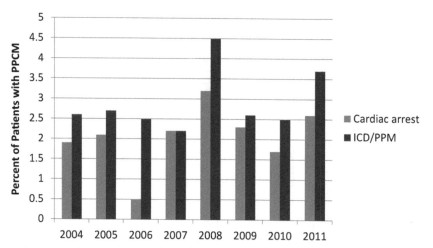

**Fig. 4.** Temporal trends in cardiac arrest and implantable cardioverter-defibrillator (ICD) and permanent pacemaker (PPM) implantation among patients with peripartum cardiomyopathy (PPCM). (*Data from* Kolte D, Khera S, Aronow WS, et al. Temporal trends in incidence and outcomes of peripartum cardiomyopathy in the United States: a nationwide population-based study. J Am Heart Assoc 2014;3(3):e001056.)

and arrhythmias refractory to medical therapy. DCCV is safe in pregnancy.[27,28] For patients requiring DCCV prior to delivery, involvement by a high-risk obstetrician is prudent because there have been rare reports of increased uterine activity after DCCV.[29] Additionally, although minimal current reaches the fetus, fetal monitoring is recommended because transient fetal arrhythmias after DCCV have been described.[28]

### Catheter Ablation

There is lack of data on catheter ablation of arrhythmias associated with PPCM. One recent report described successful mapping and ablation of sustained, unstable VT in a patient with PPCM.[30] In a woman who is still pregnant, the risks and benefits of catheter ablation must be weighed against risks to both mother and fetus, including fetal radiation exposure and maternal hemodynamic compromise with impaired placental perfusion.[23] In general, given the risks to the fetus, catheter ablation in pregnant women should be reserved for hemodynamically unstable arrhythmias refractory to medical management and DCCV, and abdominal shielding should be used.[27]

### Wearable Cardioverter-Defibrillator

Patients with PPCM are at risk for SCD, and, as with other cardiomyopathies, this risk is increased in patients with lower ejection fractions.[31] Wearable cardioverter-defibrillators (WCDs) have been used successfully in patients with nonischemic cardiomyopathy and LV ejection fraction less

than or equal to 35%, in the early period after diagnosis, and in patients with temporary or permanent contraindications to ICD placement.[32] Because some PPCM patients with depressed ejection fraction ultimately recover LV function, it is reasonable to consider a WCD as a bridge to LV recovery or to ICD.[5] Only 2 studies to date have examined WCDs in patients with PPCM; no patients died while using a WCD in either study.[33,34] In 1 small study, 3 of 7 women with PPCM using a WCD received one or more shocks for ventricular fibrillation at a median follow-up of 81 days.[33] There were no inappropriate discharges.[33] In the other study, 107 women with PPCM were followed for an average of 3 years; mortality in this cohort was low (2.8%), despite a mean baseline LV ejection fraction of 21%. No women with PPCM, however, received any appropriate or inappropriate shocks.[34]

### Implantable Cardioverter-Defibrillator

Between 2004 and 2011, 2.9% of women in the United States with PPCM had an ICD and/or permanent pacemaker placed. Data delineating the proportion of this group that received an ICD, cardiac resynchronization therapy, or a pacemaker, however, are not available.[15] Given that approximately half of women do not recover LV function, these data suggest that ICDs are underutilized in women with PPCM. In a series of 100 US women, 53 patients who did not recover LV function qualified for an ICD based on LV ejection fraction less than or equal to 35%, but only 7 women (13%) in this group received an ICD.[17] Six additional women in this series received an ICD early

**Table 2**
**Risk categorization of antiarrhythmic drugs in pregnancy and lactation**

| Drug | Vaughan-Williams Class | Food and Drug Administration Risk Category | Adverse Effects | Teratogenic | Use During Lactation |
|------|------------------------|--------------------------------------------|-----------------|-------------|----------------------|
| Quinidine | IA | C | Torsades de pointes, ototoxicity, thrombocytopenia | No | Compatible but caution advised |
| Procainamide | IA | C | Torsades de pointes, drug-induced lupus | No | Compatible but avoid long-term use |
| Disopyramide | IA | C | Torsades de pointes, uterine contractions | No | Compatible |
| Lidocaine | IB | B | Fetal bradycardia, CNS adverse effects; avoid in fetal distress | No | Compatible |
| Mexiletine | IB | C | Fetal bradycardia, CNS adverse effects, low Apgar score | No | Compatible |
| Flecainide | IC | C | Increased mortality in patients with prior MI | No | Compatible |
| Propafenone | IC | C | Similar to flecainide; mild β-blocker effects | No | Unknown |
| Propranolol | II | C | Fetal bradycardia, fetal apnea, hypoglycemia | No | Compatible |
| Metoprolol | II | C | Same as propranolol | No | Compatible |
| Sotalol | III | B | Torsades de pointes, β-blocker effects | No | Compatible but caution advised |
| Amiodarone | III | D | Fetal hypothyroidism, low birth weight, prematurity | Yes | Avoid |
| Dofetilide | III | C | Torsades de pointes | Unknown | Unknown |
| Dronedarone | III | X | Torsades de pointes | Yes | Contraindicated |
| Ibutilide | III | C | Torsades de pointes | Unknown | Unknown |
| Verapamil | IV | C | Maternal hypotension, fetal bradycardia | No | Compatible |
| Diltiazem | IV | C | Same as verapamil | Unknown | Compatible |
| Adenosine | | C | Dyspnea, bradycardia | No | Unknown |
| Digoxin | | C | Low birth weight | No | Compatible |

*Abbreviations:* CNS, central nervous system; MI, myocardial infarction.
*Data from* Enriquez AD, Economy KE, Tedrow UB. Contemporary management of arrhythmias during pregnancy. Circ Arrhythm Electrophysiol 2014;7(5):961–7; and Joglar JA, Page RL. Management of arrhythmia syndromes during pregnancy. Curr Opin Cardiol 2014;29(1):36–44.

after diagnosis of PPCM but subsequently had recovered LV function.[17]

The European Society of Cardiology guidelines advise that for women presenting with symptoms and severe LV dysfunction 6 months after initial presentation, despite optimal medical therapy and QRS duration greater than 120 ms, cardiac resynchronization therapy or ICD treatment should be strongly considered.[1] The guidelines do not comment on prevention of SCD or the use of devices in the first 6 months after diagnosis.

An ICD may be placed during pregnancy, although in most cases of PPCM, delivery prior to device implantation is advised. As with catheter ablation, efforts should be made to minimize fetal radiation exposure by limiting fluoroscopy and using abdominal shielding. Successful ICD implantation using echocardiography without fluoroscopy has been reported.[23]

## SUMMARY

Peripartum cardiomyopathy is a potentially life-threatening complication of pregnancy, occurring in the final month of gestation or up to 5 months postpartum. Management entails standard therapies for heart failure with reduced ejection fraction, with some exceptions in the antepartum period. Patients are at risk for arrhythmias and SCD. Much remains unknown about PPCM. In particular, further research is needed to elucidate the prevalence, underlying mechanism, and natural history of arrhythmias in this condition and to guide the use of devices for the prevention of SCD.

## REFERENCES

1. European Society of Gynecology (ESG), Association for European Paediatric Cardiology (AEPC), German Society for Gender Medicine (DGesGM), et al. ESC guidelines on the management of cardiovascular diseases during pregnancy: the task force on the management of cardiovascular diseases during pregnancy of the European Society of Cardiology (ESC). Eur Heart J 2011;32(24):3147–97.
2. Pearson GD, Veille JC, Rahimtoola S, et al. Peripartum cardiomyopathy: National Heart, Lung, and Blood Institute and Office of Rare Diseases (National Institutes of Health) workshop recommendations and review. JAMA 2000;283(9):1183–8.
3. Sliwa K, Hilfiker-Kleiner D, Petrie MC, et al. Current state of knowledge on aetiology, diagnosis, management, and therapy of peripartum cardiomyopathy: a position statement from the Heart Failure Association of the European Society of Cardiology working group on peripartum cardiomyopathy. Eur J Heart Fail 2010;12(8):767–78.
4. Hu CL, Li YB, Zou YG, et al. Troponin T measurement can predict persistent left ventricular dysfunction in peripartum cardiomyopathy. Heart 2007; 93(4):488–90.
5. Elkayam U. Clinical characteristics of peripartum cardiomyopathy in the United States: diagnosis, prognosis, and management. J Am Coll Cardiol 2011;58(7):659–70.
6. Hilfiker-Kleiner D, Sliwa K. Pathophysiology and epidemiology of peripartum cardiomyopathy. Nat Rev Cardiol 2014;11(6):364–70.
7. Puri A, Sethi R, Singh B, et al. Peripartum cardiomyopathy presenting with ventricular tachycardia: a rare presentation. Indian Pacing Electrophysiol J 2009;9(3):186–9.
8. Gemici G, Tezcan H, Fak AS, et al. Peripartum cardiomyopathy presenting with repetitive monomorphic ventricular tachycardia. Pacing Clin Electrophysiol 2004;27(4):557–8.
9. Tanous D, Siu SC, Mason J, et al. B-type natriuretic peptide in pregnant women with heart disease. J Am Coll Cardiol 2010;56(15):1247–53.
10. Gentry MB, Dias JK, Luis A, et al. African-American women have a higher risk for developing peripartum cardiomyopathy. J Am Coll Cardiol 2010; 55(7):654–9.
11. Kao DP, Hsich E, Lindenfeld J. Characteristics, adverse events, and racial differences among delivering mothers with peripartum cardiomyopathy. JACC Heart Fail 2013;1(5):409–16.
12. Brar SS, Khan SS, Sandhu GK, et al. Incidence, mortality, and racial differences in peripartum cardiomyopathy. Am J Cardiol 2007;100(2):302–4.
13. Harper MA, Meyer RE, Berg CJ. Peripartum cardiomyopathy: population-based birth prevalence and 7-year mortality. Obstet Gynecol 2012;120(5):1013–9.
14. Mielniczuk LM, Williams K, Davis DR, et al. Frequency of peripartum cardiomyopathy. Am J Cardiol 2006;97(12):1765–8.
15. Kolte D, Khera S, Aronow WS, et al. Temporal trends in incidence and outcomes of peripartum cardiomyopathy in the United States: a nationwide population-based study. J Am Heart Assoc 2014;3(3):e001056.
16. Loyaga-Rendon RY, Pamboukian SV, Tallaj JA, et al. Outcomes of patients with peripartum cardiomyopathy who received mechanical circulatory support. data from the Interagency Registry for Mechanically Assisted Circulatory Support. Circ Heart Fail 2014; 7(2):300–9.
17. Pillarisetti J, Kondur A, Alani A, et al. Peripartum cardiomyopathy: predictors of recovery and current state of implantable cardioverter-defibrillator use. J Am Coll Cardiol 2014;63(25 Pt A):2831–9.
18. Elkayam U, Tummala PP, Rao K, et al. Maternal and fetal outcomes of subsequent pregnancies in women with peripartum cardiomyopathy. N Engl J Med 2001;344(21):1567–71.
19. Habli M, O'Brien T, Nowack E, et al. Peripartum cardiomyopathy: prognostic factors for long-term maternal outcome. Am J Obstet Gynecol 2008; 199(4):415.e1–5.
20. Fett JD, Fristoe KL, Welsh SN. Risk of heart failure relapse in subsequent pregnancy among peripartum cardiomyopathy mothers. Int J Gynaecol Obstet 2010;109(1):34–6.
21. Hynes BJ, Luck JC, Wolbrette DL, et al. Arrhythmias in patients with heart failure. Curr Treat Options Cardiovasc Med 2002;4(6):467–85.
22. Diao M, Diop IB, Kane A, et al. Electrocardiographic recording of long duration (Holter) of 24 hours

during idiopathic cardiomyopathy of the peripartum. Arch Mal Coeur Vaiss 2004;97(1):25–30.

23. Enriquez AD, Economy KE, Tedrow UB. Contemporary management of arrhythmias during pregnancy. Circ Arrhythm Electrophysiol 2014;7(5):961–7.

24. Sliwa K, Forster O, Libhaber E, et al. Peripartum cardiomyopathy: inflammatory markers as predictors of outcome in 100 prospectively studied patients. Eur Heart J 2006;27(4):441–6.

25. Fett JD. Sudden cardiac death is still a risk for some peripartum cardiomyopathy mothers. J Card Fail 2012;18(3):262 [author reply: 262–3].

26. Joglar JA, Page RL. Management of arrhythmia syndromes during pregnancy. Curr Opin Cardiol 2014; 29(1):36–44.

27. Knotts RJ, Garan H. Cardiac arrhythmias in pregnancy. Semin Perinatol 2014;38(5):285–8.

28. Ferrero S, Colombo BM, Ragni N. Maternal arrhythmias during pregnancy. Arch Gynecol Obstet 2004;269(4):244–53.

29. Barnes EJ, Eben F, Patterson D. Direct current cardioversion during pregnancy should be performed with facilities available for fetal monitoring and emergency caesarean section. BJOG 2002;109(12):1406–7.

30. Tokuda M, Stevenson WG, Nagashima K, et al. Electrophysiological mapping and radiofrequency catheter ablation for ventricular tachycardia in a patient with peripartum cardiomyopathy. J Cardiovasc Electrophysiol 2013;24(11):1299–301.

31. Elkayam U, Akhter MW, Singh H, et al. Pregnancy-associated cardiomyopathy: clinical characteristics and a comparison between early and late presentation. Circulation 2005;111(16):2050–5.

32. Chung MK, Szymkiewicz SJ, Shao M, et al. Aggregate national experience with the wearable cardioverter-defibrillator: event rates, compliance, and survival. J Am Coll Cardiol 2010;56(3):194–203.

33. Duncker D, Haghikia A, Konig T, et al. Risk for ventricular fibrillation in peripartum cardiomyopathy with severely reduced left ventricular function-value

of the wearable cardioverter/defibrillator. Eur J Heart Fail 2014;16(12):1331–6.

34. Saltzberg MT, Szymkiewicz S, Bianco NR. Characteristics and outcomes of peripartum versus nonperipartum cardiomyopathy in women using a wearable cardiac defibrillator. J Card Fail 2012;18(1):21–7.

35. Biteker M, Ilhan E, Biteker G, et al. Delayed recovery in peripartum cardiomyopathy: an indication for long-term follow-up and sustained therapy. Eur J Heart Fail 2012;14(8):895–901.

36. Kane A, Mbaye M, Ndiaye MB, et al. Evolution and thromboembolic complications of the idiopathic peripartal cardiomyopathy at Dakar University Hospital: forward-looking study about 33 cases. J Gynecol Obstet Biol Reprod (Paris) 2010;39(6):484–9.

37. Isezuo SA, Abubakar SA. Epidemiologic profile of peripartum cardiomyopathy in a tertiary care hospital. Ethn Dis 2007;17(2):228–33.

38. Laghari AH, Khan AH, Kazmi KA. Peripartum cardiomyopathy: ten year experience at a tertiary care hospital in Pakistan. BMC Res Notes 2013;6:495.

39. Palma EC, Saxenberg V, Vijayaraman P, et al. Histopathological correlation of ablation lesions guided by noncontact mapping in a patient with peripartum cardiomyopathy and ventricular tachycardia. Pacing Clin Electrophysiol 2001;24(12):1812–5.

40. Nelson M, Moorhead A, Yost D, et al. A 35-year-old pregnant woman presenting with sudden cardiac arrest secondary to peripartum cardiomyopathy. Prehosp Emerg Care 2012;16(2):299–302.

41. Colombo J, Lawal AH, Bhandari A, et al. Case 1—2002—a patient with severe peripartum cardiomyopathy and persistent ventricular fibrillation supported by a biventricular assist device. J Cardiothorac Vasc Anesth 2002;16(1):107–13.

42. Hetey M, Preda I, Magyar I, et al. Peripartum cardiomyopathy with fatal outcome. Orv Hetil 1996; 137(41):2263–6.

43. Pearl W. Familial occurrence of peripartum cardiomyopathy. Am Heart J 1995;129(2):421–2.

# Arrhythmias in Left Ventricular Noncompaction

Christina Y. Miyake, MD, MS, Jeffrey J. Kim, MD*

## KEYWORDS

- Cardiomyopathy • Arrhythmias • Left ventricular noncompaction • Heart failure
- Electrocardiogram • Sudden death • Ventricular tachycardia • Atrial fibrillation

## KEY POINTS

- Left ventricular noncompaction (LVNC) is associated with heart failure, arrhythmias, thromboembolic events, and sudden death.
- Arrhythmias are common and may have prognostic significance in LVNC; the risk of sudden death seems to be associated with left ventricular (LV) size, systolic function, and presence of arrhythmias.
- Arrhythmias are not restricted to noncompacted myocardium and include atrial fibrillation (AF) (adults), atrioventricular (AV) accessory pathways/Wolff-Parkinson-White (WPW) syndrome (children), and ventricular tachycardia (VT).
- Management strategies include antiarrhythmic medications, ablation, and implantable cardioverter-defibrillator (ICD) implantation.

## INTRODUCTION

Since initial pathologic descriptions in the 1920s, LVNC has been identified in association with a variety of congenital heart malformations or metabolic syndromes.[1–4] More recently, it has become recognized in its isolated form as a distinct form of cardiomyopathy.[5–11] LVNC is thought to be caused by the intrauterine arrest of the normal compaction process of myocardial fibers and meshwork in the ventricular endocardium,[5,12] although recent debate regarding later development of trabeculations has arisen.[13] Clinically, it is characterized by the presence of deep intertrabecular recesses in hypertrophied segments of the LV myocardium (**Fig. 1**). Suggested diagnostic criteria are summarized in **Table 1**. Although it was initially thought to be an exceedingly rare disorder, it has recently become clear that LVNC is much more prevalent than previously recognized. Current studies in children and young adults estimate that LVNC accounts for approximately 9% of newly diagnosed cardiomyopathies.[7,14] The prevalence of LVNC in adult screening echocardiograms is reported to be approximately 0.05%.[8]

The clinical manifestations of LVNC are highly variable, ranging from asymptomatic to progressive heart failure and recurrent or life-threatening arrhythmias. Therefore, great interest has developed in characterizing the natural history of this disease and its associated arrhythmias, in order to help guide the counseling and management of this heterogeneous patient population. Both

The authors have nothing to disclose.
Section of Pediatric Cardiology, Department of Pediatrics, Baylor College of Medicine, Texas Children's Hospital, 6621 Fannin Street, Houston, TX 77030, USA
* Corresponding author. Section of Pediatric Cardiology, Texas Children's Hospital, 6621 Fannin Street, MC# 19345-C, Houston, TX 77030.
*E-mail address:* jjkim@texaschildrens.org

Card Electrophysiol Clin 7 (2015) 319–330
http://dx.doi.org/10.1016/j.ccep.2015.03.007
1877-9182/15/$ – see front matter © 2015 Elsevier Inc. All rights reserved.

A

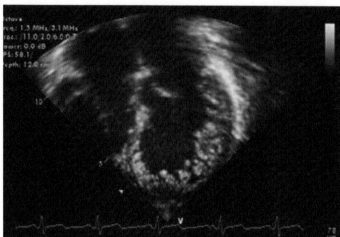

B

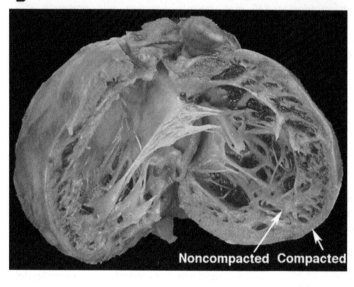

Noncompacted  Compacted

**Fig. 1.** (*A*) Echocardiographic still frame of LVNC. Noncompacted to compacted ratio of 2.3:1. (*B*) Pathologic specimen of LVNC. (*Courtesy of* Norman Silverman, MD, Palo Alto, CA.)

ventricular and supraventricular arrhythmias are now well described as prominent clinical components of LVNC.[15] Throughout the spectrum of age, they have been associated with prognosis and outcome, and thus, clinical management of these arrhythmias is an important part of patient care.[16–18] This review aims to describe the findings in literature related to arrhythmias in LVNC, allowing us to better define the presentation, history, significance, and management of rhythm abnormalities in this relatively newly defined patient population.

## GENETICS

LVNC is associated with both sporadic and familial cases, with an estimated familial recurrence rate of 23% to 33%.[16,19–22] Inheritance most commonly follows an autosomal dominant or X-linked pattern, although autosomal recessive and mitochondrial inheritance have also been observed.[23,24] As is seen with many inherited cardiac diseases, variable penetrance and phenotypic variability result in lack of clear genotype-phenotype correlation, even among family members carrying the same mutation. Although multiple genes have now been identified (**Table 2**), these mutations have not been shown to affect risk assessment, and therefore at this time there is no role for genetic testing to guide clinical management.[22–38] LVNC has been observed in case reports of patients with gene mutations involving cardiac arrhythmia syndromes including CPVT (RYR2) and long QT (KCNH2/KCNQ1)[35,36] and may be affected by SCN5a variants.[38]

**Table 1**
**Proposed diagnostic criteria for LVNC**

| Echocardiography | |
|---|---|
| Chin et al[5]<br>• Parasternal short axis, measurements at end diastole | • Two-layered structure of myocardium<br>• Determine X to Y ratio ($\leq$0.5)<br>• X = distance between epicardial surface and trough of intertrabecular recess<br>• Y = distance between epicardial surface and peak of trabeculation |
| Jenni et al[10]<br>• Short axis, measured at end systole | • Two-layered myocardium<br>• Noncompacted to compacted ratio >2.0<br>• Color Doppler of LV deep intertrabecular recesses filled with blood<br>• Absence of coexisting cardiac anomalies |
| Stöllberger et al[15,21]<br>• Apical 4-chamber view, angle views to obtain the technically best picture for differentiation between false chords/aberrant bands and trabeculations | • >3 trabeculations protruding from LV wall, located apically to papillary muscles and visible in 1 image plane<br>• Trabeculations with the same echogenicity as the myocardium and synchronous movement with ventricular contractions<br>• Perfusion of intertrabecular spaces from LV cavity<br>• Ratio of noncompacted to compacted >2 at end diastole (added subsequently) |
| van Dalen et al[74] | • Consider speckle tracking to determine LV ventricular twist |
| **Cardiac MRI** | |
| Petersen et al[26]<br>• Measured at end diastole | • Ratio between noncompacted to compacted >2.3 |
| Jacquier[27]<br>• Measured at end diastole | • Trabeculated LV mass >20% of global LV mass |

*Adapted from* Oechslin E, Jenni R. Left ventricular non-compaction revisited: a distinct phenotype with genetic heterogeneity? Eur Heart J 2011;32:1446–56.

## ELECTROCARDIOGRAPHIC FINDINGS

Electrocardiographic (ECG) abnormalities are a hallmark of many cardiomyopathies. Early findings in recent studies suggest that LVNC may be similar in this regard. An evaluation by Steffel and colleagues[39] found that only 13% of adults with diagnosed LVNC had normal results of ECGs at presentation.[39] The most common findings were intraventricular conduction delay such as left bundle branch block, voltage signs of hypertrophy, and repolarization abnormalities (**Table 3**). Over 70% of the individuals were noted to have pathologic repolarization with over 50% having prolongation in their QT intervals. No ECG findings were thought to be specific for LVNC, although conduction delay and prolongation of the QTc were associated with reduced systolic function and voltage findings of LV hypertrophy were associated with systemic embolic events ($P$<.05). Alternatively, those with normal results of ECGs at presentation were more likely to have better left ventricular ejection fractions (LVEF).

A subsequent study using a prospective noncompaction cardiomyopathy registry found early repolarization to be highly prevalent on ECG in 39% of this cohort. Early repolarization was noted to be more common in those presenting with VT/ventricular fibrillation (VF) (75%) as opposed to those without VT/VF (31%) ($P$ = .02). Long-term outcome for VT/VF also seemed to be worse in those with early repolarization ($P$ = .05).[40] Mechanistically, it was proposed that increased trabeculation with deep intramyocardial invagination, carrying the Purkinje system deeper into the myocardium, resulted in both delayed depolarization and inhomogeneous repolarization.

WPW syndrome has also been reported in association with LVNC since early descriptions.[6] Although precise estimates in adults are not delineated, it seems that WPW is more commonly seen in children, ranging from 8% to 14%.[6,16] As expected, this can be associated with the

**Table 2**
**Genes associated with LVNC**

| Gene | Protein |
|------|---------|
| ACTC1 | α-Actinin-2 |
| ACTN2 | α-Cardiac actin |
| DTNA | α-Dystrobrevin |
| DYS/nZASP | Dystrophin |
| GLA | α-Galactosidase |
| LDB3 | LIM-domain binding 3 |
| LMNA | Lamin A/C |
| MYBPC3 | Myosin-binding protein C |
| MYH7 | β-Myosin heavy chain 7 |
| TAZ | Tafazzin |
| TNNT2 | Cardiac troponin T, type 2 |
| TPM1 | α-Tropomyosin |
| TNNI3 | Cardiac troponin I |

*Data from* Refs.[22–38]

development of future episodes of supraventricular arrhythmias. It is hypothesized that in these patients, primitive AV connections persist because of the generalized arrest in cardiac development,

**Table 3**
**Baseline ECG findings at initial diagnosis in patients with LVNC**

| ECG Findings | Adults (n = 78) | Children (n = 242) |
|--------------|-----------------|---------------------|
| Normal result of ECG | 10 (13%) | 32 (13%) |
| Right bundle branch block | 2 (3%) | 10 (4%) |
| Left bundle branch block | 15 (19%) | 1 (<1%) |
| WPW | 2 (3%) | 20 (8%) |
| Left axis deviation | - | 21 (9%) |
| LV hypertrophy | 30 (38%) | 87 (36%) |
| RV hypertrophy | 5 (6%) | 13 (5%) |
| P mitrale | 20 (26%) | 17 (7%) |
| P pulmonale | 12 (15%) | 28 (12%) |
| First-degree AV block | 12 (15%) | 2 (1%) |
| Complete AV block | 2 (3%) | 2 (1%) |
| ST-segment changes | 48 (61%) | 82 (34%) |
| T-wave inversion | 32 (41%) | 78 (32%) |
| QTc prolongation | 40 (52%) | 22 (9%) |

*Data from* Steffel J, Kobza R, Oechslin E, et al. Electrocardiographic characteristics at initial diagnosis in patients with isolated left ventricular noncompaction. Am J Cardiol 2009;104:984–9; and Brescia ST, Rossano JW, Pignatelli R, et al. Mortality and sudden death in pediatric left ventricular noncompaction in a tertiary referral center. Circulation 2013;127:2202–8.

resulting in direct continuity between the atrial and ventricular myocardium across the annulus fibrosus.

With regard to children with LVNC, similar to adults, ECG abnormalities should be considered the norm. A study by Brescia and colleagues[16] found that only 13% of children had normal results of ECGs at presentation, with the majority having significant abnormalities. The most common finding in children was voltage criteria for ventricular hypertrophy, some with extreme QRS voltage similar to that seen in Pompe disease. Other common findings included repolarization abnormalities, atrial enlargement, axis deviation, and WPW syndrome (see **Table 3**). Children were less likely to have conduction abnormalities than adults, such as bundle branch block or AV block. Again, no findings were specific to LVNC; however, T-wave inversion and ST-segment changes were associated with increased mortality ($P \leq .05$).

These early descriptions highlight the fact that ECG abnormalities are indeed commonplace in LVNC and may be associated with mechanisms for arrhythmogenesis. Use of electrocardiography in this cohort may therefore be important because it may harbor both diagnostic and prognostic potential. Whether these ECG findings have more prominent implications in patient outcomes warrant further prospective investigation.

## VENTRICULAR ARRHYTHMIAS

Early descriptions of LVNC point to 3 major clinical manifestations of the disease, including heart failure, embolic events, and arrhythmias.[5,8] Although a variety of arrhythmias have subsequently been identified in association with LVNC, ventricular tachyarrhythmias have been considered the hallmark. Recent larger series have found VT in as many as 47% of affected individuals (**Table 4**), with sudden cardiac death (SCD) accounting for a significant portion of the mortality.[5,8,17,40,41] There has been wide variability, however, with some studies suggesting a much lower prevalence of ventricular arrhythmias.[42] A recent systematic overview of literature by Bhatia and colleagues,[43] including over 200 adults, found the prevalence of VT (both sustained and nonsustained) to be 38%. This finding was thought to merit special attention because SCD accounted for greater than 55% of all LVNC-related mortality in their analysis. In children, the reported prevalence of ventricular arrhythmias has varied widely, ranging from 0% to 40%.[5,6,16] The most recent description by Brescia and colleagues[16] reported an incidence of VT in 17% of children, with most developing during the course of follow-up. Owing to these

**Table 4**
**Prevalence of arrhythmias and mortality in LVNC**

| | Chin et al[5] | Ichida et al[6] | Brescia et al[16] | Ritter et al[8] | Oechslin et al[17] | Murphy et al[20] | Stöllberger & Finsterer[40] | Aras et al[21] |
|---|---|---|---|---|---|---|---|---|
| Patients (n) | 8 | 27 | 242 | 17 | 34 | 45 | 62 | 67 |
| Median age (y) | 7 | 5 | 7 (mean) | 45 | 42 | 37 (mean) | 50 (mean) | 41 |
| Median follow-up (y) | — | 6 | 4 | 2.5 (mean) | 3 (mean) | 2.7 | — | 2.5 |
| ECG abnormalities (%) | 88 | 88 | 87 | 88 | 94 | 91 | 92 | 88 |
| VT (%) | 38 | 0 | 17 | 47 | 41 | 20 | 18 | 36 |
| AF (%) | — | — | 1 | 29 | 26 | 7 | 5 | 12 |
| Atrial flutter (%) | 0 | 0 | 2 | — | — | — | — | 0 |
| Atrial tachycardia (%) | 0 | 0 | 6 | — | — | — | 3 | 0 |
| Supraventricular tachycardia (%) | 13 | 7 | 8 | — | — | — | 0 | 0 |
| Mortality (%) | 38 | 7 | 13 | 47 | 35 | 2 | — | 15 |
| Sudden death (%) | 13 | 0 | 6 | 18 | 18 | 2 | — | 9 |

The symbol "—" denotes unreported.

findings, several investigators recommend routine monitoring for arrhythmias with regimented follow-up, as well as aggressive management including antiarrhythmic therapy and consideration for implantation of cardioverter-defibrillators.

Although the primary form of ventricular arrhythmia reported in studies remains sustained or nonsustained monomorphic VT, specific morphologic descriptions have not been carried out and series to date have emphasized the broad spectrum of presentation. Indeed, case reports have found a variety of ventricular arrhythmias in association with LVNC, including bundle branch reentry, right ventricular outflow tract (RVOT) origin, apparent idiopathic VT, left bundle branch and right bundle branch morphologies, fascicular VT, bidirectional VT, polymorphic VT, and VF.[44–48] Despite overarching lack of specificity, on case-by-case bases, morphologic assessment may be helpful in determining possible therapeutic approaches as discussed below. In addition, the arrhythmias may be a diagnostic trigger where LVNC was not considered before, pointing to the need for a high index of suspicion.

The precise mechanism for ventricular arrhythmias in patients with LVNC is not delineated. However, it is postulated that developmental arrest of conduction and the presence of intratrabecular crypts may create pathways for reentrant circuits. In addition, relatively decreased perfusion and ischemia-related fibrosis at subendocardial noncompacted regions can cause electrical inhomogeneity and microreentry resulting in ventricular arrhythmias.[45,49] Histologic examination has demonstrated evidence of increased subendocardial fibrosis within areas of noncompacted myocardium supporting this theory.[5] The presence of late potentials or prolonged QT dispersion has also been described, which may play a role in the substrate for ventricular arrhythmias and sudden death.

The prognostic implications of ventricular arrhythmias in LVNC are being evaluated. Although results are limited to date, the presence of ventricular arrhythmias seems to be associated with an increased risk of death or transplantation. A recent study of 65 adults found a history of sustained VT (>30 seconds) to be an independent risk factor for cardiovascular death or heart transplantation based on multivariate analysis, with a hazard ratio (HR) of 10.1 (P = .004).[19] In children, the presence of VT was similarly found to be a risk factor for death or transplantation with an HR of 4.0 (P = .001).[16] Further study is warranted, but early data suggest, as might be expected, that ventricular arrhythmias may be a harbinger of poor prognosis.

## SUPRAVENTRICULAR ARRHYTHMIAS

Recent reports suggest that supraventricular arrhythmias are also implicated in the natural history of LVNC. In adults, this seems to be primarily manifested by AF. Studies by Weiford and colleagues[18] and Ritter and colleagues[8] describe a prevalence of AF in their cohorts of as high as 29% (see **Table 4**). Other evaluations, however, found a slightly lower prevalence of AF in LVNC, ranging from 5% to 26%.[20,21,50] The mechanistic role of LVNC in the development of AF remains unclear; it may be related to atrial dilation secondary to cardiac dysfunction and relative AV valve regurgitation or primary myocardial involvement because of underlying myopathy and affected ion channels. When patients with LVNC and AF were investigated by cardiac MRI, however, no areas of fibrosis in the atria were reported.[51]

Prognostically, in patients with LVNC, the presence of AF was associated with increased symptoms of heart failure, higher New York Heart Association (NYHA) class, and worse systolic function (P<.01). In addition, based on log rank testing, patients with AF had higher mortality rates than patients without AF (P = .012).[50] In one study, multivariate analysis found AF to be an independent predictor of mortality in LVNC with an HR of 3.3, causing the investigators to question whether more aggressive AF therapy would potentially improve prognosis.[52]

In children, the mechanisms for supraventricular arrhythmias seem to be more related to AV reentrant tachycardia or focal atrial tachycardia than primary intra-atrial pathology. Pediatric studies to date show a low prevalence of AF or atrial flutter, but describe a 7% to 13% prevalence of supraventricular tachycardia (SVT) (see **Table 4**). Recent assessment by Brescia and colleagues[16] found macroreentrant SVT in 8% and focal atrial tachycardia in 6% of their cohort. This higher incidence of SVT in children may be related to the relatively common association with WPW, as mentioned previously. Although the presence of any arrhythmia in children with LVNC seems to increase the risk of cardiac death (HR, 2.8; P = .002),[16] it is thought that ventricular arrhythmias remain the predominant player and it is unclear what prognostic contribution supraventricular arrhythmias might have.

## SUDDEN DEATH

In current reports, rates of sudden death have varied significantly, ranging from 0% to 18%, possibly because of differences in selection of patient population (isolated vs nonisolated LVNC) and length of follow-up.[5,6,8,16,17,19–21,52] In the largest pediatric study of isolated LVNC to date, the risk of sudden death was reported to be 6%.[16] In the scheme of all-cause mortality, sudden death may account for up to 50% of deaths, suggesting the possible importance of primary or secondary prevention schemes.[5,8,16,17,19,21] Unfortunately, definitive risks of sudden death have not been well defined as of yet. However, several factors including age at presentation and presence of cardiac and extracardiac manifestations have been suggested to contribute to the overall risk profile. In particular, decreased LV systolic function, abnormal LV dimensions, and the presence of ventricular arrhythmias seem to contribute to sudden death rates.[16,17,19,21]

In pediatric patients, dysmorphic features (in particular a prominent forehead, low-set ears, strabismus, micrognathia) and the presence of AV bypass tracts have also been associated with increased risk of ventricular arrhythmias and sudden death.[5,53–55] An electrophysiology (EP) study, risk assessment, and ablation procedure should therefore be considered in the presence of WPW. In addition, an ICD may be considered in certain subsets of patients as described below.[5,53–55]

## RISK ASSESSMENT

The ability to identify predictors of outcome is important in the effective and optimal management of all patients with cardiomyopathy. Unfortunately, determining risk factors for mortality or sudden death in LVNC has been complicated by several factors including: (1) phenotypic heterogeneity of disease, (2) varying diagnostic criteria, and (3) lack of randomized controlled studies. Thus, definitive risk factors remain lacking. Nonetheless, as mentioned above, increased mortality does seem to be associated with increased LV size, decreased LV systolic function, and the presence of ventricular arrhythmias.[16,17,19,21] In addition, symptomatic heart failure (ie, NYHA class III/IV) and AF in adults and repolarization abnormalities (ST changes and T-wave inversion) in pediatric patients may also be harbingers of poor outcome.[16,17,19,21,52] As such, periodic echocardiography and ambulatory monitoring for arrhythmias at regular intervals is recommended, likely at minimum on an annual basis.[16] Age has not been implicated as a risk factor unless presentation occurs at less than 1 year of age.[16,17,21] Gender, location, and degree of noncompaction also do not seem to be risk factors. Risk factors suggested in the literature are demonstrated in **Box 1**.

Data regarding the utility of programmed electrical stimulation (PES) in LVNC is limited, and there are no guidelines or recommendations regarding

---

**Box 1**
**Risk factors for increased mortality in LVNC**

*Risk factors for mortality (death, OHT)*

All patients

- Increased LV dimensions
- Decreased LV systolic function
- NYHA class III/IV
- Ventricular arrhythmias
- AF

Pediatric patients

- Age at presentation less than 1 year
- ECG changes (ST changes or T-wave inversions)
- Dysmorphic facies (prominent forehead, strabismus, low-set ears, micrognathia, high arched palate)

---

its use. In the largest adult study to date, Steffel and colleagues[56] demonstrated inducible ventricular arrhythmias in 9 of 24 patients (38%) referred for PES. Among 7 patients with inducible VT who underwent ICD implantation, 3 received appropriate device therapy during a follow-up period of 30 ± 19 months. Among 13 patients without inducible VT, symptomatic tachyarrhythmias were not seen in follow-up. Nevertheless, there have been several case reports of patients with documented atrial and ventricular tachyarrhythmias (including polymorphic VT) and even sudden death that did not have inducible arrhythmias at the EP study, suggesting that the negative predictive value may be inadequate.[48,57,58] Thus, the usefulness of PES for risk stratification in this population remains to be determined.[56]

Characterization of myocardial fibrosis by cardiac MRI has been prognostic in some forms of cardiomyopathy; however, in LVNC, late gadolinium enhancement has a heterogeneous distribution and has neither been shown to be of prognostic value in patients with arrhythmias nor been shown to correlate with mortality.[59]

## THERAPEUTIC APPROACHES

Proposed therapeutic strategies for arrhythmias in LVNC are summarized in **Table 5**.

### Supraventricular Arrhythmias

In adult patients, treatment of AF should be based on published guidelines. Owing to the increased risk of embolic events in this patient population, aggressive anticoagulation strategies may be

**Table 5**
**Proposed diagnostic evaluation and therapeutic strategies for LVNC**

| Diagnostic evaluation | |
|---|---|
| Echocardiogram | • See **Table 1** for criteria |
| Cardiac MRI | • Ratio of noncompacted to compacted >2.3<br>• Trabeculated mass >20% global mass |
| Neurologic examination | |
| Family screening (first degree) | • Echocardiogram and/or genetic testing |
| Genetic testing | |
| Electrophysiology study | • Symptomatic arrhythmias or unexplained syncope |
| **Therapeutic strategies** | |
| If normal LV size and function and without arrhythmias | • Children: yearly echocardiogram and Holter<br>• Adults: every 2 y |
| Heart failure | • Follow standard guidelines |
| Anticoagulation | • Consider aspirin if LVEF $\geq$40% and <55%<br>• If LVEF <40% or history of AF, goal INR 2–3 |
| Supraventricular arrhythmias | • Standard treatment of AF<br>• Risk stratification of WPW syndrome and ablation in symptomatic (and/or asymptomatic) WPW syndrome<br>• Consider Holter q 6 mo |
| Ventricular arrhythmias | • Antiarrhythmic medications ($\beta$-blockers, sotalol, amiodarone)<br>• Consider PES and/or ablation<br>• Consider ICD if history of aborted arrest, refractory to medications or ablation<br>• Consider Holter q 6 mo |
| ICD | • Secondary prevention and/or primary prevention based on current published guidelines |
| Biventricular resynchronization | • LVEF <35% with dyssynchrony |

*Abbreviation:* INR, international normalized ratio.

warranted. Case reports of successful ablation with pulmonary vein isolation, in AF with rapid ventricular response, have been described.[60] Pediatric patients with reentrant SVT due to AV bypass tracts (WPW and concealed) can also be managed with antiarrhythmic medications or ablation. Patients with WPW may warrant risk stratification with an EP study given the risks of rapid antegrade conduction and sudden death. Also, because of possible associations with dyssynchrony from anomalous AV excitation and progressive cardiac dysfunction, WPW in the presence of LVNC may merit more assertive approaches to ablation. Reentrant SVT due to accessory bypass tracts as well as focal atrial tachycardia have been successfully ablated in LVNC.[16,21]

## Ventricular Arrhythmias

There have been no controlled studies to determine efficacy of antiarrhythmic treatment of ventricular tachyarrhythmias in LVNC. $\beta$-Blockade as a single agent for nonsustained VT has been used; however, most reports suggest that combination therapy or more potent antiarrhythmics may be necessary, with amiodarone being the most frequently used medication among adults and in those with severely depressed function. Amiodarone seems to have good efficacy in this scenario; however, incomplete control has also been described.[61,62] Monomorphic ventricular arrhythmias, particularly those that are sustained, have been successfully mapped and ablated using radiofrequency energy in patients with LVNC.[16,45,62] Arrhythmogenic substrate (most often microreentrant or focal) can be located within the noncompacted endocardium, noncompacted myocardium, or compacted epicardium. VT ablation, therefore, although typically amenable to endocardial approach, may require epicardial ablation in certain cases.[63,64]

## Implantable Cardioverter-Defibrillator

Patients with a history of aborted cardiac arrest, ventricular arrhythmias refractory to antiarrhythmic therapy or not amenable to ablation, may benefit from ICD implantation. There are no specific guidelines for primary prevention ICD implantation in patients with LVNC; however, extrapolation from current guidelines based on underlying substrate (hypertrophic or dilated) may be effective to some degree until more definitive data are available.[65,66] As such, it may be reasonable to use documented risk factors for HCM (hypertrophic cardiomyopathy) in patients with LVNC and a hypertrophic phenotype or corollary ejection fractions and cardiac dimensions believed to be risk factors in DCM for patients with a dilated phenotype. Small studies have demonstrated appropriate shocks in both secondary and primary prevention, suggesting the potential utility of ICDs in this cohort. In nearly all reported cases, ICDs have been shown to be an effective treatment strategy,[16,19,65,67,68] with only 1 reported case of a patient death due to recalcitrant VT despite an ICD.[17] Conversely, inappropriate shock rates in this population have been reported to be 13% to 20%.[65,66] Therefore, because of the high prevalence of supraventricular arrhythmias in this cohort of patients, dual-chamber devices with enhanced detection and discrimination algorithms should be considered.

## Sympathetic Denervation

Information and long-term follow-up of left cardiac sympathetic denervation in patients with LVNC is lacking. Based on short-term follow-up of 2 patients with LVNC, sympathetic denervation may be an adjunct therapy if there are poorly controlled ventricular arrhythmias; however, further studies are needed.[69]

## Bradyarrhythmias

Although less common, patients with LVNC have been reported to demonstrate a wide variety of bradyarrhythmias including sinus bradycardia and varying degrees of AV block including complete heart block.[21,61,70] Pacemakers have been implanted successfully with good results.[5,19,21,61]

## Biventricular Resynchronization Therapy

Data regarding the use of biventricular pacing and cardiac resynchronization therapy (CRT) in patients with LVNC are limited. In adult patients in whom a biventricular pacemaker or ICD was implanted based on existing heart failure guidelines, improvement in LVEF, LV end diastolic volume, and functional capacity has been reported.[71–73] However, response is not uniform, and to date there are no data to differentiate responders from nonresponders. Data regarding CRT in the pediatric LVNC population are not available.

## SUMMARY

LVNC is a newly recognized form of cardiomyopathy that has been associated with heart failure, arrhythmias, thromboembolic events, and sudden death. Both ventricular and supraventricular arrhythmias are now well described as prominent clinical components of LVNC. Arrhythmias are not restricted to noncompacted myocardium and can include AF (adults), AV accessory pathways/WPW and SVT (children), and VT. Throughout the spectrum of age, these arrhythmias have been associated with prognosis and outcome, and their clinical management is therefore an important aspect of patient care. The risk of sudden death seems to be associated with ventricular dilation, systolic dysfunction, and the presence of arrhythmias. Proposed management strategies shown to have efficacy include antiarrhythmic therapy, ablation techniques, and ICD implantation.

## REFERENCES

1. Betrián Blasco P, Gallardo Agromayor E. Ebstein's anomaly and left ventricular noncompaction association. Int J Cardiol 2007;119:264–5.
2. Feldt RH, Rahimtoola SH, Davis GD, et al. Anomalous ventricular myocardial patterns in a child with complex congenital heart disease. Am J Cardiol 1969;23:732–4.
3. Freedom RM, Patel RG, Bloom KR, et al. Congenital absence of the pulmonary valve associated with imperforate membrane type of tricuspid atresia, right ventricular tensor apparatus and intact ventricular septum: a curious developmental complex. Eur J Cardiol 1979;10:171–96.
4. Ichida F, Tsubata S, Bowles KR, et al. Novel gene mutations in patients with left ventricular noncompaction or Barth syndrome. Circulation 2001;103:1256–63.
5. Chin TK, Perloff JK, Williams RG, et al. Isolated noncompaction of left ventricular myocardium. A study of eight cases. Circulation 1990;82:507–13.
6. Ichida F, Hamamichi Y, Miyawaki T, et al. Clinical features of isolated noncompaction of the ventricular myocardium: long-term clinical course, hemodynamic properties, and genetic background. J Am Coll Cardiol 1999;34:233–40.
7. Pignatelli RH, McMahon CJ, Dreyer WJ, et al. Clinical characterization of left ventricular noncompaction in children: a relatively common form of cardiomyopathy. Circulation 2003;108:2672–8.
8. Ritter M, Oechslin E, Sütsch G, et al. Isolated noncompaction of the myocardium in adults. Mayo Clin Proc 1997;72:26–31.
9. Wald R, Veldtman G, Golding F, et al. Determinants of outcome in isolated ventricular noncompaction in childhood. Am J Cardiol 2004;94:1581–4.

10. Jenni R, Rojas J, Oechslin E. Isolated noncompaction of the myocardium. N Engl J Med 1999;340: 966–7.

11. Hook S, Ratliff NB, Rosenkranz E, et al. Isolated noncompaction of the ventricular myocardium. Pediatr Cardiol 1996;17:43–5.

12. Pepper MS. Transforming growth factor-beta: vasculogenesis, angiogenesis, and vessel wall integrity. Cytokine Growth Factor Rev 1997;8:21–43.

13. Oechslin E, Jenni R. Left ventricular non-compaction revisited: a distinct phenotype with genetic heterogeneity? Eur Heart J 2011;32:1446–56.

14. Nugent AW, Daubeney PE, Chondros P, et al. National Australian Childhood Cardiomyopathy Study. Clinical features and outcomes of childhood hypertrophic cardiomyopathy: results from a national population-based study. Circulation 2005; 112:1332–8.

15. Steffel J, Duru F. Rhythm disorders in isolated left ventricular noncompaction. Ann Med 2012;44: 101–8.

16. Brescia ST, Rossano JW, Pignatelli R, et al. Mortality and sudden death in pediatric left ventricular noncompaction in a tertiary referral center. Circulation 2013;127:2202–8.

17. Oechslin EN, Attenhofer Jost CH, Rojas JR, et al. Long-term follow-up of 34 adults with isolated left ventricular noncompaction: a distinct cardiomyopathy with poor prognosis. J Am Coll Cardiol 2000; 36:493–500.

18. Weiford BC, Subbarao VD, Mulhern KM. Noncompaction of the ventricular myocardium. Circulation 2004;109:2965–71.

19. Lofiego C, Biagini E, Pasquale F, et al. Wide spectrum of presentation and variable outcomes of isolated left ventricular non-compaction. Heart 2007; 93:65–71.

20. Murphy RT, Thaman R, Blanes JG, et al. Natural history and familial characteristics of isolated left ventricular non-compaction. Eur Heart J 2005;26: 187–92.

21. Aras D, Tufekcioglu O, Ergun K, et al. Clinical features of isolated ventricular noncompaction in adults long-term clinical course, echocardiographic properties, and predictors of left ventricular failure. J Card Fail 2006;12:726–33.

22. Gimeno JR, Lacunza J, García-Alberola A, et al. Penetrance and risk profile in inherited cardiac diseases studied in a dedicated screening clinic. Am J Cardiol 2009;104:406–10.

23. Digilio MC, Marino B, Bevilacqua M, et al. Genetic heterogeneity of isolated noncompaction of the left ventricular myocardium. Am J Med Genet 1999;85:90–1.

24. Towbin JA. Left ventricular noncompaction: a new form of heart failure. Heart Fail Clin 2010;6: 453–69, viii.

25. Sasse-Klaassen S, Gerull B, Oechslin E, et al. Isolated noncompaction of the left ventricular myocardium in the adult is an autosomal dominant disorder in the majority of patients. Am J Med Genet A 2003;119A:162–7.

26. Towbin JA. Inherited cardiomyopathies. Circ J 2014; 78:2347–56.

27. Wessels MW, Herkert JC, Frohn-Mulder IM, et al. Compound heterozygous or homozygous truncating MYBPC3 mutations cause lethal cardiomyopathy with features of noncompaction and septal defects. Eur J Hum Genet 2014. [Epub ahead of print].

28. Bagnall RD, Molloy LK, Kalman JM, et al. Exome sequencing identifies a mutation in the ACTN2 gene in a family with idiopathic ventricular fibrillation, left ventricular noncompaction, and sudden death. BMC Med Genet 2014;15:99.

29. Klaassen S, Probst S, Oechslin E, et al. Mutations in sarcomere protein genes in left ventricular noncompaction. Circulation 2008;117:2893–901.

30. Probst S, Oechslin E, Schuler P, et al. Sarcomere gene mutations in isolated left ventricular noncompaction cardiomyopathy do not predict clinical phenotype. Circ Cardiovasc Genet 2011;4:367–74.

31. Luedde M, Ehlermann P, Weichenhan D, et al. Severe familial left ventricular non-compaction cardiomyopathy due to a novel troponin T (TNNT2) mutation. Cardiovasc Res 2010;86:452–60.

32. Chang B, Nishizawa T, Furutani M, et al. Noncompaction study collaborators. Identification of a novel TPM1 mutation in a family with left ventricular non-compaction and sudden death. Mol Genet Metab 2011;102:200–6.

33. Teekakirikul P, Kelly MA, Rehm HL, et al. Inherited cardiomyopathies: molecular genetics and clinical genetic testing in the postgenomic era. J Mol Diagn 2013;15:158–70.

34. Shieh JT. Implications of genetic testing in noncompaction/hypertrabeculation. Am J Med Genet C Semin Med Genet 2013;163C:206–11.

35. Szentpáli Z, Szili-Torok T, Caliskan K. Primary electrical disorder or primary cardiomyopathy? A case with a unique association of noncompaction cardiomyopathy and cathecolaminergic polymorphic ventricular tachycardia caused by ryanodine receptor mutation. Circulation 2013;127:1165–6.

36. Nakashima K, Kusakawa I, Yamamoto T, et al. A left ventricular noncompaction in a patient with long QT syndrome caused by a KCNQ1 mutation: a case report. Heart Vessels 2013;28:126–9.

37. Ogawa K, Nakamura Y, Terano K, et al. Isolated noncompaction of the ventricular myocardium associated with long QT syndrome: a report of 2 cases. Circ J 2009;73:2169–72.

38. Shan L, Makita N, Xing Y, et al. SCN5A variants in Japanese patients with left ventricular noncompaction and arrhythmia. Mol Genet Metab 2008;93:468–74.

39. Steffel J, Kobza R, Oechslin E, et al. Electrocardiographic characteristics at initial diagnosis in patients with isolated left ventricular noncompaction. Am J Cardiol 2009;104:984–9.

40. Stöllberger C, Finsterer J. Arrhythmias and left ventricular hypertrabeculation/noncompaction. Curr Pharm Des 2010;16:2880–94.

41. Rigopoulos A, Rizos IK, Aggeli C, et al. Isolated left ventricular noncompaction: an unclassified cardiomyopathy with severe prognosis in adults. Cardiology 2002;98:25–32.

42. Fazio G, Corrado G, Zachara E, et al. Ventricular tachycardia in non-compaction of left ventricle: is this a frequent complication? Pacing Clin Electrophysiol 2007;30:544–6.

43. Bhatia NL, Tajik AJ, Wilansky S, et al. Isolated noncompaction of the left ventricular myocardium in adults: a systematic overview. J Card Fail 2011;17:771–8.

44. Güvenç TS, Ilhan E, Alper AT, et al. Exercise-induced right ventricular outflow tract tachycardia in a patient with isolated left ventricular noncompaction. ISRN Cardiol 2011;2011:729040–4.

45. Derval N, Jais P, O'Neill MD, et al. Apparent idiopathic ventricular tachycardia associated with isolated ventricular noncompaction. Heart Rhythm 2009;6:385–8.

46. Barra S, Moreno N, Providência R, et al. Incessant slow bundle branch reentrant ventricular tachycardia in a young patient with left ventricular noncompaction. Rev Port Cardiol 2013;32:523–9.

47. Santoro F, Manuppelli V, Brunetti ND. Multiple morphology ventricular tachycardia in noncompaction cardiomyopathy: multi-modal imaging. Europace 2013;15:304.

48. Serés L, Lopez J, Larrousse E, et al. Isolated noncompaction left ventricular myocardium and polymorphic ventricular tachycardia. Clin Cardiol 2003;26:46–8.

49. Junga G, Kneifel S, Smekal Von A, et al. Myocardial ischaemia in children with isolated left ventricular noncompaction. Eur Heart J 1999;20:910–6.

50. Stöllberger C, Blazek G, Winkler-Dworak M, et al. Atrial fibrillation in left ventricular noncompaction with and without neuromuscular disorders is associated with a poor prognosis. Int J Cardiol 2009;133:41–5.

51. Ivan D, Flamm SD, Abrams J, et al. Isolated ventricular non-compaction in adults with idiopathic cardiomyopathy: cardiac magnetic resonance and pathologic characterization of the anomaly. J Heart Lung Transplant 2005;24:781–6.

52. Stöllberger C, Blazek G, Wegner C, et al. Heart failure, atrial fibrillation and neuromuscular disorders influence mortality in left ventricular hypertrabeculation/noncompaction. Cardiology 2011;119:176–82.

53. Yasukawa K, Terai M, Honda A, et al. Isolated noncompaction of ventricular myocardium associated with fatal ventricular fibrillation. Pediatr Cardiol 2001;22:512–4.

54. Fichet J, Legras A, Bernard A, et al. Aborted sudden cardiac death revealing isolated noncompaction of the left ventricle in a patient with Wolff-Parkinson-White syndrome. Pacing Clin Electrophysiol 2007;30:444–7.

55. Nihei K, Shinomiya N, Kabayama H, et al. Wolff-Parkinson-White (WPW) syndrome in isolated noncompaction of the ventricular myocardium (INVM). Circ J 2004;68:82–4.

56. Steffel J, Kobza R, Namdar M, et al. Electrophysiological findings in patients with isolated left ventricular non-compaction. Europace 2009;11:1193–200.

57. Seethala S, Knollman F, McNamara D, et al. Exercise-induced atrial and ventricular tachycardias in a patient with left ventricular noncompaction and normal ejection fraction. Pacing Clin Electrophysiol 2011;34:e94–7.

58. Coppola G, Guttilla D, Corrado E, et al. ICD implantation in noncompaction of the left ventricular myocardium: a case report. Pacing Clin Electrophysiol 2009;32:1092–5.

59. Nucifora G, Aquaro GD, Pingitore A, et al. Myocardial fibrosis in isolated left ventricular noncompaction and its relation to disease severity. Eur J Heart Fail 2011;13(2):170–6.

60. Kato Y, Horigome H, Takahashi-Igari M, et al. Isolation of pulmonary vein and superior vena cava for paroxysmal atrial fibrillation in a young adult with left ventricular non-compaction. Europace 2010;12:1040–1.

61. Celiker A, Ozkutlu S, Dilber E, et al. Rhythm abnormalities in children with isolated ventricular noncompaction. Pacing Clin Electrophysiol 2005;28:1198–202.

62. Fiala M, Januska J, Bulková V, et al. Septal ventricular tachycardia with alternating LBBB-RBBB morphology in isolated ventricular noncompaction. J Cardiovasc Electrophysiol 2010;21:704–7.

63. Lim HE, Pak HN, Shim WJ, et al. Epicardial ablation of ventricular tachycardia associated with isolated ventricular noncompaction. Pacing Clin Electrophysiol 2006;29:797–9.

64. Chinushi M, Iijima K, Furushima H, et al. Suppression of storms of ventricular tachycardia by epicardial ablation of isolated delayed potential in noncompaction cardiomyopathy. Pacing Clin Electrophysiol 2013;36:e115–9.

65. Kobza R, Steffel J, Erne P, et al. Implantable cardioverter-defibrillator and cardiac resynchronization therapy in patients with left ventricular noncompaction. Heart Rhythm 2010;7:1545–9.

66. Caliskan K, Szili-Torok T, Theuns DA, et al. Indications and outcome of implantable cardioverter-defibrillators

for primary and secondary prophylaxis in patients with noncompaction cardiomyopathy. J Cardiovasc Electrophysiol 2011;22:898–904.

67. Amadieu R, Acar P, Séguéla PE. Implantable cardioverter defibrillator in a young child with left ventricular noncompaction. Arch Cardiovasc Dis 2011;104: 417–8.

68. Celiker A, Kafali G, Doğan R. Cardioverter defibrillator implantation in a child with isolated noncompaction of the ventricular myocardium and ventricular fibrillation. Pacing Clin Electrophysiol 2004;27:104–8.

69. Coleman MA, Bos JM, Johnson JN, et al. Videoscopic left cardiac sympathetic denervation for patients with recurrent ventricular fibrillation/malignant ventricular arrhythmia syndromes besides congenital long-QT syndrome. Circ Arrhythm Electrophysiol 2012;5:782–8.

70. Nascimento BR, Vidigal DF, De Carvalho Bicalho Carneiro R, et al. Complete atrioventricular block as the first manifestation of noncompaction of the ventricular myocardium. Pacing Clin Electrophysiol 2013;36:e107–10.

71. Okubo K, Sato Y, Matsumoto N, et al. Cardiac resynchronization and cardioverter defibrillation therapy in a patient with isolated noncompaction of the ventricular myocardium. Int J Cardiol 2009;136: e66–8.

72. Kobza R, Jenni R, Erne P, et al. Implantable cardioverter-defibrillators in patients with left ventricular noncompaction. Pacing Clin Electrophysiol 2008;31:461–7.

73. Kubota S, Nogami A, Sugiyasu A, et al. Cardiac resynchronization therapy in a patient with isolated noncompaction of the left ventricle and a narrow QRS complex. Heart Rhythm 2006;3:619–20.

74. van Dalen BM, Caliskan K, Soliman OI, et al. Left ventricular solid body rotation in non-compaction cardiomyopathy: a potential new objective and quantitative functional diagnostic criterion? Eur J Heart Fail 2008;10:1088–93.

# Arrhythmias in Takotsubo Cardiomyopathy

Kathleen Hayes Brown, MD, Richard G. Trohman, MD, MBA, Christopher Madias, MD*

## KEYWORDS

- Taskotsubo • Ventricular fibrillation • Torsades de pointes • Stress-induced cardiomyopathy
- Arrhythmia

## KEY POINTS

- Although takotstubo cardiomyopathy (TCM) is a reversible cardiomyopathy with a generally favorable prognosis, it can be associated with life-threatening ventricular arrhythmias.
- Catecholamine excess has been implicated as the precipitant of left ventricular dysfunction, and cardioprotective cellular signaling is among the mechanisms responsible for electrical derangements leading to arrhythmogenesis.
- Based on the pattern of electrocardiographic changes, the mechanism of ventricular arrhythmias during the subacute phase is likely distinct from that at the time of presentation.
- Because of the risk of severe QT prolongation during the subacute phase resulting in pause-dependent torsades de pointes, patients should be monitored in a telemetry setting until the QT interval normalizes.
- Genetic and gender-specific associations have been described, but further study is required to confirm a basis for arrhythmic susceptibility in these patients.

## INTRODUCTION

Takotsubo cardiomyopathy (TCM) is a distinct, usually reversible, form of myocardial stunning that most commonly occurs in the setting of severe emotional or physical stress. The exact mechanism of the cardiomyopathy remains undefined; however, it is thought that ventricular dysfunction is induced by catecholamine-mediated myocardial toxicity.[1–3]

The clinical profile of TCM has been well described. Although the ventricular dysfunction in TCM is reversible, the syndrome can be associated with significant morbidity and, uncommonly, mortality. Cardiac arrhythmias are among the complications associated with TCM. A gamut of arrhythmias has been reported, ranging from benign atrial arrhythmias to conduction abnormalities, including heart block, and life-threatening ventricular tachyarrhythmias. Notable electrocardiogram (ECG)

repolarization abnormalities have been established as a cardiac manifestation of the syndrome. Most patients with typical left ventricular (LV) apical involvement develop diffuse T-wave inversions (TWI), often associated with marked QT prolongation. It is clear that TCM should be considered among the causes of the acquired long QT syndrome (LQTS) and that patients can be at risk for sudden cardiac death (SCD) from the distinctive reentrant polymorphic ventricular tachyarrhythmias, torsades de pointes (TdP) and ventricular fibrillation (VF). Despite the increased recognition of the arrhythmic complications associated with TCM, the mechanism of arrhythmias remains incompletely understood, and the true risk is still ill defined. This article describes the arrhythmic burden associated with TCM and explores the pathogenesis underlying arrhythmias in the setting of this transient cardiomyopathy.

The authors have nothing to disclose.
Clinical Cardiac Electrophysiology Service, Division of Cardiology, Department of Medicine, Rush University Medical Center, Chicago, IL, USA
* Corresponding author. Division of Cardiology, Department of Medicine, Rush University Medical Center, 1750 West Harrison Street, Suite 983 Jelke, Chicago, IL 60612.
E-mail address: christopher_madias@rush.edu

Card Electrophysiol Clin 7 (2015) 331–340
http://dx.doi.org/10.1016/j.ccep.2015.03.015
1877-9182/15/$ – see front matter © 2015 Elsevier Inc. All rights reserved.

## BACKGROUND AND DEFINITION OF TAKOTSUBO CARDIOMYOPATHY

TCM, also known as stress cardiomyopathy, was first described in Japan by Sato in 1991.[1,3,4] It is defined as transient LV dysfunction typically after severe emotional or physical stress, with regional wall motion abnormalities that are confined to apical (70%–80% of cases), mid, or basal sections of the myocardium in the absence of obstructive coronary artery disease.[5] The modified Mayo Clinic Criteria for Diagnosis published in 2008 are generally accepted for the diagnosis of TCM (**Box 1**).[6] The LV dysfunction commonly extends beyond the territory associated with a single coronary artery distribution. Initial descriptions were limited to apical hypokinesis or apical ballooning; however, it is now understood that the disease encompasses isolated apical, basal, or even mid cardiac dyskinesis. Given the extent of regional wall motion abnormality, cardiac biomarker elevations are disproportionately low in comparison with patients with acute myocardial infarction (MI).[2,6,7] A diagnosis of TCM is unlikely in patients with troponin T greater than 6 ng/mL or troponin I greater than 15 ng/mL.[8]

Although typically considered benign in comparison with acute ST-elevation MI, the disease does carry significant risk, with a mortality rate of 2% to 8 %[3,9,10] associated with acute cardiogenic shock, fatal cardiac arrhythmias, or mechanical complications such as myocardial rupture.[5,9,11] Additional morbidity resulting from embolization of intraventricular thrombi, or acute severe mitral regurgitation and LV outflow tract obstruction, is not insignificant.[1,5,9,11,12]

TCM comprises 1% to 2.5 %[1,5,12] of patients presenting with acute coronary syndrome and represents 2% of patients presenting with ST elevation, typically resembling acute anterior MI, on ECG.[2,10] Most cases occur in postmenopausal women. There is no significant age difference in incidence between men and women, but men are more likely to have a physical stressor as an inciting factor as opposed to women, in whom emotional stress plays a more dominant role[5,9]; however, in some cases there is no obvious identifiable trigger.

## MECHANISMS OF TAKOTSUBO CARDIOMYOPATHY

The primary mechanism of TCM is thought to be catecholamine-mediated myocardial toxicity. Circulating levels of epinephrine and norepinephrine have been reported to be 2 to 3 times higher in TCM patients than those with acute MI.[10,11,13] Catecholaminergic injury is further supported by the description of TCM induced with the administration of agents such as epinephrine in the management of respiratory compromise, phenylephrine during noncardiac surgery, dobutamine during stress testing, and even intranasal phenylephrine for refractory epistaxis.[9,14] The exact mechanism of cardiac myocyte dysfunction is controversial.[1] Hyperadrenergic theories attribute catecholamine excess to direct myocardial toxicity and/or activation of α- and β-adrenergic receptors, leading to microvascular dysfunction or coronary spasm. The variable distribution of cardiac β receptors- might be responsible for regional variations in myocyte dysfunction.[10,14] Myocardial biopsies in patients with TCM demonstrate contraction band necrosis, infiltration of inflammatory cells, and localized fibrosis, all evidence of direct catecholamine toxicity.[15] Because there is a higher density of β adrenoreceptors in the apical aspect and higher nerve density in the basal myocardium,[14] the mechanisms of disease might be different in the various patterns of dyskinesis. Initial occurrence is a known risk factor for recurrence, suggesting that certain individuals are predisposed to cardiac effects of a hypercatecholaminergic state.[16,17]

Ongoing studies are being conducted establish a genetic predisposition to TCM. High catecholamine levels are known to increase the expression and enzymatic activity of G-protein–coupled receptor kinases (GRKs). GRKs are ultimately responsible for the downregulation of β adrenoreceptors, leading to uncoupling of G proteins and negative inotropy.[10,14] The prevailing hypothesis

---

**Box 1**
**Modified Mayo Clinic Criteria for diagnosis of takotsubo cardiomyopathy**

1. Transient hypokinesis, akinesis, or dyskinesis of the left ventricle mid segments with or without apical involvement; the regional wall motion abnormalities extend beyond a single epicardial vascular distribution; a stressful trigger is often, but not always present

2. Absence of obstructive coronary disease or angiographic evidence of acute plaque rupture

3. New electrocardiographic abnormalities (either ST-segment elevation and/or T-wave inversion) or modest elevation in cardiac troponin

4. Absence of pheochromocytoma or myocarditis

(*From* Prasad A, Lerman A, Rihal CS. Apical ballooning syndrome (Tako-tsubo or stress cardiomyopathy): a mimic of acute myocardial infarction. Am Heart J 2008;155(3):408–17; with permission.)

is that this downregulation is cardioprotective in the setting of catecholamine excess, as ongoing presence of the activated form of the G protein, G$_s$, results in apoptosis.[11,14] One of the most commonly expressed protein kinases in the heart is GRK5, which is linked to the L41Q gene polymorphism. In a study of 20 patients with TCM and 22 controls, Novo and colleagues[10] demonstrated that a variant of L41Q was present in 40% of patients with TCM and only 8% of controls, suggesting that patients with a genetic predisposition might have more sensitivity to catecholamine effects on G-protein coupling.

## EVOLUTION OF ELECTROCARDIOGRAPHIC CHANGES

The ECG in TCM evolves with the clinical progression of the syndrome. Typically the ECG reveals ST elevation, predominantly in the precordial leads, at the time of presentation in 53% to 90% of patients and concomitant QT prolongation within the first few hours.[1–3,16] In a series evaluating presenting ECGs of 33 TCM patients, the ECGs displayed a lower maximal ST elevation, but showed a greater overall number of leads with ST-segment elevation, compared with patients presenting with acute anterior ST-elevation MI. Specifically, ST elevation in TCM was more frequently seen in leads I, II, III, aVF, and especially aVR. By contrast, TCM was less frequently associated with ST-segment elevation in leads aVL and particularly V1. In addition,

presenting ECGs in TCM displayed reciprocal changes and pathologic Q waves significantly less frequently.[18] Low QRS voltage and attenuation of the amplitude of the QRS complexes is also highly prevalent in TCM, and might be another means of differentiating this syndrome from MI.[19] Occasionally, patients with TCM present with TWI on the first ECG. It is postulated that in such patients a brief phase of ST elevation might have been missed at the onset of the episode.[19]

As the clinical course progresses to the subacute phase (days 1–3 after admission), ST elevation is typically replaced by deep TWI, most prominent in leads V2 to V6 and I, II, and aVL.[2,3,16] TCM is associated with a wider distribution and greater maximal amplitude of negative T waves in comparison with acute MI.[7] Similarly to acute MI, some patients show a bimodal occurrence of T-wave deepening, at 24 to 48 hours and again at 2 to 3 weeks.[16] Transient Q waves are also present in approximately 10% of patients and are most likely to be present in V2 and V3.[2,3,16]

The progression of QT prolongation in TCM parallels the evolution of TWIs. QT prolongation is present in up to 86% of patients, most of whom have no risk factors or prior history of LQTS, and can persist for weeks.[3,16] In a study by Bennett and colleagues,[3] the mean peak QTc interval in 145 TCM patients was 515.8 ± 61.1 milliseconds within the first 24 hours. Even when increased on admission, the QT interval prolongs further, usually peaking at 2 to 3 days (the subacute phase; **Fig. 1**).[4,7,20] During

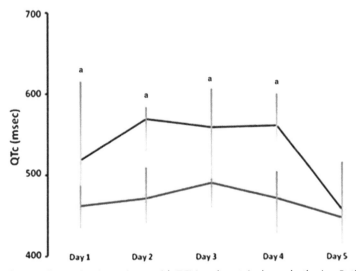

**Fig. 1.** Time course of QT prolongation in patients with TCM and ventricular arrhythmias. Patients with TCM and ventricular arrhythmias (*blue*) show longer QTc intervals on presentation compared with TCM patients without ventricular arrhythmias (*red*). During the subacute phase (days 2 and 3), QTc intervals are further prolonged significantly in patients with ventricular arrhythmias. By day 5, QTc intervals return to similar levels in both groups. Data shown are median QTc with interquartile range ([a]P<.05). (*From* Madias C, Fitzgibbons TP, Alsheikh-Ali AA, et al. Acquired long QT syndrome from stress cardiomyopathy is associated with ventricular arrhythmias and torsades de pointes. Heart Rhythm 2011;8:555–61; with permission.)

this phase, the combination of TWI and QT prolongation, which can be substantial, can produce the pattern of giant TWI, especially if bradycardia is also present.[4,21] QT prolongation gradually resolves in conjunction with resolution of TWIs; however, the ECG changes in TCM often resolve significantly later than the ECG demonstration of LV wall motion recovery.[7,20] The QT has been described to lengthen again in patients that display a biphasic TWI pattern, but the degree of prolongation is not as severe as that seen during the subacute phase of the syndrome.[7,20] The mechanisms of ECG changes associated with TCM are not well understood; however, it has been suggested that myocardial edema might be among the causes underlying the commonly observed repolarization abnormalities.[22] Cardiac magnetic resonance imaging is emerging as a useful tool to differentiate acute ischemic MI from TCM and to document progression of disease via the pattern of edema. Reproducible studies have demonstrated the appearance and resolution of segmental edema using cardiac magnetic resonance imaging with late gadolinium enhancement, with clearly delineated segmental wall motion abnormalities that cross the distribution of more than 1 coronary artery perfusion territory. The pattern of edema, and its progression and resolution, has been seen to parallel TWI and QTc prolongation in this patient population, including its biphasic pattern.[9,22] Of note, the ECG findings in rarer, variant forms of TCM, namely midventricular and reverse TCM, are less well defined and appear to differ from those in patients with typical apical ballooning patterns. ST elevation and TWI are less frequent and QT prolongation is often not as severe.[23,24]

## PREVALENCE OF ARRHYTHMIAS

There is an increased incidence of both atrial and ventricular arrhythmias among TCM patients. The true arrhythmic burden in TCM remains poorly defined and is likely to be underestimated. Despite the severe repolarization abnormalities observed in TCM and the heightened adrenergic milieu, the reported arrhythmic risk is surprisingly low. In a comprehensive literature review encompassing 816 cases, Syed and colleagues[25] reported a range of arrhythmias including atrial fibrillation (4.7% of cases), sinus node dysfunction (1.3% of cases), and atrioventricular nodal dysfunction (including heart block in 2.9% of cases). The frequency of life-threatening ventricular arrhythmias, including VF or sustained ventricular tachycardia (VT), was 3.4% (28 of 816 cases). Analysis of data from 16,450 patients with TCM in the Nationwide Inpatient Sample database established an overall arrhythmic burden of 26%. Atrial arrhythmias were

most common, with atrial fibrillation and flutter accounting for 8.8% of arrhythmias overall. Paroxysmal supraventricular tachycardia was reported in 0.8% of cases. The overall incidence of life-threatening ventricular arrhythmias was 4.2%.[26]

## MECHANISMS OF VENTRICULAR ARRHYTHMIA

Studies of the mechanisms of ventricular arrhythmia in TCM are ongoing, although patterns suggest broad mechanisms for arrhythmogenesis. In addition to the direct effects of catecholamines, oxidative stress leading to dysregulation of calcium homeostasis is also thought to contribute to myocyte dysfunction in addition to cardiac arrhythmias.[5,13,14] Early afterdepolarizations from catecholamine surge, as evidenced by giant T-U waves notable on ECG tracings, are likely inciting factors.[4] The risk for ventricular arrhythmias resides in the acute and subacute phases of the disease process, although the mechanisms seem to differ.[4] VT and VF have been described in the acute phase, before QT-interval prolongation, but are rare and typically associated with episodes of cardiac arrest or cardiogenic shock during the highest levels of circulating catecholamines (**Fig. 2**). The stress of cardiac arrest and subsequent resuscitation could itself be a trigger for TCM. Catecholamine excess is known to promote calcium entry into cardiac myocytes by stimulation of receptor-mediated calcium channels.[27] Increased cardiac ryanodine receptor-dependent diastolic sarcoplasmic reticulum calcium leak is present in heart failure and under conditions whereby adrenergic tone is high, with increased calcium leak from the sarcoplasmic reticulum resulting in spontaneous calcium wave formation, which in turn activates the inward sodium/calcium exchange current causing early afterdepolarizations potentially leading to arrhythmias.[28] This effect has been demonstrated in animal models using isoproterenol exposure, which may replicate the effects of catecholamines on cardiac signaling. In TCM patients with significant ST elevation during this phase, a mechanism similar to that in an acute ischemic event is potentially a protective response to increased calcium surge. This ECG change is likely related to action potential shortening, preferentially in the subepicardium, leading to a reduction in calcium influx and depressed contraction to conserve oxygen consumption.[29]

In the subacute phase, QT prolongation with pause-dependent TdP or VF seems to be the most likely cause of SCD, and TCM should be recognized as a cause of acquired LQTS (**Fig. 3**). The concept of catecholamine excess leading to

**A**

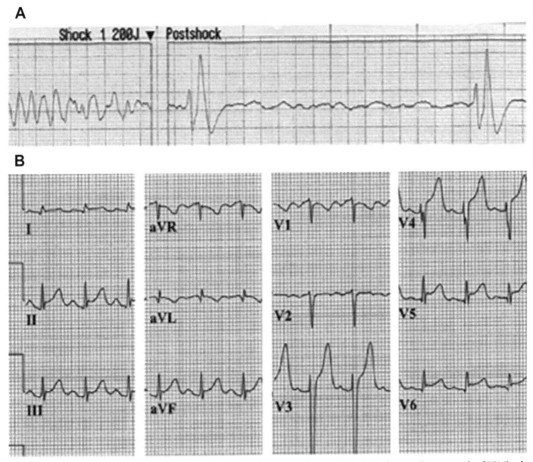

**Fig. 2.** Electrocardiograms (ECGs) and telemetry strips from a patient with takotsubo cardiomyopathy (TCM) who presented after being resuscitated in the field for VF arrest. (*A*) Defibrillator strips demonstrating resuscitation from VF. (*B*) Twelve-lead ECG at the time of presentation with ST elevations in V3 to V6, II, III, and aVF.

LV dysfunction, QT prolongation, and TdP is not limited to TCM, and is described in other hyperadrenergic states such as pheochromocytoma.[30] and subarachnoid hemorrhage.[31] Comparisons of patients with pheochromocytoma and SCD demonstrate similar patterns of QT prolongation, although in pheochromocytoma the QT prolongation and the extent of LV remodeling are slowly progressive over time, in contrast to the rapid changes seen in TCM.[30] Similarly, sympathetic nervous system–mediated QT-interval prolongation plays a role in the pathophysiology of congenital LQTS. Stimulation of the left stellate ganglion has been demonstrated to prolong the QT interval, and left cardiac sympathetic denervation remains a treatment option for intractable arrhythmias in LQTS.[32] Calcium overload leading to augmentation of ionic currents and the generation of afterdepolarizations instigating ventricular arrhythmia has been established in heart failure, LQTS, and

catecholaminergic VT from ryanodine receptor mutations. It has also been linked to prolongation of the action potential, and is likely a cause of arrhythmogenesis in TCM.[27]

TdP is infrequent after MI, and notably the timing appears to be similar to that of TCM, occurring in the subacute period (>48 hours after presentation). In a series documenting pause-dependent TdP following acute MI, TdP occurred only after the third hospitalization day, and the pattern of QT prolongation was similar to that seen in TCM. Diffuse TWI and severe QT prolongation were observed in each case. Despite absence of obstructive coronary disease in TCM, a shared mechanism is likely at play during TCM and infarct-related pause-dependent TdP. Because the ECG pattern in TCM is consistent with circumferential subepicardial ischemia (as evidenced by the nonsegmental pattern of TWI),[33] and the tachyarrhythmic risk seems to correlate with the extent of QT prolongation and TWI, other

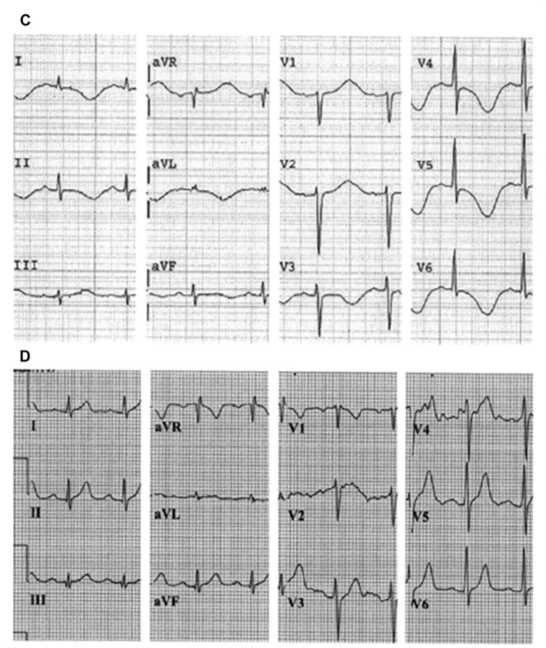

**Fig. 2.** (*continued*). (*C*) Subacute phase with deep T-wave inversions and dramatically prolonged QTc. (*D*) Post-recovery ECG demonstrating normalization of PR and QT intervals and resolution of T-wave inversions. (*From Madias C, Fitzgibbons TP, Alsheikh-Ali AA, et al. Acquired long QT syndrome from stress cardiomyopathy is associated with ventricular arrhythmias and torsades de pointes. Heart Rhythm 2011;8:555–61; with permission.*)

studies have sought to use imaging modalities to better understand and predict arrhythmic propensity in these patients.[29] A series of case studies has demonstrated transient LV myocardial edema, assessed with contrast-enhanced cardiac magnetic resonance, in patients with reversible LV dysfunction, either ischemic or nonischemic. These imaging findings resolve in parallel to the Wellens-like pattern of deep TWI seen in patients with TCM and independently of LV wall motion abnormalities, leading to speculation that cardiac arrhythmias could be linked to intramyocardial repolarization gradients between endocardial and epicardial layers (dispersion of refractoriness), providing a propensity for

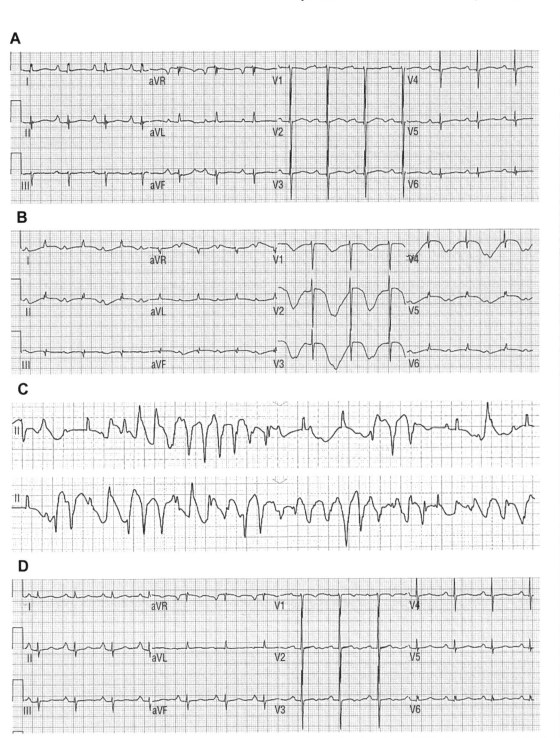

**Fig. 3.** ECGs and telemetry strips from a patient with TCM and torsades de pointes (TdP) who experienced TCM secondary to sepsis and epinephrine infusion for hypotension. (*A*) Admission ECG demonstrates first-degree atrioventricular block with QT prolongation and diffuse nonspecific T-wave abnormalities. (*B*) ECG 24 hours after epinephrine infusion shows long first-degree atrioventricular block with diffuse T-wave inversions and marked QT prolongation. (*C*) Telemetry strips show heart block and junctional escape rhythm with premature ventricular contractions triggering runs of TdP. (*D*) ECG several months later shows resolution of T-wave inversions and normalization of PR and QT intervals. *From* Madias C, Trohman RG. Ventricular arrhythmias in takotsubo cardiomyopathy. In: Zipes DP, Jalife J, editors. Cardiac electrophysiology from cell to bedside. 6th edition. Philadelphia: Elsevier; 2014. p. 919–24; with permission.

arrhythmia initiation and propagation.[22] Mammalian animal studies have demonstrated a disparity in catecholaminergic effects on subendocardial and subepicardial tissues, with a larger long-term resistance of the subepicardium in premenopausal women. This disparity is thought to be due to female sex hormone regulatory effects on calcium distribution in the sarcomere in an effort to preserve diastolic function and prevent subepicardial damage in response to the stresses of pregnancy and delivery. The reversal of this hormonal protection has been theorized among the causes of the preponderance of postmenopausal women in TCM.[29]

Abnormal repolarization reserve was first implicated as the mechanism of QT-prolonging drugs in predisposed individuals carrying silent mutations in congenital LQTS.[34] An underlying genetic basis for long QT and TdP in the setting of MI has recently been explored.[35] In 13 post-MI patients who developed TdP in the setting of deep TWI and QT prolongation, 2 (15%) were found to carry long QT mutations (KCNH2-R744X and SCN5A-E446K). Nine of the remaining 11 patients (82%) carried the KCNH2-K897T polymorphism. The KCNH2-K897T polymorphism has previously been shown to act as a modifier of arrhythmic risk in congenital LQTS. These data suggest that an enabling genetic arrhythmic substrate, which might be subclinical throughout an individual's life, could be unmasked by MI, and that common polymorphisms that act as modifiers of arrhythmic risk in LQTS might reduce the repolarization reserve and increase arrhythmic risk in the subacute phase of MI. A similar unmasking of subclinical LQTS might be responsible for the pronounced QT prolongation in patients with TCM.[36,37] Interestingly there have been reports of persistent QT prolongation after TdP events in the setting of TCM,[35,36,38,39] with an LQTS mutation identified in 1 case (mutation in the KCNH2 gene).[38] These reports suggest that, similar to TdP occurring in the subacute phase of MI, TCM might unmask a reduced repolarization reserve and an underlying predisposition toward repolarization abnormality in certain patients. Studies examining the genetic basis of arrhythmic risk in TCM are ongoing.

## MANAGEMENT

Medical management of TCM is typically similar to that of other forms of systolic heart failure, including the use of β-blockers and angiotensin-converting enzyme inhibitors, although there is no consensus on the duration of treatment. Some disease-specific medications can be considered on a case-by-case basis. Prophylactic use of anticoagulation might be considered in patients who are at higher risk of stroke, given the propensity of these patients to develop apical thrombi and subsequent embolic sequelae. In addition, in patients with evidence of LV outflow tract obstruction, the use of a β-blocker to decrease the LV outflow pressure gradient might be considered.

Regarding prevention of ventricular arrhythmia, physicians should be keenly aware of the time course of arrhythmic risk associated with TCM. Patients should be monitored in a telemetry setting for at least 3 days or until resolution of QT prolongation, with serial ECGs performed at least daily (**Box 2**). A QTc interval of greater than 500 milliseconds should alert physicians to arrhythmic risk, and has been demonstrated to have sensitivity of 82% and specificity of 85% for the risk of TdP.[40] QT-prolonging agents should be strictly avoided in all patients with TCM, regardless of their presenting QT interval. Although early use of β-blockers remains the mainstay of therapy because of catecholamine excess, judicious use of β-blockers is advised for all TCM patients and should be avoided in patients with severe QT prolongation or bradycardia, owing to the risk of pause-dependent TdP.[2,41] β-Blocker therapy can be initiated when QT intervals normalize. β-Blockade does not seem to be protective for either the initial or recurrent episodes of TCM; therefore, it remains controversial as to how long β-blockade should be continued in these patients.[9] Based on

---

**Box 2**
**Management of ventricular arrhythmias in takotsubo cardiomyopathy (TCM)**

Patients should be monitored in a telemetry setting for at least 3 days or until QTc normalizes

Cautious use of β-blockers is advised in most patients

β-Blockers should be avoided in patients with QTc greater than 500 milliseconds

QT-prolonging agents should be strictly avoided in all patients with TCM

Rapid and aggressive potassium and magnesium repletion to high to normal levels in patients with QTc greater than 500 milliseconds is recommended

In patients with pause-dependent torsades de pointes, therapies to limit bradycardia should be pursued, preferably with temporary pacing

experiences with other QT-prolonging diseases, the authors recommend potassium and magnesium supplementation to maintain high to normal levels, with rapid and aggressive supplementation provided to those patients with severe QT prolongation, TdP, or VF.[42–44] Antiarrhythmic therapy, including amiodarone, is often used to manage VT or VF associated with acute cardiac arrest; however, its use should be avoided in patients with TCM who develop prolonged QT interval, as the risk of further QT prolongation and pause-dependent TdP could be increased.

If TdP is observed, therapies to limit bradycardia and long-short extrasystolic pauses should be pursued. In light of evidence indicating that catecholamine excess is associated with TCM, the use of temporary pacing should likely be favored over isoproterenol infusion. Indications for implantable defibrillators are controversial and should be based on clinical judgment in the absence of class I indications, such as SCD. For patients with persistent bradycardia or QT prolongation, a dual-chamber permanent pacemaker or defibrillator might also be considered.

## REFERENCES

1. Roshanzamir S, Showkathali R. Takotsubo cardiomyopathy: a short review. Curr Cardiol Rev 2013;9(3): 191–6.

2. Sharkey S, Lesser JR, Menon M, et al. Spectrum and significance of electrophysiologic patterns, troponin levels, and thrombolysis in myocardial infarction frame count in patients with stress (tako-tsubo) cardiomyopathy and comparison to those in patients with ST-elevation anterior wall myocardial infarction. Am J Cardiol 2008;100:1723–8.

3. Bennett J, Fedinande B, Kayaert P, et al. Time course of electrocardiographic changes in transient left ventricular ballooning syndrome. Int J Cardiol 2013;169:276–80.

4. Madias C, Fitzgibbons TP, Alsheikh-Ali AA, et al. Acquired long QT syndrome from stress cardiomyopathy is associated with ventricular arrhythmias and torsades de pointes. Heart Rhythm 2011;8(4): 555–61.

5. Andrade AA, Stainback RF. Takotsubo cardiomyopathy. Tex Heart Inst J 2014;41:299–303.

6. Prasad A, Lerman A, Rihal CS. Apical ballooning syndrome (tako-tsubo or stress cardiomyopathy): a mimic of acute myocardial infarction. Am Heart J 2008;155(3):408–17.

7. Kurisu S, Inoue I, Kawagoe T, et al. Time course of electrocardiographic changes in patients with tako-tsubo syndrome—comparison with acute myocardial infarction with minimal enzymatic release. Circ J 2004;68:77–81.

8. Ramaraj R, Sorrell VL, Movahed MR. Levels of troponin release can aid in the early exclusion of stress-induced (takotsubo) cardiomyopathy. Exp Clin Cardiol 2009;14(1):6–8.

9. Sharkey S, Windenburg DC, Lesser JR, et al. Natural history and expansive clinical profile of stress (takotsubo) cardiomyopathy. J Am Coll Cardiol 2010; 55(4):333–41.

10. Novo G, Giambanco S, Guglielmo M, et al. G-protein-coupled receptor kinase 5 polymorphism and takotsubo cardiomyopathy. J Cardiovasc Med (Hagerstown) 2014. [Epub ahead of print].

11. Komamura K, Fukui M, Iwasaku T, et al. Takotsubo cardiomyopathy: pathophysiology, diagnosis and treatment. World J Cardiol 2014;6(7):602–9.

12. Nileshkumar J, Patel KD, Prasad A, et al. Burden of arrhythmias in patients with takotsubo cardiomyopathy (apical ballooning syndrome). Int J Cardiol 2013; 170(1):64–8.

13. Wittstein IS, Thiemann DR, Lima JA, et al. Neurohumoral features of myocardial stunning due to sudden emotional stress. N Engl J Med 2005;352: 539–48.

14. Wright PT, Tranter MH, Morley-Smith AC, et al. Pathophysiology of takotsubo syndrome- temporal phases of cardiovascular responses to extreme stress. Circ J 2014;78:1550–8.

15. Nef HM, Mollmann H, Kostin S, et al. Takotsubo cardiomyopathy: intraindividual structural analysis in the acute phase and after functional recovery. Eur Heart J 2007;28:2456–64.

16. Chaparro-Muñoz M, Recio-Mayoral A, Carlos Kaski J, et al. Myocardial stunning identified by using strain/strain rate imaging during dobutamine stress echocardiography in a rare late recurrence of tako–tsubo syndrome. Int J Cardiol 2010;145(1): E9–12.

17. Kosuge M, Ebina T, Hibi K, et al. Simple and accurate electrocardiographic criteria to differentiate takotsubo cardiomyopathy from anterior acute myocardial infarction. J Am Coll Cardiol 2010;55: 2514–6.

18. Madias JE. Transient attenuation of the amplitude of the QRS complexes in the diagnosis of Takotsubo syndrome. Eur Heart J Acute Cardiovasc Care 2014;3:28–36.

19. Kosuge M, Ebina T, Hibi K, et al. Differences in negative T waves between takotsubo cardiomyopathy and reperfused anterior acute myocardial infarction. Circ J 2012;76:462–8.

20. Mitsuma W, Kodama M, Ito M, et al. Serial electrocardiographic findings in women with Takotstubo cardiomyopathy. Am J Cardiol 2007;100: 106–9.

21. Thakar S, Chandra P, Hollander G, et al. Electrocardiographic changes in Takotsubo cardiomyopathy. Pacing Clin Electrophysiol 2011;34:1278–82.

22. Migliori F, Zorzi A, Marra MP, et al. Myocardial edema underlies dynamic T-wave inversion (Wellens' ECG pattern) in patients with reversible left ventricular dysfunction. Heart Rhythm 2011;10:1629–34.

23. Hahn JY, Gwon HC, Park SW, et al. The clinical features of transient left ventricular nonapical ballooning syndrome: comparison with apical ballooning syndrome. Am Heart J 2007;154:1166–73.

24. Kurisu S, Kato Y, Mitsuba N, et al. Comparison of electrocardiographic findings between the midventricular ballooning form and the apical ballooning form of takotsubo cardiomyopathy. Clin Cardiol 2011;34:555–9.

25. Syed FF, Asirvatham SJ, Francis J. Arrhythmia occurrence with takotsubo cardiomyopathy: a literature review. Europace 2011;13(6):780–8.

26. Pant S, Deshmukh A, Mehta K, et al. Burden of arrhythmias in patients with Takotsubo cardiomyopathy (apical ballooning syndrome). Int J Cardiol 2013;170(1):64–8.

27. Zipes DP, Rubart M. Neural modulation of cardiac arrhythmias and sudden cardiac death. Heart Rhythm 2006;3:108–13.

28. Curran J, Hayes Brown K, Santiago DJ, et al. Spontaneous Ca$^{2+}$ waves in ventricular myocytes from failing hearts depend on Ca$^{2+}$-calmodulin-dependent protein kinase II. J Mol Cell Cardiol 2010; 49(1):25–32.

29. Sclarovsky S, Nikus K. The electrocardiographic paradox of tako-tsubo cardiomyopathy—comparison with acute ischemic syndromes and consideration of molecular biology and electrophysiology to understand the electrical-mechanical mismatching. J Electrocardiol 2010;43(2):173–6.

30. Choi SY, Cho KI, You JH, et al. Impact of pheochromocytoma on left ventricular hypertrophy and QTc prolongation: comparison with takotsubo cardiomyopathy. Korean Circ J 2014;44(2):88–9.

31. Hakem A, Marks AD, Bhatti S, et al. When the worse headache becomes the worst heartache! Stroke 2007;38:3292–5.

32. Schwartz PJ. Efficacy of left cardiac sympathetic denervation has an unforeseen side effect: medicolegal complications. Heart Rhythm 2010;7:1330–2.

33. Halkin A, Roth A, Luri I, et al. Pause-dependent torsade de pointes following acute myocardial infarction: a variant of the acquired long QT syndrome. J Am Coll Cardiol 2001;38:1168–74.

34. Crotti L, Hu D, Barajas-Martinez H, et al. Torsades de pointes following acute myocardial infarction: evidence for a deadly link with a common genetic variant. Heart Rhythm 2012;9:1104–12.

35. Mahida S, Dalageorgou C, Behr ER. Long-QT syndrome and torsades de pointes in a patient with Takotsubo cardiomyopathy: an unusual case. Europace 2009;11:376–8.

36. Roden DM. Long QT syndrome: reduced repolarization reserve and the genetic link. J Intern Med 2006; 259:59–69.

37. Wedekind H, Muller JG, Ribbing M, et al. A fatal combination in an old lady: Tako-Tsubo cardiomyopathy, long QT syndrome, and cardiac hypertrophy. Europace 2009;11:820–2.

38. Grilo LS, Pruvot E, Grobety M, et al. Takotsubo cardiomyopathy and congenital long QT syndrome in a patient with a novel duplication in the Per-Arnt-Sim (PAS) domain of hERG1. Heart Rhythm 2010; 7:260–5.

39. Ahn JH, Park SH, Shin WY, et al. Long QT syndrome and torsade de pointes associated with Takotsubo cardiomyopathy. J Korean Med Sci 2011;26:959–61.

40. Behr ER, Mahida S. Takotsubo cardiomyopathy and the long-QT syndrome: an insult to repolarization reserve. Europace 2009;11:697–700.

41. Eitel I, von Knobelsdorff-Brekenhoff F, Bernhardt P, et al. Clinical characteristics and cardiovascular magnetic resonance findings in stress (takotsubo) cardiomyopathy. JAMA 2011;306:277–86.

42. Madias JE, Shah B, Chintalapally G, et al. Admission serum potassium in patients with acute myocardial infarction: its correlates and value as a determinant of in-hospital outcome. Chest 2011;118:904–13.

43. Morton AP. Takotsubo cardiomyopathy: a role for magnesium? Heart Rhythm 2010;7:e1.

44. Kannankeril PJ, Roden DM. Drug-induced long QT and torsades de pointes: recent advances. Curr Opin Cardiol 2007;22:39–43.

# QT Prolongation and Oncology Drug Development

Michael G. Fradley, MD[a],*, Javid Moslehi, MD[b,c,d]

## KEYWORDS

- QT prolongation • Cardiotoxicity • Cardio-oncology • Chemotherapy • Cancer treatment
- Torsades de pointes

## KEY POINTS

- Many pharmaceutical agents interact with cardiac ion channels resulting in prolongation of the QT interval, which is associated with the development of torsades de pointes.
- QT interval monitoring is an essential part of pharmaceutical development and significant increases in the QT interval may prevent a drug from gaining approval.
- Given that QT interval prolongation does not always translate into an increased clinical risk of arrhythmia, current guidelines may be too restrictive for novel oncology drugs.
- New strategies should be considered for monitoring the QT interval and risk of abnormal ventricular repolarization in anticancer pharmaceutical agents.
- Given the significant influx of novel oncology pharmaceutical agents with associated QT prolongation, experience in both cardio-oncology and electrophysiology is necessary to provide appropriate clinical guidance.

## INTRODUCTION

QT prolongation has been associated with the development of a dangerous and potentially life-threatening form of polymorphic ventricular tachycardia known as torsades de pointes (TdP). Despite this association, the QT interval has been shown to be a poor predictor for the development of TdP. Unfortunately, there are few other readily available methods to better determine risk of TdP. Multiple factors have been implicated in QT interval prolongation, including electrolyte abnormalities or underlying genetic disorders. In addition, pharmaceutical agents have been shown to prolong the QT interval and in rare circumstances lead to TdP. As a result, QT monitoring has become an essential part of drug development. This issue has become particularly of concern given the explosion of novel targeted cancer therapies in the last decade, which have revolutionized oncology treatment. Although it is essential to mitigate risk when developing novel pharmaceutical agents, cancer drugs represent a unique challenge as they are developed to treat a life-threatening condition for which there may not be other treatment options. Given that QT interval prolongation does not always translate into increased clinical risk of arrhythmia, current guidelines may be too restrictive for novel oncology drugs. In this review, the unique challenges of QT

The authors have nothing to disclose.
[a] Division of Cardiovascular Medicine, Morsani College of Medicine, University of South Florida, 2 Tampa General Circle, Tampa, FL 33606, USA; [b] Division of Cardiovascular Medicine, Department of Medicine, Vanderbilt-Ingram Cancer Center, Vanderbilt University School of Medicine, 2220 Pierce Avenue, Nashville, TN 37232, USA; [c] Division of Hematology-Oncology, Department of Medicine, Vanderbilt-Ingram Cancer Center, Vanderbilt University School of Medicine, 2220 Pierce Avenue, Nashville, TN 37232, USA; [d] Cardio-Oncology Program, Vanderbilt University School of Medicine, Nashville, TN 37232, USA
* Corresponding author.
E-mail address: mfradley@health.usf.edu

Card Electrophysiol Clin 7 (2015) 341–355
http://dx.doi.org/10.1016/j.ccep.2015.03.013
1877-9182/15/$ – see front matter © 2015 Elsevier Inc. All rights reserved.

interval monitoring in the development of cytotoxic oncology drugs are discussed and agents are identified that may require more intensive evaluation when given to patients. It is also posited that given the relative target specificity of some of these novel therapies, QT prolongation may provide insight into basic electrophysiology.

## BASIC ELECTROPHYSIOLOGY OF THE QT INTERVAL AND TORSADES DE POINTES

On a surface electrocardiogram (ECG), the QT interval is measured from the beginning of the QRS complex to the end of the T wave and represents the entirety of ventricular depolarization and repolarization (**Fig. 1**).[1] At a cellular level, this electrical process, also known as the action potential, is mediated by channels in the myocardial cell membrane that regulate the flow of ions into and out of the cardiac cells (**Fig. 2**).[2] Normal depolarization is due to the rapid inflow of positively charged ions (sodium and calcium), whereas repolarization is due to outflow of potassium ions. The action potential consists of 5 distinct phases. Phase 0 (depolarization) occurs with the opening and closing of $Na^+$ channels, represented by a sharp initial upstroke. Phase 1 begins the repolarization process with the rapid transient outflow of $K^+$ ions. Phase 2 (plateau phase) is the result of a balance between inward $Ca^{2+}$ current and outward flow through $K^+$ channels (particularly the slow delayed rectifier potassium channel $IK_s$). During phase 3 (rapid repolarization), the $Ca^{2+}$ channels close and the $K^+$ channels remain open. The channel predominantly responsible for phase 3 is the rapid

delayed rectifier potassium channel, $IK_r$. Phase 4 is a return to baseline (resting membrane potential) when the cell is not being stimulated.[3,4]

Sustained inflow of $Na^+$ ions or impaired outflow of $K^+$ ions leads to delay in the action potential and thus QT interval prolongation. In the 1950s and 1960s, genetic syndromes of QT prolongation were first identified, most of which are due to mutations in these ion channels involved in the cardiac action potential.[5,6] In addition, electrolyte abnormalities and specific drug effects can also lead to QT prolongation. Most pharmaceutical agents that prolong the QT interval do so by impacting the function of the $IK_r$ channel, which is encoded by the gene KCNH2. This gene is also referred to as the human ether-a-go-go gene (HERG). This channel is known to interact with a variety of structurally diverse compounds.[4]

Afterdepolarizations are abnormal oscillatory changes in cell membrane voltage that disrupt normal repolarization. They are called early afterdepolarizations (EAD) when they occur during phase 2 or 3 of the action potential and delayed afterdepolarizations when they occur during phase 4. EADs most frequently occur in the setting of a baseline prolonged action potential duration.[7] The resulting myocardial electrical heterogeneity renders it vulnerable to the development of TdP, typically occurring after a salvo of several EADs; this is manifested by long-short sequences on the ECG.[7,8] Although transmural dispersion of repolarization is a significantly better predictor for TdP compared with QT prolongation, it is not easily measured, and the QT interval is a frequently

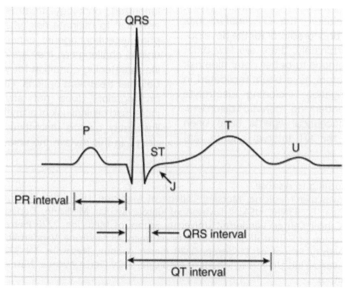

**Fig. 1.** Surface electrocardiogram with QT interval representation. (*From* Goldberger AL. Clinical electrocardiography: a simplified approach. 7th edition. St. Louis (MO): CV Mosby; 2006; with permission.)

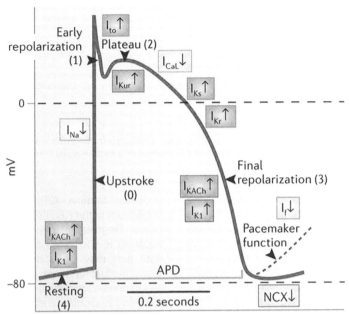

**Fig. 2.** Ventricular myocyte action potential curve with associated ion channels. APD, action potential duration; NCX, sodium-calcium exchanger. (*From* Nattel S, Carlsson L. Innovative approaches to anti-arrhythmic drug therapy. Nat Rev Drug Discov 2006;5:1034–49; with permission.)

used surrogate to determine risk.[8,9] Certain cell populations within the heart, specifically those constituting the Purkinje fibers and the midmyocardium (M cells), are particularly vulnerable to this phenomenon.[10,11]

## QT INTERVAL MEASUREMENT AND ANALYSIS

Accurate measurement of the QT interval can be challenging (**Box 1**). One study revealed that less than 25% of cardiologists and only 62% of "arrhythmia experts" could accurately identify QT prolongation.[12] When measuring the QT interval, the longest QT interval should be used (typically in the limb leads); however, if this measurement differs by more than 40 ms from other leads, it may be erroneous and measurement from other leads should be considered. It is recommended

that this measurement should be averaged over 3 to 5 beats. It can be particularly challenging to determine the end of the T wave to appropriately measure the QT interval. One recommendation is to draw a tangent from the steepest slop of the descending end of the T wave to the isoelectric line, typically in lead II or V5 (**Fig. 3**).[13] In addition, measurement of the QT interval should not include U waves unless they clearly merge with the T wave. It is essential to manually validate the QT measurement recorded by an electronic ECG machine because errors frequently occur.[3,14,15]

Atrial fibrillation and wide QRS complexes (due to either conduction defects/bundle branch blocks or ventricular pacing) pose unique problems for accurately assessing the corrected QT (QTc) interval. There is no consensus as to the correct way to measure and interpret QTc intervals in the setting

---

**Box 1**
**Key points for accurate QT measurements**

1. Measure longest QT interval

2. Average measurement over several beats

3. Use tangent method to determine the end of the T wave

4. Avoid measuring U waves in most circumstances

5. During atrial fibrillation, average the QT interval more than 10 beats

6. Use the JT interval in patients with bundle branch blocks or ventricular pacing

7. Always manually verify electronic QT measurements

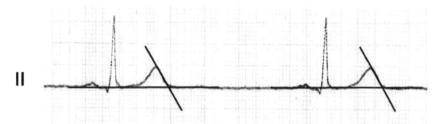

**Fig. 3.** QT interval measurement using the tangent method. (*Adapted from* Anttonen O, Junttila MJ, Rissanen H, et al. Prevalence and prognostic significance of short QT interval in a middle-aged Finnish population. Circulation 2007;116(7):714–20; with permission.)

of atrial fibrillation. Because of the variability of the R-wave intervals during atrial fibrillation, the QT interval can change in each beat. Some experts recommend averaging QTc measurements greater than 10 beats; others suggest averaging the QTc measurements associated with the shortest and longest R-R intervals.[3,16] Similarly, there is no clear consensus for the measurement of the QTc in the setting of wide QRS complexes. Experts recommend using the JT interval (QTc-QRS duration); however, this can be confusing and cumbersome especially for noncardiologists.[14,17] It has been suggested to avoid initiation of a drug if the QTc interval is greater than 500 ms in the setting of ventricular conduction delay.[3]

The QT interval is longer at slower heart rates and shorter at faster heart rates. Several formulae have been developed to adjust for this variation (**Table 1**). The Bazett formula, in which the QT interval is divided by the square root of the RR interval, is most frequently used in clinical practice; however, this method is inaccurate at slower and faster heart rates.[18] Other formulae include the

Fridericia formula (QT interval divided by the cubed root of the RR interval) and the Framingham Linear Regression Equation. The Framingham equation is supported by empiric epidemiologic data and may be a more accurate approach when evaluating large populations. The Bazett and Fridericia formulas are based on mathematical modeling/reasoning and are most often used for drug development monitoring. Unfortunately, none of these methods have been evaluated and compared with one another to determine which is most accurate at predicting risk of TdP.[14,19]

## RISK FACTORS FOR CORRECTED QT PROLONGATION AND TORSADES DE POINTES

Multiple pharmaceutical agents are known to prolong the QT interval, typically by inhibiting or modulating the function of the HERG channel. Nevertheless, most episodes of drug-induced TdP occur in the setting of other patient-specific or acquired risk factors. For example, genetic conditions (long QT syndrome [LQTS]) have been

| Table 1 | | | | |
|---|---|---|---|---|
| **QT correction formulae** | | | | |
| | **Bazett** | **Fridericia** | **Framingham** | **Hodges** |
| Mathematical formula | $QTc = QT/(RR^{1/2})$ | $QTc = QT/(RR^{1/3})$ | $QTc = QT + 0.154$ $(1000 - RR)$ | $QTc = QT + 1.75$ $(HR-60)$ |
| Type | Nonlinear | Nonlinear | Linear | Linear |
| Advantages | Simple; most widely used in practice | More accurate at slower HR (risk of TdP is greater at slower HR) | Adaptable across genders; population-based formula | Useful with multiple populations |
| Disadvantages | Overcorrects at fast HRs and undercorrects at slow HRs | Overcorrects at high HRs | Uncertain validity in populations other than Framingham Heart Study; overcorrects at high HRs | Less correlation with HR variability; overcorrects at high HRs |

*Abbreviations:* HR, heart rate; QT, QT interval; QTc, QT correction; RR, RR interval.

*Adapted from* Curigliano G, Spitaleri G, Fingert HJ, et al. Drug-induced QTc interval prolongation: a proposal towards an efficient and safe anticancer drug development. Eur J Cancer 2008;44(4):494–500.

identified that phenotypically present with QT prolongation and an increased risk of sudden cardiac death, typically due to mutations that affect the ions channels responsible for the action potential. Most forms are due to either a reduction in the outward potassium currents (LQTS-1: $IK_s$; LQTS-2: $IK_r$) or an enhancement of the inward sodium current (LQTS-3: $I_{Na}$). Other forms of LQTS are due to abnormalities in proteins that affect ion channel trafficking or function. When these patients are treated with certain drugs, the additive QT prolonging effect can be substantial.[20,21]

Nonpharmacologic factors can also impact the QT interval (**Box 2**). Electrolyte abnormalities (hypokalemia or hypomagnesemia), bradycardia, left ventricular hypertrophy and congestive heart failure, intracranial pathologic abnormality, HIV infection, connective tissue disorders, and hypothermia are also all known to prolong the QT interval.[19] Age and gender also impact normal QT/QTc intervals. It is thought that sex hormone levels play a role in these QT interval changes.[22–25] After puberty, men have shorter QT intervals than women, which may be related to increased testosterone levels. As both genders age, the QT interval gradually increases. Progesterone has been reported to affect HERG trafficking, and postmenopausal women treated with estrogen demonstrated prolonged QT intervals compared with controls.[26,27] In addition, female hearts have fewer ion channels, which render them more susceptible to repolarization abnormalities.[28] For these reasons, using the Bazett formula, a normal QTc is less than 450 ms for men and less than 460 to 470 ms for women. It has been reported that approximately 70% of all cases of TdP occur in women.[20,29–31] Although no absolute threshold has been determined to confer excess risk of TdP, most cases occur when the QTc exceeds 500 ms. Therefore, caution should be exercised when evaluating patients with QT intervals greater than 500 ms.[9,32]

For patients with prolonged QT intervals, treatment is focused on correcting the underlying cause. In particular, medications that are known to prolong the QT interval should be stopped if at all possible. In addition, potassium and magnesium should both be regularly evaluated and aggressively corrected. Magnesium repletion has been shown to shorten the QT interval as has potassium repletion with a goal serum concentration of 4.5 to 5 mmol/L.[33–35]

## HISTORY OF DRUG-INDUCED QT PROLONGATION AND TORSADES DE POINTES

Antiarrhythmic medications were the first class of medications found to prolong the QT interval and increase the risk of TdP. Syncope associated with quinidine exposure was first observed in the 1920s; however, TdP was not identified as the causative mechanism until the 1960s.[36] The term TdP was first used by the French cardiologist Dessertenne[37] in 1966 to describe this unique arrhythmia. Over the next several decades, the association of QTc prolongation and TdP was identified. It was found to occur relatively frequently during the administration of class III antiarrhythmic medications, which are known to block $IK_r$, with rates exceeding 1% in some series.[38,39] At the same time, other classes of pharmaceutical agents, including psychiatric medications and antibiotics, were reported to cause TdP; however, the rates were quite low and little attention was paid to the arrhythmogenic potential of noncardiac drugs.

The landscape changed dramatically in the fall of 1989 when the first case of QT prolongation and TdP associated with terfenadine administration was reported. Terfenadine was a widely prescribed nonsedating antihistamine. Although it had potent HERG-channel blocking effects, its impact on the QTc at standard clinical doses was insignificant. Further studies revealed that terfenadine underwent extensive first-pass hepatic metabolism by cytochrome P450 3A4 to its active metabolite, which has no effect on the HERG channel. In patients with impaired hepatic metabolism, systemic terfenadine levels were significantly elevated, leading to marked QTc prolongation.[40,41] Although the exact number of cases of TdP and death from terfenadine is not certain, one review cited at least 125 deaths in the United States from this drug.[42] Given that this medication treated a benign condition and there were other safer alternatives, it was ultimately withdrawn from the market in 1997. Since then, 6 additional drugs have been removed from the market for increased rates of TdP and death,

| Box 2 |
|---|
| **Risk factors for QT prolongation** |

| | |
|---|---|
| Increasing age (>65 y) | Female gender |
| Bradycardia | Congestive heart failure |
| Left ventricular hypertrophy | Congenital long QT syndromes (ion channelopathies) |
| Drugs | Electrolyte disturbances (potassium and magnesium) |
| Hypothermia | HIV infection |
| Intracranial pathologic abnormality | Connect tissue disorders |

including the antibiotic grepafloxacin (at least 13 arrhythmia-associated deaths[43]) and the gastro-prokinetic cisapride (80 arrhythmia-associated deaths reported to the US Food and Drug Administration [FDA])[44,45] and many others have received updated labeling and/or black box warnings.

## CORRECTED QT MONITORING AND REGULATION IN DRUG DEVELOPMENT

Because of the significant consequences associated with the QT prolonging effects of the aforementioned drugs, regulatory agencies were developed to provide guidance and oversight in the drug development process. In 2005, the International Committee on Harmonization (ICH), a multinational regulatory body, published guidelines for QT monitoring of novel non-antiarrhythmic pharmaceutical agents in both the preclinical and the clinical settings.[46,47] These guidelines have since been adopted by regulatory agencies in both the United States and the European Union.

### Preclinical Assessment

ICH safety guideline 7B (S7B) is the portion of the ICH document that deals with drug development before human administration. The goal of these preclinical studies is to identify the potential of a drug and its metabolites to delay ventricular repolarization. The recommendation is to conduct both in vitro $IK_r$ and HERG assays and in vivo QT analyses using laboratory animals such as canines or nonhuman primates. The choice of species is important because some animals, for example mice and rats, have very different mechanisms of repolarization compared with humans.[46] Tests may be also conducted to evaluate action potential effects in Purkinje or ventricular muscle fibers. When conducting in vitro assays, appropriate positive controls must be used and testing of metabolites (separate from the parent compound) should be considered.[48] Despite significant improvements in these tests, there are several limitations. No gold standard has been established and although the sensitivity of these nonclinical tests is quite good, the specificity of these tests has been questioned.[49] The degree in which a drug interacts with the HERG channel poorly correlates with the likelihood and extent to which the QT interval will be prolonged in the clinical setting. In fact, recent data suggest that simply screening for $IK_r$ inhibition may not be sufficient; rather, arrhythmogenic potential may more closely linked to inhibition of the phosphatidylinositide 3-kinase pathway and augmentation of the late sodium current ($I_{Na-L}$).[50,51] Last, drugs that do not increase transmural dispersion of repolarization are unlikely to cause TdP regardless of HERG inhibition or QT prolongation. The issue of transmural dispersion of repolarization is not discussed or recommended in these documents.[52,53]

### Clinical Assessment and the "Thorough QT/Corrected QT Study"

ICH efficacy guideline 14 (E14) is the portion of the ICH document that provides guidance about the clinical evaluation of a drug's effect on ventricular repolarization and the QT interval. A specific trial, coined the "Thorough QT/QTc Study (TQTS)" should be conducted early in clinical development of the pharmaceutical agents. This study is typically conducted in healthy volunteers to determine if a drug has a threshold effect on cardiac repolarization. The goal of the TQTS is to exclude a drug prolongs the QTc interval by 10 ms or more at the one-sided upper 95% confidence limit. The results of this study will help determine if further testing and evaluation is required during later phases of development (ie, if a drug effect exceeding 10 ms cannot be excluded). A TQTS is required as a part of drug development even if preclinical testing is negative for HERG inhibition or QT prolongation. Until the QT effects of the drug are delineated, certain exclusion criteria have been established for study volunteers. Those individuals with a prolonged baseline QTc interval (>450 ms) or those with a history of additional risk factors for TdP (such as cardiac disease, congenital syndromes, or electrolyte abnormalities) should be excluded from the TQTS.[4,47,54]

Healthy volunteers receive placebo, a positive control that prolongs the QT interval slightly, the study drug at the therapeutic dose as well as at a supratherapeutic dose. This trial is conducted in either a randomized crossover or a parallel fashion. Given that there is less intrasubject variability, the crossover study design is preferable and requires a smaller sample size to exclude a QT prolongation effect. The parallel design may be preferred if the drug must be dosed for an extended period of time to achieve appropriate serum levels.[4,47,54] The placebo drug is included to account for random variability associated with the study. The positive control is included to ensure adequate sensitivity. It is necessary for the study to detect changes in the QT interval as small as 5 ms; changes smaller than this are unlikely to cause TdP.[47,54] The fluoroquinolone moxifloxacin is used as the positive control in the overwhelming majority of TQTS cases.[55] Ideally, the positive control should have a QT prolonging effect of about 5 ms; however, moxifloxacin typically prolongs the QTc by 8 to 15 ms. This excess QT prolonging effect of a positive control is considered acceptable provided that it is not so long as to hinder the study's ability to detect small QTc changes. In addition, the QT prolonging effect of the positive control should be similar to values obtained in prior TQTS. If the effect of the positive control is substantially different, the sensitivity of the current TQTS would be questioned.[54]

Recent updates to the ICH E14 recommendations have focused on issues of gender representation in these studies and the appropriate algorithm for QT correction. It is well known that women have longer QT intervals compared with men, but the exact cause for this difference is not completely understood. The current recommendations suggest equal representation of genders in TQTS and to perform subgroup analysis whenever a TQTS is positive. Regarding QTc assessment, earlier iterations of the ICH E14 document did not specifically address which correction formula should be used during a TQTS. Although the current document does not go so far as to recommend one specific method, they do suggest that the Fridericia formula is likely to be appropriate in most situations.[56,57]

It is important to note that the TQTS is not designed to determine the likelihood that a new pharmaceutical will cause TdP. In fact, a positive study cannot adequately determine the proarrhythmia effects of a drug because there is not a linear relationship between the QT interval and the risk of TdP.[9] Rather, the TQTS is conducted to identify those drugs that will require more thorough ECG and safety evaluation.

## QT/CORRECTED QT MONITORING IN ONCOLOGY DRUG DEVELOPMENT

It is well recognized that the TQTS cannot be applied to every new pharmaceutical agent in development. This reasoning holds particularly true for oncology drugs and other cytotoxic agents. The E14 guidelines acknowledge that the administration of chemotherapeutic agents to healthy volunteers would be unethical.[47] As an alternative, TQTS-like studies are sometimes conducted in target patient populations as part of phase 1 oncology trials. This can still be a significant challenge because most oncology patients enrolled in phase 1 trials have advanced malignancies. These patients are often elderly and have comorbid conditions such as underlying cardiovascular disease that would otherwise exclude them from a TQTS. They are also frequently taking other drugs such as antiemetics and antibiotics,

which can also prolong the QT interval, thus making accurate interpretation challenging.[4,58]

Determining reasonable and appropriate inclusion and exclusion criteria for these modified QT monitoring studies for oncology drugs is of significant importance. The guidelines set forth for TQTS is likely far too restrictive for oncology drug studies. As already indicated, many of these patients have concomitant medical conditions that can prolong the QT interval, which would otherwise exclude them from a TQTS. They may also be taking other medications with a QT prolonging effect, which cannot be safely stopped.[58] In addition, the QTc cutoff of 450 ms may be too restrictive for this population. There appears to be greater variability in the QT interval among patients with cancer compared with healthy controls. These data suggest that if the current QT/QTc exclusion of 450 ms is applied to oncology trials, more than 10% of potential study participants would be excluded.[59,60]

Phase 1 oncology trials often have multiple protocol issues that make QTc evaluation challenging. Conversely, the rigorous QTc protocols outlined in the ICH E14 document can be applied to healthy volunteer populations but are not appropriate when treating patients with advanced cancer. For example, oncology trials are often not randomized and the administration of either a placebo or a positive control drug would be completely inappropriate for patients with advanced cancer. It should also be recognized that oncology patients themselves may be either physically or psychologically incapable of participating in the intensive time-sensitive ECG collection and cardiac monitoring necessary for these types of studies.[4,58]

With this in mind, the E14 document suggests that when a TQTS is impossible, other methods of monitoring the QTc must be developed so as to ensure safety and mitigate risk. This method can include extensive preclinical assessment for HERG inhibition and QT prolongation as well as robust ECG collection at different time points during the trial itself.[4] Some experts suggest applying the National Cancer Institute's toxicity criteria for QTc prolongation (Version 4 of the Common Terminology Criteria for Adverse Cardiac Events [CTCAE.v4]) to guide decision-making during these studies.[61]

Based on these criteria, it is recommended to define dose-limiting toxicity as grade 2 or higher QTc prolongation. These definitions, however, may be too restrictive to guide dosing in oncology patients. For example, diurnal variation of more than 60 ms has frequently been observed in oncology patients, and oncology patients have a wider range of QTc intervals compared with healthy controls.[4,62,63] Because the QT interval is so poorly correlated with the development of TdP, these parameters may unnecessarily prevent patients with cancer from receiving life-saving therapy. Although it is still mandatory to determine the QT prolonging effects of cytotoxic agents to ensure appropriate patient safety, it is clear that the current guidelines cannot be uniformly applied to oncology drug development.

Despite all of this, there remains little uniformity in the definition, management, and monitoring of QT interval prolongation in the realm of oncology drug development. The authors recommend liberalizing the definition of dose-limiting QTc prolongation for oncology trials to grade 3 toxicity or higher, especially because the overwhelming majority of TdP cases occur at QTc values greater than 500 ms and those with substantial QT changes (>100 ms) from baseline. In addition, patients with baseline QTc measurements of 480 ms or less should be considered for enrollment in these trials. Frequent ECG monitoring has not been shown to provide significant improvement in the prediction or diagnosis of future cardiac events.[64,65] It would be reasonable therefore to obtain an ECG at baseline (before the initiation of the drug), and at least 2 consecutive measurements within 48 hours of receiving the drug. Finally, pharmaceutical companies should standardize the method used for QT correction. Given the current data, the authors would advocate for universal use of the Fridericia formula in oncology drug development.

## CORRECTED QT PROLONGATION ASSOCIATED WITH SPECIFIC CHEMOTHERAPEUTIC AGENTS
### Arsenic Trioxide

The medicinal properties of arsenic were first identified by the Chinese as early as the first century BC; however, arsenic's toxicity profile and association as a poison have limited its medical use in the modern era and led to substantial regulations.[66] In the 1990s, arsenic trioxide was identified as an effective therapy for patients with relapsed or refractory acute promyelocytic leukemia (APL). APL accounts for 10% to 15% of all adult acute myeloid leukemias, and although first-line therapy with all-trans-retinoic acid has substantially improved survival, 20% to 30% of patients will relapse.[67–71] Initial single-center studies reported complete remission rates between 85% and 93% for patients with relapsed APL treated with arsenic, and these results were confirmed in a multicenter study that reported similar complete remission rates of 85% in patients treated with arsenic.[69,72–74]

QTc prolongation and TdP are known cardiovascular complications associated with arsenic poisoning.[75] Several early studies suggested only minor asymptomatic ECG abnormalities in APL patients treated with arsenic trioxide; however, multiple case reports were published of patients with TdP in the setting of arsenic trioxide treatment.[72,76,77] Several studies have been conducted to more systematically evaluate arsenic associated cardiotoxicity. In a smaller study from Japan, 8 patients treated with arsenic were monitored with continuous ambulatory ECG during infusion of the drug. Although all patients in this trial experienced QT prolongation, there were no episodes of sustained VT or TdP.[78] In a larger study evaluating 99 patients from several different phase 1 and phase 2 trials, the risk was significantly lower with 38% demonstrating QT prolongation, and 26% having a QT greater than 500 ms. Only one patient had TdP and that was in the setting of significant hypokalemia. In all arsenic trials, the median daily dose was 0.15 mg/kg with a dose range of 0.06 mg/kg to 0.35 mg/kg.[79] A recent study evaluating more than 3000 ECGs in 113 patients treated with arsenic for non-APL malignancies produced similar results: QT prolongation occurred in 26% of patients with 12% demonstrating a QT interval greater than 500 ms. Despite this, no clinically significant cardiac events were noted.[80]

Although arsenic clearly prolongs the QT interval, these studies demonstrate that the risk of TdP is quite low. Given the great success arsenic has had against relapsed APL, it would be a disservice to withhold this medication based solely on QTc criteria outlined in regulatory committee documents. At this time, labeling instructions recommend that arsenic trioxide should be stopped if the absolute QT interval exceeds 500 ms or if the patient develops symptoms suggestive of ventricular arrhythmias, but it can be resumed if the QT interval decreases to less than 460 ms. In addition, the potassium should remain greater than 4 meq/L and the magnesium greater than 1.8 meq/L.[81] Arsenic trioxide represents an excellent example of successful risk mitigation strategies for a necessary therapeutic.

### Molecularly Targeted Agents

#### Tyrosine kinase inhibitors
Protein kinases are a family of enzymes that regulates cellular signaling and function by transferring a phosphate group, typically from ATP, and attaching it to amino acids with a free hydroxyl group.[82] One group of protein kinases act on tyrosine, whereas the other group acts on serine and

threonine, with a minority of enzymes acting on all 3 amino acids. Because of their aberrant activation in multiple types of cancers, protein kinases have become important targets for oncology drug development.[82–84] Specifically, small molecules inhibit tyrosine kinase (TK) enzymes by interfering with ATP or substrate binding of TKs, thus inhibiting their catalytic activity. Such tyrosine kinase inhibitors (TKIs) are relatively nonselective and generally have potency against more than one receptor TK. In 2001, imatinib (Gleevec), an inhibitor of BCR-ABL1 chimeric TK aberrantly active in chronic myeloid leukemia (CML), became the first success story using this strategy by dramatically changing the prognosis of CML patients.[85] Since then, more than 30 TKIs have already been FDA approved for various cancers with many more TKIs currently in clinical trials. Although TKIs have been generally well tolerated, specific classes have been associated with cardiotoxicity.[86] For example, TKIs that target vascular endothelial growth factor receptor (VEGFR) and platelet-derived grown factor (PDGFR) signaling have been associated with hypertension, thrombosis, and, less frequently, heart failure.[87] In 2013, ponatinib, which had potent activity against BCR-ABL1 kinase, but also against other TKs (including VEGFR), was temporarily withdrawn from the market because of vascular toxicity.[88] Nilotinib, a TKI with potent activity against BCR-ABL1 kinase and FDA approved for treatment of CML, has been associated with peripheral vascular atherosclerotic disease.[89]

Several TKIs have been associated with QT prolongation, although incidence of TdP is exceedingly rare.[84] For example, nilotinib was associated with a 5- to 15-ms prolongation of the corrected QT internal in a subset of patients in early clinical trials.[90] Subsequent follow-up revealed no evidence of TdP.

Interestingly, QT prolongation associated with TKIs may be more complex than simple inhibition of the HERG subunit of the $IK_r$ channel. Lu and colleagues[50] showed that 3 TKIs associated with QT prolongation in early clinical trials, dasatinib, sunitinib, and nilotinib, prolonged the action potential of the cardiac myocytes via inhibition of the phosphoinositide 3-kinase (PI3K) signaling pathway. Dasatinib, sunitinib, and nilotinib caused an increase in action potential duration that was reversed by intracellular infusion of phosphatidylinositol 3,4,5-triphosphate in a study using canine myocytes. PI3K inhibition has downstream effects on many ion channels, including increases in the late sodium current, $I_{Na-L}$, as well as decreases in the potassium current via $IK_r$. Experiments using specific PI3K inhibitors and transgenic mice with

reduced PI3K signaling, which had prolonged QT intervals at baseline compared with wild-type controls, supported a critical role for PI3K signaling. Despite these data, there is no clear class-related QT prolonging effect of TKIs. The chemical structure of the TKI may be the only feature that can predict the likelihood that the drug will prolong the QT interval. It has been observed that the presence of a fluorinated phenyl ring on the TKI may lead to an increased risk of QT prolongation and should lead to more intensive monitoring.[84,91]

As mentioned previously, the results of preclinical data on cardiac repolarization do not always translate into QT prolongation in the clinical arena. As was the case with nilotinib, this concept applies to several other drugs in this class. At least 9 of the TKIs carry either standard or black box warnings regarding QT prolongation. Among the TKIs, nilotinib, vandetanib, and sunitinib are frequently implicated for their QT prolonging effects. Sunitinib, a small-molecule TKI, affects the VEGFR, PDGFR, and c-kit and has been FDA approved in the treatment of gastrointestinal stromal tumors and metastatic renal cell carcinoma. Preclinical studies indicated significant effects on cardiac repolarization, interacting with HERG, and prolonging AP duration in Purkinje fibers and the QT interval in primate studies. In clinical trials, QT prolongation was only observed with high concentrations of the drug; however, no clinical events were reported. The mean increase in the QTc using the Fridericia formula was 15.4 ms (90% confidence interval 8.4–22.4 ms). Other clinical studies with sunitinib failed to show any impact on the QT interval. Some experts suggest that the FDA warnings are too restrictive for this medication given the clinical findings.[84,92,93]

Vandetanib is a potent TKI, which affecting VEGFR-2, RET, and endothelial growth factor receptor, is FDA approved for the treatment of locally advanced or metastatic medullary thyroid cancer. Preclinical studies suggested the potential for QTc prolongation; this was confirmed in multiple clinical trials.[58,94] Several phase 1 trials reported QTc prolongation rates between 9% and 61%.[95,96] In a phase 2 trial assessing vandetanib in combination with docetaxel for patients with drug refractory non-small-cell lung cancer (NSCLC), the rate of QT prolongation was 15% and all events were classified as grade 1 or 2. No clinical events were observed and each episode was effectively managed with dose reduction or interruption.[97] Several other phase 2 trials confirmed these results.[98,99] In a phase 3 trial evaluating vandetanib in patients with advanced NSCLC, QTc prolongation occurred in 5.1% of patients. Although most events were asymptomatic, one patient developed TdP leading to cessation of the drug. QT prolongation was defined as a single measurement of greater than 550 ms or an increase of greater than 100 ms from baseline, 2 consecutive measurements (within 48 hours) that were greater than 500 ms but less than 550 ms, or an increase of greater than 60 ms but less than 100 ms from baseline to a value of greater than 480 ms.[100,101] A large meta-analysis of 9 vandetanib trials reported an incidence of all-grade QTc prolongation of 16.4% and high-grade QTc prolongation of 3.7% in patients with nonthyroid cancer compared with 18% and 12% in patients with thyroid cancer.[102] Given these data, vandetanib has a black box warning for QTc prolongation, and physicians must complete the Vandetanib Risk Evaluation and Mitigation Strategy Program to prescribe this medication.[84]

As discussed above, nilotinib is used in the treatment of Philadelphia chromosome-positive CML. It targets the BCR-ABL fusion protein, c-Kit, and PDGFR receptors. In preclinical studies, cardiac repolarization was affected with this drug, and clinical studies suggested substantial QT prolonging effects. In healthy volunteers, the mean QTc change was 18 ms; however, prolongation of more than 60 ms (using the Fridericia formula) was reported in 1.9% of CML-chronic phase patients and 2.5% of CML-accelerated phase patients.[58,103] Sudden cardiac death has been reported in approximately 0.3% of patients treated with nilotinib. Abnormal ventricular repolarization is thought to have contributed to these events, and as a result, nilotinib has received a black box warning for QTc prolongation.[104]

### Histone deacetylase inhibitors

Histone deacetylase inhibitors (HDI) are group of molecularly targeted pharmaceutical agents that modulate the posttranscriptional activity of proteins by inactivating histone deacetylase enzymes. The resultant abnormal proteins are stuck in $G_1$ and $G_2$ of the cell cycle, leading to apoptosis.[105] QTc prolongation has been observed with some HDIs and is thought to be due to interaction with the HERG channel. A recent study confirmed that the pharmacophere for HERG and histone deacetylase-1 is quite similar, suggesting one possible reason for the QT prolonging effects of some HDIs.[106] Vorinostat is an HDI with FDA approval for the treatment of cutaneous T-cell lymphoma. In a phase II study, 3 patients were observed to have grade 1 or 2 QTc prolongation without any clinical sequelae or need for dose adjustment.[107] There is one case report of a severely prolonged QT interval leading to polymorphic ventricular tachycardia in a patient treated with vorinostat; however, this patient also had

concomitant hypokalemia.[108] Depsipeptide, also known as romidepsin, is an HDI used to treat a variety of malignancies including T-cell lymphoma. Romidepsin can cause QT prolongation, and although sudden cardiac death has been reported in several studies, this association with QT prolongation is not certain because most patients had multiple risk factors for sudden cardiac arrest and the QT interval was not clearly documented before the event.[58,60,93] In a study of patients with T-cell lymphoma, the mean QTc prolongation (using the Bazett formula) was 14 ms in patients receiving romidepsin.[60] Oral panobinostat is another HDI known to impact HERG activity and increase the Fridericia QTc up to 20 ms in a dose-related fashion without clinical sequelae.[93] Although these data confirm HDI-associated QTc prolongation, this has not translated into increased clinical risk.

### Other Chemotherapeutic Agents

Left ventricular dysfunction is the most commonly recognized cardiotoxicity of anthracyclines; however, these chemotherapeutics can also cause QTc prolongation. In a study evaluating patients with non-Hodgkin lymphoma treated with epirubicin, all patients experienced some degree of QTc prolongation. The QTc prolonging effects were mitigated when concomitant dexrazoxane was given to the patients, however.[109] In a Finnish study, 18% of patients exposed to doxorubicin experienced QTc prolongation of greater than 50 ms. These changes were independent of LV function.[110] Tamoxifen has also been shown to cause QTc prolongation in both clinical and preclinical studies, likely related to HERG interaction.[111]

Several other classes of molecularly targeted agents are still relatively early in their development. Certain vascular disruption agents such as CA4P (combrestatin) have been shown to prolong the QTc in clinical trials, whereas others (plinabulin) have not shown this effect.[58,112] Therefore, QTc prolongation does not appear to be a class-related effect of the vascular disruption agents. A similar finding has been observed with farnesyl protein transferase inhibitors. The agent L-778123 has been shown in several trials to induce QTc prolongation without clinical sequelae.[113–115] In contrast, there are conflicting data regarding lonafarnib because QTc prolongation has been noted in some studies but not others.[93] Last, inhibitors of the serine/threonine kinase, protein kinase C (PKC), have been shown to cause QT prolongation. Overexpression of PKC has been implicated in many different malignancies including hepatocellular cancer, colon cancer, and diffuse large B-cell lymphoma.[58] Enzastaurin is a potent selective inhibitor of PKC; however, phase I and II studies have documented dose-limiting QTc prolongation without clinical consequence.[116,117]

## SUMMARY

Safety and efficacy are the 2 paramount aspects of drug development. In general, the benefits of the pharmaceutical agent should outweigh any risk associated with it. In most instances, even a small risk of a serious complication cannot be tolerated. QTc monitoring is a central part of the drug-approval process, and most pharmaceutical agents are subjected to the TQTS, a protocol established by the ICH to ensure appropriate QTc evaluation. Although it is well known that the QT interval is a poor surrogate for TdP, the potential for this life-threatening arrhythmia in the setting of a prolonged QTc has led to the withdrawal of several drugs from the market and more intense labeling and warnings for many others. This issue becomes more complex when dealing with oncology pharmaceutical agents because the disease is often life threatening and alternative therapies may not exist. A true TQTS cannot typically be performed with cytotoxic agents and oncology patients are not an ideal population in which to rigorously test these drugs. Although the TQTS has been adapted to evaluate the QT interval and provide oversight for new chemotherapeutics, it will be necessary to develop dedicated protocols to appropriately evaluate cancer therapeutics. Many of these drugs have been shown to have excellent antitumor efficacy, and although QTc prolongation may be present, implementing appropriate risk mitigation strategies allow these patients to receive life-saving therapies without exposure to serious increased risk.[118]

## REFERENCES

1. Goldberger AL. Clinical electrocardiography. 7th edition. Philadelphia: C.V. Mosby Co; 2006.
2. Grant AO. Cardiac ion channels. Circ Arrhythm Electrophysiol 2009;2(2):185–94.
3. Al-Khatib SM, LaPointe NM, Kramer JM, et al. What clinicians should know about the QT interval. JAMA 2003;289(16):2120–7.
4. Curigliano G, Spitaleri G, Fingert HJ, et al. Drug-induced QTc interval prolongation: a proposal towards an efficient and safe anticancer drug development. Eur J Cancer 2008;44(4):494–500.
5. Jervell A, Lange-Nielsen F. Congenital deaf-mutism, functional heart disease with prolongation

of the Q-T interval and sudden death. Am Heart J 1957;54(1):59–68.
6. Ward OC. A new familial cardiac syndrome in children. J Ir Med Assoc 1964;54:103–6.
7. Zipes DP. Mechanisms of clinical arrhythmias. J Cardiovasc Electrophysiol 2003;14(8):902–12.
8. Gupta A, Lawrence AT, Krishnan K, et al. Current concepts in the mechanisms and management of drug-induced QT prolongation and torsade de pointes. Am Heart J 2007;153(6):891–9.
9. Roden DM. Drug-induced prolongation of the QT interval. N Engl J Med 2004;350(10):1013–22.
10. Roden DM, Hoffman BF. Action potential prolongation and induction of abnormal automaticity by low quinidine concentrations in canine Purkinje fibers. Relationship to potassium and cycle length. Circ Res 1985;56(6):857–67.
11. Sicouri S, Antzelevitch C. Drug-induced afterdepolarizations and triggered activity occur in a discrete subpopulation of ventricular muscle cells (M cells) in the canine heart: quinidine and digitalis. J Cardiovasc Electrophysiol 1993;4(1):48–58.
12. Viskin S, Rosovski U, Sands AJ, et al. Inaccurate electrocardiographic interpretation of long QT: the majority of physicians cannot recognize a long QT when they see one. Heart Rhythm 2005;2(6):569–74.
13. Anttonen O, Junttila MJ, Rissanen H, et al. Prevalence and prognostic significance of short QT interval in a middle-aged Finnish population. Circulation 2007;116(7):714–20.
14. Rautaharju PM, Surawicz B, Gettes LS, et al. AHA/ACCF/HRS recommendations for the standardization and interpretation of the electrocardiogram: part IV: the ST segment, T and U waves, and the QT interval: a scientific statement from the American Heart Association Electrocardiography and Arrhythmias Committee, Council on Clinical Cardiology; the American College of Cardiology Foundation; and the Heart Rhythm Society: endorsed by the International Society for Computerized Electrocardiology. Circulation 2009;119(10):e241–50.
15. Postema PG, De Jong JS, Van der Bilt IA, et al. Accurate electrocardiographic assessment of the QT interval: teach the tangent. Heart Rhythm 2008;5(7):1015–8.
16. Anderson ME, Al-Khatib SM, Roden DM, et al. Cardiac repolarization: current knowledge, critical gaps, and new approaches to drug development and patient management. Am Heart J 2002;144(5):769–81.
17. Rautaharju PM, Zhang ZM, Prineas R, et al. Assessment of prolonged QT and JT intervals in ventricular conduction defects. Am J Cardiol 2004;93(8):1017–21.

18. Milne JR, Ward DE, Spurrell RA, et al. The ventricular paced QT interval—the effects of rate and exercise. Pacing Clin Electrophysiol 1982;5(3):352–8.

19. Curigliano G, Spitaleri G, de Braud F, et al. QTc prolongation assessment in anticancer drug development: clinical and methodological issues. Ecancermedicalscience 2009;3:130.

20. Heist EK, Ruskin JN. Drug-induced arrhythmia. Circulation 2010;122(14):1426–35.

21. Roden DM. Clinical practice. Long-QT syndrome. N Engl J Med 2008;358(2):169–76.

22. Rautaharju PM, Zhou SH, Wong S, et al. Sex differences in the evolution of the electrocardiographic QT interval with age. Can J Cardiol 1992;8(7): 690–5.

23. Sides GD. QT interval prolongation as a biomarker for torsades de pointes and sudden death in drug development. Dis Markers 2002;18(2):57–62.

24. Zhang Y, Ouyang P, Post WS, et al. Sex-steroid hormones and electrocardiographic QT-interval duration: findings from the third National Health and Nutrition Examination Survey and the Multi-Ethnic Study of Atherosclerosis. Am J Epidemiol 2011; 174(4):403–11.

25. van Noord C, Dorr M, Sturkenboom MC, et al. The association of serum testosterone levels and ventricular repolarization. Eur J Epidemiol 2010;25(1):21–8.

26. Cheng J. Evidences of the gender-related differences in cardiac repolarization and the underlying mechanisms in different animal species and human. Fundam Clin Pharmacol 2006;20(1):1–8.

27. Wu ZY, Yu DJ, Soong TW, et al. Progesterone impairs human ether-a-go-go-related gene (HERG) trafficking by disruption of intracellular cholesterol homeostasis. J Biol Chem 2011;286(25):22186–94.

28. Gaborit N, Varro A, Le Bouter S, et al. Gender-related differences in ion-channel and transporter subunit expression in non-diseased human hearts. J Mol Cell Cardiol 2010;49(4):639–46.

29. Antzelevitch C, Shimizu W. Cellular mechanisms underlying the long QT syndrome. Curr Opin Cardiol 2002;17(1):43–51.

30. Bednar MM, Harrigan EP, Ruskin JN. Torsades de pointes associated with nonantiarrhythmic drugs and observations on gender and QTc. Am J Cardiol 2002;89(11):1316–9.

31. Makkar RR, Fromm BS, Steinman RT, et al. Female gender as a risk factor for torsades de pointes associated with cardiovascular drugs. JAMA 1993;270(21):2590–7.

32. Priori SG, Schwartz PJ, Napolitano C, et al. Risk stratification in the long-QT syndrome. N Engl J Med 2003;348(19):1866–74.

33. Zipes DP, Camm AJ, Borggrefe M, et al. ACC/AHA/ESC 2006 guidelines for management of patients with ventricular arrhythmias and the prevention of sudden cardiac death: a report of the American College of Cardiology/American Heart Association Task Force and the European Society of Cardiology Committee for Practice Guidelines (Writing Committee to Develop Guidelines for Management of Patients with Ventricular Arrhythmias and the Prevention of Sudden Cardiac Death). J Am Coll Cardiol 2006;48(5):e247–346.

34. Choy AM, Lang CC, Chomsky DM, et al. Normalization of acquired QT prolongation in humans by intravenous potassium. Circulation 1997;96(7): 2149–54.

35. McBride BF, Min B, Kluger J, et al. An evaluation of the impact of oral magnesium lactate on the corrected QT interval of patients receiving sotalol or dofetilide to prevent atrial or ventricular tachyarrhythmia recurrence. Ann Noninvasive Electrocardiol 2006;11(2):163–9.

36. Selzer A, Wray HW. Quinidine syncope. Paroxysmal ventricular fibrillation occurring during treatment of chronic atrial arrhythmias. Circulation 1964; 30:17–26.

37. Dessertenne F. Ventricular tachycardia with 2 variable opposing foci. Arch Mal Coeur Vaiss 1966; 59(2):263–72 [in French].

38. Lehmann MH, Hardy S, Archibald D, et al. Sex difference in risk of torsade de pointes with d,l-sotalol. Circulation 1996;94(10):2535–41.

39. Singh S, Zoble RG, Yellen L, et al. Efficacy and safety of oral dofetilide in converting to and maintaining sinus rhythm in patients with chronic atrial fibrillation or atrial flutter: the symptomatic atrial fibrillation investigative research on dofetilide (SAFIRE-D) study. Circulation 2000;102(19): 2385–90.

40. Honig PK, Woosley RL, Zamani K, et al. Changes in the pharmacokinetics and electrocardiographic pharmacodynamics of terfenadine with concomitant administration of erythromycin. Clin Pharmacol Ther 1992;52(3):231–8.

41. Monahan BP, Ferguson CL, Killeavy ES, et al. Torsades de pointes occurring in association with terfenadine use. JAMA 1990;264(21):2788–90.

42. Flockhart DA. Drug interactions, cardiac toxicity, and terfenadine: from bench to clinic? J Clin Psychopharmacol 1996;16(2):101–3.

43. Mandell L, Tillotson G. Safety of fluoroquinolones: an update. Can J Infect Dis 2002;13(1):54–61.

44. Wysowski DK, Bacsanyi J. Cisapride and fatal arrhythmia. N Engl J Med 1996;335(4):290–1.

45. Richter JE. Cisapride: limited access and alternatives. Cleve Clin J Med 2000;67(7):471–2.

46. European Agency for the Evaluation of Medicinal Products (EMEA). ICH topic S7B: note for guidance on the nonclinical evaluation of the potential for delayed ventricular repolarization (QT interval prolongation) by human pharmaceuticals. (CPMP/ICH/423/02). 2005.

47. Dethlefsen C, Hojfeldt G, Hojman P. The role of intratumoral and systemic IL-6 in breast cancer. Breast Cancer Res Treat 2013;138(3):657–64.

48. Pugsley MK, Authier S, Curtis MJ. Principles of safety pharmacology. Br J Pharmacol 2008; 154(7):1382–99.

49. Gintant GA, Limberis JT, McDermott JS, et al. The canine Purkinje fiber: an in vitro model system for acquired long QT syndrome and drug-induced arrhythmogenesis. J Cardiovasc Pharmacol 2001; 37(5):607–18.

50. Lu Z, Wu CY, Jiang YP, et al. Suppression of phosphoinositide 3-kinase signaling and alteration of multiple ion currents in drug-induced long QT syndrome. Sci Transl Med 2012;4(131):131ra150.

51. Yang T, Chun YW, Stroud DM, et al. Screening for acute IKr block is insufficient to detect torsades de pointes liability: role of late sodium current. Circulation 2014;130(3):224–34.

52. Antzelevitch C. Role of transmural dispersion of repolarization in the genesis of drug-induced torsades de pointes. Heart Rhythm 2005;2(2 Suppl):S9–15.

53. Belardinelli L, Shryock JC, Wu L, et al. Use of preclinical assays to predict risk of drug-induced torsades de pointes. Heart Rhythm 2005;2(2 Suppl): S16–22.

54. Darpo B. The thorough QT/QTc study 4 years after the implementation of the ICH E14 guidance. Br J Pharmacol 2010;159(1):49–57.

55. Bloomfield DM, Kost JT, Ghosh K, et al. The effect of moxifloxacin on QTc and implications for the design of thorough QT studies. Clin Pharmacol Ther 2008;84(4):475–80.

56. Committee for Medicinal Products for Human Use. ICH topic E14: the clinical evaluation of QT/QTc interval prolongation and proarrhythmic potential for non-arrhythmic drugs questions and answers (EMA/CHMP/ICH/310133/2008). London: EMEA; 2012. Available at: http://www.ema.europa.eu/docs/en_GB/document_library/Scientific_guideline/2009/09/WC500002878.pdf. Accessed August 27, 2014.

57. Shah RR, Morganroth J. ICH E14 Q & A (R1) document: perspectives on the updated recommendations on thorough QT studies. Br J Clin Pharmacol 2013;75(4):959–65.

58. Locatelli M, Criscitiello C, Esposito A, et al. QT prolongation induced by targeted biotherapies used in clinical practice and under investigation: a comprehensive review. Target Oncol 2015;10(1): 27–43.

59. Varterasian M, Meyer M, Fingert H, et al. Baseline heart rate-corrected QT and eligibility for clinical trials in oncology. J Clin Oncol 2003;21(17):3378–9.

60. Piekarz RL, Frye AR, Wright JJ, et al. Cardiac studies in patients treated with depsipeptide, FK228, in a phase II trial for T-cell lymphoma. Clin Cancer Res 2006;12(12):3762–73.

61. US Department of Health and Human Services: common terminology criteria for adverse events (CTCAE), version 4.0, DHHS, NIH, NCI. 2009. Available at: http://evs.nci.nih.gov/ftp1/CTCAE/Archive/CTCAE_4.02_2009-09-15_QuickReference_8.5x11.pdf. Accessed March 9, 2015.

62. Fingert H, Varterasian M. Safety biomarkers and the clinical development of oncology therapeutics: considerations for cardiovascular safety and risk management. AAPS J 2006;8(1):E89–94.

63. Varterasian M, Fingert H, Agin M, et al. Consideration of QT/QTc interval data in a phase I study in patients with advanced cancer. Clin Cancer Res 2004;10(17):5967–8 [author reply: 5968–9].

64. Naing A, Veasey-Rodrigues H, Hong DS, et al. Electrocardiograms (ECGs) in phase I anticancer drug development: the MD Anderson Cancer Center experience with 8518 ECGs. Ann Oncol 2012; 23(11):2960–3.

65. Kim PY, Ewer MS. Chemotherapy and QT prolongation: overview with clinical perspective. Curr Treat Options Cardiovasc Med 2014;16(5):303.

66. Rust DM, Soignet SL. Risk/benefit profile of arsenic trioxide. Oncologist 2001;6(Suppl 2):29–32.

67. Castaigne S, Chomienne C, Daniel MT, et al. All-trans retinoic acid as a differentiation therapy for acute promyelocytic leukemia. I. Clinical results. Blood 1990;76(9):1704–9.

68. Frankel SR, Eardley A, Heller G, et al. All-trans retinoic acid for acute promyelocytic leukemia. Results of the New York Study. Ann Intern Med 1994;120(4):278–86.

69. Hu J, Shen ZX, Sun GL, et al. Long-term survival and prognostic study in acute promyelocytic leukemia treated with all-trans-retinoic acid, chemotherapy, and As2O3: an experience of 120 patients at a single institution. Int J Hematol 1999;70(4):248–60.

70. Stone RM, Mayer RJ. The unique aspects of acute promyelocytic leukemia. J Clin Oncol 1990;8(11): 1913–21.

71. Warrell RP Jr, Maslak P, Eardley A, et al. Treatment of acute promyelocytic leukemia with all-trans retinoic acid: an update of the New York experience. Leukemia 1994;8(6):929–33.

72. Shen ZX, Chen GQ, Ni JH, et al. Use of arsenic trioxide (As2O3) in the treatment of acute promyelocytic leukemia (APL): II. Clinical efficacy and pharmacokinetics in relapsed patients. Blood 1997;89(9):3354–60.

73. Soignet SL, Frankel SR, Douer D, et al. United States multicenter study of arsenic trioxide in relapsed acute promyelocytic leukemia. J Clin Oncol 2001;19(18):3852–60.

74. Soignet SL, Maslak P, Wang ZG, et al. Complete remission after treatment of acute promyelocytic leukemia with arsenic trioxide. N Engl J Med 1998;339(19):1341–8.

75. Weinberg SL. The electrocardiogram in acute arsenic poisoning. Am Heart J 1960;60:971–5.

76. Niu C, Yan H, Yu T, et al. Studies on treatment of acute promyelocytic leukemia with arsenic trioxide: remission induction, follow-up, and molecular monitoring in 11 newly diagnosed and 47 relapsed acute promyelocytic leukemia patients. Blood 1999;94(10):3315–24.

77. Unnikrishnan D, Dutcher JP, Varshneya N, et al. Torsades de pointes in 3 patients with leukemia treated with arsenic trioxide. Blood 2001;97(5):1514–6.

78. Ohnishi K, Yoshida H, Shigeno K, et al. Prolongation of the QT interval and ventricular tachycardia in patients treated with arsenic trioxide for acute promyelocytic leukemia. Ann Intern Med 2000; 133(11):881–5.

79. Barbey JT, Pezzullo JC, Soignet SL. Effect of arsenic trioxide on QT interval in patients with advanced malignancies. J Clin Oncol 2003; 21(19):3609–15.

80. Roboz GJ, Ritchie EK, Carlin RF, et al. Prevalence, management, and clinical consequences of qt interval prolongation during treatment with arsenic trioxide. J Clin Oncol 2014;32(33):3723–8.

81. Barbey JT. Cardiac toxicity of arsenic trioxide. Blood 2001;98(5):1632 [author reply: 1633–4].

82. Krause DS, Van Etten RA. Tyrosine kinases as targets for cancer therapy. N Engl J Med 2005; 353(2):172–87.

83. Chen MH, Kerkela R, Force T. Mechanisms of cardiac dysfunction associated with tyrosine kinase inhibitor cancer therapeutics. Circulation 2008; 118(1):84–95.

84. Shah RR, Morganroth J, Shah DR. Cardiovascular safety of tyrosine kinase inhibitors: with a special focus on cardiac repolarisation (QT interval). Drug Saf 2013;36(5):295–316.

85. Druker BJ, Talpaz M, Resta DJ, et al. Efficacy and safety of a specific inhibitor of the BCR-ABL tyrosine kinase in chronic myeloid leukemia. N Engl J Med 2001;344(14):1031–7.

86. Ky B, Vejpongsa P, Yeh ET, et al. Emerging paradigms in cardiomyopathies associated with cancer therapies. Circ Res 2013;113(6):754–64.

87. Bair SM, Choueiri TK, Moslehi J. Cardiovascular complications associated with novel angiogenesis inhibitors: emerging evidence and evolving perspectives. Trends Cardiovasc Med 2013;23(4): 104–13.

88. Groarke JD, Cheng S, Moslehi J. Cancer-drug discovery and cardiovascular surveillance. N Engl J Med 2013;369(19):1779–81.

89. Tefferi A, Letendre L. Nilotinib treatment-associated peripheral artery disease and sudden death: yet another reason to stick to imatinib as front-line therapy for chronic myelogenous leukemia. Am J Hematol 2011;86(7):610–1.

90. Kantarjian H, Giles F, Wunderle L, et al. Nilotinib in imatinib-resistant CML and Philadelphia chromosome-positive ALL. N Engl J Med 2006; 354(24):2542–51.

91. Morgan TK Jr, Sullivan ME. An overview of class III electrophysiological agents: a new generation of antiarrhythmic therapy. Prog Med Chem 1992;29: 65–108.

92. Submission control no 102788Product monograph: sutent, sunitimib malate capsules. Kirkland (WA); Quebec (Canada): Pfizer Canada Inc; 2006.

93. Strevel EL, Ing DJ, Siu LL. Molecularly targeted oncology therapeutics and prolongation of the QT interval. J Clin Oncol 2007;25(22):3362–71.

94. Miller KD, Trigo JM, Wheeler C, et al. A multicenter phase II trial of ZD6474, a vascular endothelial growth factor receptor-2 and epidermal growth factor receptor tyrosine kinase inhibitor, in patients with previously treated metastatic breast cancer. Clin Cancer Res 2005;11(9):3369–76.

95. Holden SN, Eckhardt SG, Basser R, et al. Clinical evaluation of ZD6474, an orally active inhibitor of VEGF and EGF receptor signaling, in patients with solid, malignant tumors. Ann Oncol 2005; 16(8):1391–7.

96. Tamura T, Minami H, Yamada Y, et al. A phase I dose-escalation study of ZD6474 in Japanese patients with solid, malignant tumors. J Thorac Oncol 2006;1(9):1002–9.

97. Heymach JV, Johnson BE, Prager D, et al. Randomized, placebo-controlled phase II study of vandetanib plus docetaxel in previously treated non small-cell lung cancer. J Clin Oncol 2007;25(27): 4270–7.

98. Kiura K, Nakagawa K, Shinkai T, et al. A randomized, double-blind, phase IIa dose-finding study of Vandetanib (ZD6474) in Japanese patients with non-small cell lung cancer. J Thorac Oncol 2008;3(4):386–93.

99. Kovacs MJ, Reece DE, Marcellus D, et al. A phase II study of ZD6474 (Zactima, a selective inhibitor of VEGFR and EGFR tyrosine kinase in patients with relapsed multiple myeloma–NCIC CTG IND.145. Invest New Drugs 2006;24(6):529–35.

100. Wells SA Jr, Gosnell JE, Gagel RF, et al. Vandetanib for the treatment of patients with locally advanced or metastatic hereditary medullary thyroid cancer. J Clin Oncol 2010;28(5):767–72.

101. Natale RB, Thongprasert S, Greco FA, et al. Phase III trial of vandetanib compared with erlotinib in patients with previously treated advanced non-small-cell lung cancer. J Clin Oncol 2011;29(8):1059–66.

102. Zang J, Wu S, Tang L, et al. Incidence and risk of QTc interval prolongation among cancer patients treated with vandetanib: a systematic review and meta-analysis. PLoS One 2012;7(2):e30353.

103. Tam CS, Kantarjian H, Garcia-Manero G, et al. Failure to achieve a major cytogenetic response by 12 months defines inadequate response in patients receiving nilotinib or dasatinib as second or subsequent line therapy for chronic myeloid leukemia. Blood 2008;112(3):516–8.

104. US Food and Drug Administration. Safety information: tasigna (nilotinib) capsule. 2014. Available at: http://www.fda.gov/Safety/MedWatch/SafetyInformation/ucm218929.htm. Accessed November 17, 2014.

105. Johnstone RW. Histone-deacetylase inhibitors: novel drugs for the treatment of cancer. Nat Rev Drug Discov 2002;1(4):287–99.

106. Shultz MD, Cao X, Chen CH, et al. Optimization of the in vitro cardiac safety of hydroxamate-based histone deacetylase inhibitors. J Med Chem 2011; 54(13):4752–72.

107. Olsen EA, Kim YH, Kuzel TM, et al. Phase IIb multicenter trial of vorinostat in patients with persistent, progressive, or treatment refractory cutaneous T-cell lymphoma. J Clin Oncol 2007;25(21):3109–15.

108. Lynch DR Jr, Washam JB, Newby LK. QT interval prolongation and torsades de pointes in a patient undergoing treatment with vorinostat: a case report and review of the literature. Cardiol J 2012;19(4): 434–8.

109. Galetta F, Franzoni F, Cervetti G, et al. Effect of epirubicin-based chemotherapy and dexrazoxane supplementation on QT dispersion in non-Hodgkin lymphoma patients. Biomed Pharmacother 2005;59(10):541–4.

110. Nousiainen T, Vanninen E, Rantala A, et al. QT dispersion and late potentials during doxorubicin therapy for non-Hodgkin's lymphoma. J Intern Med 1999;245(4):359–64.

111. Liu XK, Katchman A, Ebert SN, et al. The anti-estrogen tamoxifen blocks the delayed rectifier potassium current, IKr, in rabbit ventricular myocytes. J Pharmacol Exp Ther 1998;287(3): 877–83.

112. Dowlati A, Robertson K, Cooney M, et al. A phase I pharmacokinetic and translational study of the novel vascular targeting agent combretastatin a-4 phosphate on a single-dose intravenous schedule in patients with advanced cancer. Cancer Res 2002;62(12):3408–16.

113. Britten CD, Rowinsky EK, Soignet S, et al. A phase I and pharmacological study of the farnesyl protein transferase inhibitor L-778,123 in patients with solid malignancies. Clin Cancer Res 2001;7(12):3894–903.

114. Hahn SM, Bernhard EJ, Regine W, et al. A Phase I trial of the farnesyltransferase inhibitor L-778,123 and radiotherapy for locally advanced lung and head and neck cancer. Clin Cancer Res 2002; 8(5):1065–72.

115. Martin NE, Brunner TB, Kiel KD, et al. A phase I trial of the dual farnesyltransferase and geranylgeranyltransferase inhibitor L-778,123 and radiotherapy for locally advanced pancreatic cancer. Clin Cancer Res 2004;10(16):5447–54.

116. Robertson MJ, Kahl BS, Vose JM, et al. Phase II study of enzastaurin, a protein kinase C beta inhibitor, in patients with relapsed or refractory diffuse large B-cell lymphoma. J Clin Oncol 2007;25(13): 1741–6.

117. Carducci MA, Musib L, Kies MS, et al. Phase I dose escalation and pharmacokinetic study of enzastaurin, an oral protein kinase C beta inhibitor, in patients with advanced cancer. J Clin Oncol 2006; 24(25):4092–9.

118. Camm AJ, Malik M, Yap YG. Acquired long QT syndrome. New York: Wiley-Blackwell; 2004.

# Arrhythmia in Stem Cell Transplantation

Shone O. Almeida, MD[a], Rhys J. Skelton[a,b], Sasikanth Adigopula, MD[a], Reza Ardehali, MD, PhD[a,c],*

## KEYWORDS

- Arrhythmia • Stem cell • Coupling • Cardiomyocyte • Regeneration • Paracrine
- Electromechanical

## KEY POINTS

- Candidates for cardiac cell therapy include autologous sources such as bone marrow progenitor cells, skeletal myoblasts, and resident cardiac stem cells. Human pluripotent stem cells, including embryonic stem cells and induced pluripotent stem cells, are additional candidates with vast differentiation potential, although no clinical trial has yet tested their efficacy.
- Cell coupling and engraftment are vital to improved myocardial function.
- Mechanisms for arrhythmia in stem cell transplantation include reentrant rhythms, automaticity that is at least in part dependent on host heart rate, noncardiac graft contaminates and noncellular features involving nerve sprouting and increased sympathetic innervation.
- Paracrine effects may serve a protective role.
- The method of stem cell transplantation also contributes to arrhythmogenicity, in that intramyocardial injection carries a higher rate of arrhythmia caused by disruption of the native architecture of the heart.

## INTRODUCTION

The human heart has limited regenerative capacity, and there is an unmet demand for improved therapies for cardiovascular disease. Both adult stem cells (ASCs) and human pluripotent stem cells (hPSCs) have the potential to facilitate development of cell-based therapies. ASCs have been used in clinical trials,[1,2] and hPSCs have been used extensively to regenerate injured mammalian hearts, including a recent report of nonhuman primates.[3] However, full clinical translation of stem cell–based therapies has been limited by numerous challenges, including the proarrhythmic

nature of stem cell–derived cardiac grafts. The potential arrhythmic risk may be attributed to differences in electrophysiologic maturity,[4–6] gap junction isotypes, cell orientation, and wave propagation between graft and the host myocardium. In vivo, the normal myocardial architecture has a unique three-dimensional extracellular matrix, offering cyclic mechanical stress (from rhythmic heart beating), electric stimulation, cell-cell signaling, and topographic cues among the cardiomyocytes (CMs). On injury, the normal architecture is disrupted, and CMs are replaced by scar tissue and proliferating fibroblasts, which in turn results in compromise of the structural integrity

Dr R. Ardehali is supported by the NIH Director's New Innovator's Award (DP2HL127728) and the California Institute for Regenerative Medicine (RC1-00354-1). The other authors have nothing to disclose.
a Division of Cardiology, Department of Medicine, David Geffen School of Medicine, University of California, Los Angeles, 100 UCLA Medical Plaza, Suite 630 East, Los Angeles, CA 90095, USA; b Murdoch Children's Research Institute, The Royal Children's Hospital, Cardiac Development, 50 Flemington Road, Parkville, Victoria 3052, Australia; c Eli and Edyth Broad Stem Cell Research Center, University of California, 675 Charles E Young Drive South, MRL Room 3780, Los Angeles, CA 90095, USA
* Corresponding author. Division of Cardiology, Department of Medicine, Eli and Edyth Broad Center for Regenerative Medicine and Stem Cell Research, University of California, 675 Charles E Young Drive South, MRL Room 3780, Los Angeles, CA 90095.
E-mail address: rardehali@mednet.ucla.edu

Card Electrophysiol Clin 7 (2015) 357–370
http://dx.doi.org/10.1016/j.ccep.2015.03.012
1877-9182/15/$ – see front matter © 2015 Elsevier Inc. All rights reserved.

and adverse remodeling of the heart. These structural changes cause anisotropy, which provides substrates for reentrant arrhythmias. In addition, the action potential duration prolongation may potentially produce early afterdepolarizations or delayed afterdepolarizations. Any attempt to introduce exogenous cells for regenerative purposes should take into consideration the hostile environment, the lack of normal myocardial structure, and the potential for the introduction of cells in a microenvironment in which normal CM fibers are replaced by scar. The electromechanical integration of the transplanted cells into such an environment may be a far-fetched reality but warrants critical analysis and intense research.

In the following sections, candidates for stem cell therapies, the mechanisms of stem cell cardiac graft–induced arrhythmogenicity, and the requirements for successful integration and electrophysiologic coupling of the hPSC cardiac graft to the damaged heart are discussed.

## CANDIDATES FOR CARDIAC REPAIR

There are 2 schools of thought regarding cell therapy for cardiac regeneration: (1) delivery of cells into the heart with the goal of survival, maturation, and integration of the transplanted cells for regeneration and replacement of the scar tissue, and (2) delivery of therapeutic cells into the heart, where cells may not survive to physically replace the damaged tissue, but which leads to regeneration via a paracrine effect and recruitment of endogenous cells to repair the scar. Although both scenarios could introduce arrhythmia, survival and engraftment of transplanted cells may dangerously serve as a nidus for arrhythmias.

Potential cell candidates to replace CMs in the injured heart must generate an action potential, couple this electrical stimulus to contraction, and form the necessary gap junctions for action potential propagation and integration with host myocytes.[7] A variety of cell types have been studied as potential candidates for cardiac regeneration (Table 1). Properties such as propensity for electromechanical integration, arrhythmogenicity, and risk of teratoma formation are important considerations in selecting the appropriate cell. Cell sources for cardiac cell therapy include skeletal myoblasts (SMs), bone marrow progenitors, resident cardiac stem cells (CSCs), human embryonic stem cell (hESCs) and induced pluripotent stem cells (iPSCs).[7–9] Human ESCs, iPSCs, and resident cardiac progenitor cells have all been reported to differentiate into CMs in both in vivo and in vitro studies, whereas bone marrow

mesenchymal stem cells (MSCs) and SMs rely on transdifferentiation.[10]

In addition to selecting the appropriate cell candidate for transplantation, other concerns include the quantity of transplanted cells needed to achieve a clinically reasonable graft size, potential for proliferation in vivo and the degree of cell retention.[7] Methods for transplantation include intracoronary and direct intramyocardial via a surgical or catheter-based approach.[11] The degree of cell retention is largely dependent on the method of transplantation, whereas cell viability and survival after transplantation also depend on the cell type and the microenvironment. Widimsky and colleagues[11] reported that after intracoronary injection of bone marrow cells (BMCs) into large-animal models and humans, retention rates ranged 1.3% to 5.3% 2 hours after transplantation. Various methods of transplantation may also directly influence the arrhythmogenicity of stem cell therapy, as discussed in later sections.

Another aspect important for successful hPSC integration is graft alignment. If not patterned correctly, engrafted cells have a propensity to integrate randomly into the host heart and thereby increase electric heterogeneity and arrhythmogenic foci. Applications such as tissue engineering need to be used to ensure optimal graft alignment.

### Skeletal Myoblasts

SMs are a reservoir for skeletal muscle cell regeneration in cases of muscle injury.[12,13] A major source of SMs is satellite cells, resident muscle stem cells responsible for muscle growth, repair, and homeostasis.[14] The potential for in vitro amplification of satellite stem cells and their ability to self-renew make SMs a desirable target for CSC therapy. There are several features unique to SMs. These cells are committed to a myogenic lineage and become functional myocytes regardless, or rather despite, environmental cues.[12] Further, SMs continue to proliferate in vivo with a high degree of resistance to tissue ischemia, leading to larger graft sizes. In early mice studies, grafts were shown to be viable for as long as 3 months after transplantation.[15]

SMs were used in some of the first clinical trials for cardiac regeneration. Despite modest improvements in left ventricular ejection fraction, the increased incidence of sustained ventricular tachycardia in cell-treated patients led to increased concerns regarding cardiac cell therapy.[13,16,17] SMs do not express the gap junctions, connexin-43 (Cx43) in particular, necessary for electrical coupling with host CMs[18–20] discussed in more detail later. Roell and colleagues[20] have

**Table 1**
Selected active clinical trials in cardiac cell therapy

| Title | Cell Type | Method | Enrollment | Objective | Primary Outcome |
|---|---|---|---|---|---|
| Allogeneic Heart Stem Cells to Achieve Myocardial Regeneration (ALLSTAR) | C-DC | Intracoronary | 274 | Determine whether allogeneic cardiosphere-derived cells are safe and effective in decreasing infarct size in patients with MI | Infarct size assessed by MRI |
| Intramyocardial Transplantation of Bone Marrow Stem Cells in Addition to CABG Surgery (PERFECT) | BM-MNC | Intramyocardial | 142 | Determine whether intramyocardial injection of autologous CD133+ bone marrow stem cells yields a functional benefit in addition to CABG in patients with chronic ischemic CAD | LVEF at rest, measured by MRI |
| Effects of Intracoronary Progenitor Cell Therapy on Coronary Flow Reserve After AMI (REPAIR-ACS) | BM-MNC | Intracoronary | 100 | Determine whether intracoronary application of autologous bone marrow–derived progenitor cells benefits coronary flow reserve in NSTEMI | Improvement of coronary flow reserve in the infarct vessel |
| Autologous Bone Marrow Mononuclear Cells in the Combined Treatment of Coronary Heart Disease | BM-MNC | Intramyocardial, intravenous | 100 | Evaluate the effect of the method of administration of BM-MNCs for the duration of functioning aortocoronary bypass grafts in the surgical treatment of CAD | All-cause mortality associated with the progression of basic disease |
| Trial of Hematopoietic Stem Cells in Acute Myocardial Infarction (TECAM2) | BM-MNC | Intracoronary | 120 | Comparing intracoronary transplantation of autologous bone marrow stem cells in ventricular postinfarction remodeling to conventional treatment or mobilization of bone marrow stem cells with GCSF | Change in LVEF and left ventricular end-systolic volume relative to baseline measured by MRI |
| The Effect of Intracoronary Reinfusion of Bone Marrow–Derived Mononuclear Cells on All Cause Mortality in Acute MI (BAMI) | BM-MNC | Intracoronary | 3000 | Demonstrate that a single intracoronary infusion of autologous bone marrow–derived mononuclear cells is safe and reduces all-cause mortality in patients with reduced LVEF ($\leq$45%) after successful reperfusion for AMI | Time from randomization to all-cause death |

(continued on next page)

**Table 1**
*(continued)*

| Title | Cell Type | Method | Enrollment | Objective | Primary Outcome |
|---|---|---|---|---|---|
| Compare the Effects of Single vs Repeated IC Application of Autologous BM-MNC on Mortality in Patients With Chronic Post-Infarction Heart Failure (REPEAT) | BM-MNC | Intracoronary | 676 | Compare the effects of single vs repeated application of autologous bone marrow–derived stem cells to treat chronic postinfarction heart failure | Mortality at 2 y after inclusion in the study |
| Intracardiac CD133+ Cells in Patients With No-Option Resistant Angina | CD133+ stem cells | Intramyocardial | 60 | Evaluate the efficacy of autologous CD133+ cells in patients with resistant angina without the possibility of effective revascularization | Myocardial perfusion change assessed by perfusion scintigraphy |
| Intra-coronary Versus Intramyocardial Application of Enriched CD133pos Autologous Bone Marrow Derived Stem Cells (AlsterMACS) | CD133+ stem cells | Intracoronary | 64 | Compare the effect of intracoronary vs intramyocardial application of enriched CD133+ autologous bone marrow–derived stem cells for improving left ventricular function in chronic ischemic cardiomyopathy | Change in global LVEF measured via echocardiography |
| Repetitive Intramyocardial CD34+ Cell Therapy in Dilated Cardiomyopathy (REMEDIUM) | CD34+ PSC | Intramyocardial | 80 | Determine if repetitive administration of cell therapy would allow for long-lasting improvements in heart function | Change in LVEF measured at baseline and 1 y |
| The Enhanced Angiogenic Cell Therapy - Acute Myocardial Infarction Trial (ENACT-AMI) | EPC | Intracoronary | 100 | Assess the safety and efficacy of cell and gene therapy for patients with moderate to large anterior STEMI after revascularization with stent implantation to the infarct-related artery | Change in global LVEF by cardiac MRI |
| Intracoronary Autologous MSC Implantation in Patients With Ischemic Dilated Cardiomyopathy | MSC | Intracoronary | 80 | Test the differentiation potential and therapeutic capacity of mesenchymal stem cells in patients with severe CAD after intracoronary implantation | Serial monitoring of change in LVEF as measured by echocardiogram and MRI |

| Study | Cell Type | Delivery | Number | Objective | Outcome |
|---|---|---|---|---|---|
| Percutaneous Stem Cell Injection Delivery Effects On Neomyogenesis in Dilated Cardiomyopathy (the POSEIDON-DCM study) | MSC | Transendocardial | 36 | Compare the safety and efficacy of transendocardial injection of autologous MSCs vs allogeneic MSCs in patients with nonischemic dilated cardiomyopathy | Incidence of any treatment-emergent serious adverse events 1 mo after catheterization |
| To Evaluate Efficacy and Safety of Allogeneic Mesenchymal Precursor Cells (CEP-41750) for the Treatment of CHF | MSC | Transendocardial | 1730 | Evaluate the efficacy and safety of allogeneic mesenchymal precursor cells for the treatment of chronic heart failure | Time to first heart failure–related major adverse cardiac events |
| A Randomized, Open Labeled, Multicenter Trial for Safety and Efficacy of Intracoronary Adult Human MSCs in AMI (RELIEF) | MSC | Intracoronary | 135 | Verify the long-term efficacy and safety of the first cell treatment using Hearticellgram-AMI (autologous human bone marrow–derived mesenchymal stem cells) in patients with acute MI | LVEF measured 13 mo after the cell treatment with MRI |
| Safety Study of Allogeneic Mesenchymal Precursor Cell Infusion in Myocardial Infarction (AMICI) | MSC | Intracoronary | 225 | Determine the safety and feasibility of the intracoronary infusion of investigational mesenchymal precursor cells in patients with de novo anterior MI caused by a lesion of the LAD | Frequency of the total major adverse cardiac and cerebrovascular events |

*Abbreviations:* AMI, acute myocardial infarction; BM-MNC, bone marrow mononuclear cells; CABG, coronary artery bypass graft; CAD, coronary artery disease; C-DC, cardiosphere-derived cells; CHF, congestive heart failure; EPC, endothelial progenitor cells; GCSF, granulocyte colony-stimulating factor; IC, intracoronary; LAD, left anterior descending; LVEF, left ventricular ejection fraction; MI, myocardial infarction; MRI, magnetic resonance imaging; MSC, mesenchymal stem cells; NSTEMI, non-ST segment elevation myocardial infarction; PSC, peripheral stem cells; STEMI, ST segment elevation myocardial infarction.

*Data from* clinicaltrials.gov.

shown that large grafts, if uncoupled with host CMs, essentially act as a conduction block and thereby serve as a substrate for ventricular arrhythmias.[21] Using lentiviral-mediated transduction with Cx43, 1 study showed that genetically modified SMs had increased electrical stability and decreased arrhythmogenicity.[22] Future research into this approach will undoubtedly provide useful information.

### Bone Marrow Progenitors

BMCs have been used extensively as a candidate for cardiac regenerative therapy. Clinical trials using unfractionated BMCs, mononuclear BMCs, BMC-derived hematopoietic progenitors, and MSCs have reported the safety of these cells, but the clinical benefit has been debated. Several explanations have been suggested, including that endothelial precursors within bone marrow expressing CD34 and CD133, hematopoietic lineage markers, induce formation of new blood vessels within the infarct bed as well as proliferation of preexisting vasculature.[23] Bone marrow–derived cells that express CD133 have been hypothesized in several studies to be the critical cell type involved in cardiac functional recovery.[24] One in particular found that in patients with refractory critical limb ischemia treated with BMCs that include CD133+ cells, there was a strong association with increased endothelial proliferation locally and angiogenesis.[25] Neoangiogenesis within the infarct bed is especially important, as previous work has shown that after infarct, the capillary network within the heart is unable to keep up with increased myocardial demand because of hypertrophy and remodeling, leading to infarct extension and further loss of viable tissue. This situation is mediated by marrow-secreted factors such as vascular endothelial growth factor and macrophage chemoattractant protein 1,[26] serving to prevent cell apoptosis and reduce collagen deposition and scar formation as well as improve left ventricular function.[23]

The second explanation involves the plasticity of bone marrow-derived cells where it is proposed that these cells may have the potential to generate CMs. Although this situation has been reported as a mechanism by which transplanted BMCs exert their beneficial effect, scientific data supporting transdifferentiation to CMs is lacking. Several investigators have shown that in vitro and in small animal models, BMC-derived progenitors indeed do give rise to new CMs in addition to contributing to neoangiogenesis in myocardial infarct models.[23,27,28] Other groups have proposed a third mechanism for improved cardiac function,

showing fusion of BMCs with somatic cells in in vitro and in vivo studies.[29] These fusion cells phenotypically function like the recipient cell. Fusion of bone marrow–derived cells has also been seen with hepatocytes in the liver and neurons in the brain. This phenomenon may explain the generation of CMs observed after BMC transplantation.[29]

Human clinical trials using bone marrow progenitor cells and MSCs were met with fears over arrhythmogenesis given results of previous work with SMs. However, numerous studies have observed no increase in ventricular arrhythmogenicity in patients treated with MSC and bone marrow progenitor cells.[30–33] Recent studies have suggested a protective effect from an arrhythmia perspective after MSC transplantation, with 1 study suggesting reversal of cardiac potassium channel remodeling as a possible mechanism.[34] This finding may also be the result of poor engraftment, with most cells being cleared or otherwise lost from the host heart, thereby eliminating the chance of these cells acting as an arrhythmogenic substrate.[35,36] Furthermore, it has been postulated that paracrine effects of the MSCs may have a beneficial effect in suppressing the arrhythmogenic substrate. Perin and colleagues[37] reported that endocardial injection of autologous bone marrow mononuclear cells in patients with end-stage ischemic heart disease led to improved perfusion and myocardial contractility. Others showed similar results with intracoronary delivery of bone marrow mononuclear cells,[38] consistent with findings in the TOPCARE-AMI (Transplantation of Progenitor Cells and Regeneration Enhancement in Acute Myocardial Infarction) trial, which showed significant improvement in global left ventricular ejection fraction and reduced end-systolic volumes.[30] Although data from the BMC trials have been encouraging, no study has yet confirmed presence of functioning CMs derived from BMCs that have integrated into the host myocardium. Future trials and basic research will shed light on this controversial field.

### Resident Cardiac Stem Cells

Historically, the heart has been regarded as a terminally differentiated organ, incapable of regeneration. Cardiac growth was believed to be caused by increase in CM size rather than number. However, this dogma has been challenged by several recent studies. Taking advantage of carbon 14 dating technology, researchers have shown that CM renewal does occur, albeit at a slow rate of 1% annually at the age of 25 years and decaying over time.[39] Using a mosaic analysis with a double-marker mouse model, a recent study[40] found that postnatal CM generation is a rare occurrence and that this capacity is limited to a small population of CMs, so-called resident CSCs. Although some have shown increased cardiomyogenesis after cardiac infarct and injury,[41] this remains controversial. CSCs retain stem cell–like properties, including self-renewal and multipotency with a myocardial-restricted phenotype.[42] They can give rise to CMs, smooth muscle, and endothelial cells, with the ability to replenish the coronary microcirculation in some cases.[43] This small pool of progenitor cells also take part in myocardial homeostasis, serving to replenish CMs after injury and participating in the remodeling process.[43]

Although the existence of resident CSCs in adult mammalian heart has not been entirely characterized, several populations have been well studied. One such population is the c-kit+/Lin population, which was first described by Beltrami and colleagues[44] and was shown to give rise to myocytes, smooth muscle, and endothelial cells. Since then, CSCs have gained the intrigue of several groups studying their role in cardiac regeneration. One of the first human trials was SCIPIO (Cardiac Stem Cell Infusion in Patients With Ischemic CardiOmyopathy), a phase 1 randomized trial of autologous c-kit+ CSCs in ischemic heart failure.[45] CSCs were isolated from the right atrial appendage and expanded in culture and after coronary artery bypass grafting, the treatment arm underwent intracoronary CSC infusion. Compared with control, CSC-treated patients showed improvements in ejection fraction and a reduction in infarct size at 4 months after infusion. Despite these promising outcomes, challenges such as poor survival and retention of CSCs after transplantation regardless of delivery method have yet to be overcome.[46]

Another increasing source of autologous derived CMs is cardiospheres (CSps), a term first coined by Messina and colleagues[47] in 2004. CSps are a mixture of various cell types, including resident CSCs, spontaneously differentiated CMs, and even vascular cells. These self-assembling multicellular clusters are obtained from postnatal biopsy specimens and have properties of adult CSCs.[48] CSp-derived cells (CDCs) have been used in animal studies and clinically with promising results, particularly in the CADUCEUS (Cardiosphere-Derived Autologous Stem Cells to Reverse Ventricular Dysfunction) trial.[49] Although primarily designed as a safety trial, preliminary data show that intracoronary infusion of CDCs led to decrease in scar size and improved function of infarcted myocardium without a significant difference in rates of ventricular arrhythmia between control and treatment arms. This finding has led to the ALLSTAR (Allogeneic Heart Stem Cells to Achieve Myocardial Regeneration) trial, which aims to determine the safety and effectiveness of allogeneic CDCs in decreasing infarct size in patients with myocardial infarction (MI).[50]

## Human Pluripotent Stem Cells

hESCs and iPSCs, collectively known as hPSCs, have the potential to be an unlimited source for a variety of tissue-specific cell types. hPSCs can be efficiently differentiated toward a cardiovascular lineage, hence making them an enticing candidate for cell therapy to regenerate the damaged myocardium. iPSCs overcome the ethical and social concerns raised with hESCs. hPSCs have the advantage of yielding a variety of phenotypes, including atrial, nodal, and ventricular CMs. Although recent studies have seen major improvements in the efficiency of cardiac differentiation,[51,52] shortcomings persist, including teratoma formation with both iPSCs and hESCs and prolonged time to procure and derive iPSCs.[53]

Cardiac cells derived from hPSCs can readily engraft into the injured heart and generate a spontaneous action potential.[3] Although this characteristic makes hPSCs ideal candidates for cell therapy, it also raises legitimate concerns over their arrhythmogenicity. Several studies have reported that PSC-derived CMs show immature and fetal-like electrical activities, which would make the electromechanical coupling of these cells with the host CMs a challenge.[4–6] In addition, there still remains a significant challenge in isolating a pure population of chamber-specific CMs from an in vitro differentiation assay. Generally, hPSC differentiation does not yield 100% purity for CMs, and moreover, the generated myocytes represent a heterogeneous population, which includes ventricular, atrial, and nodal cells. It has been suggested that transplanted hESC-derived CMs show afterdepolarizations caused by a low expression of the iK1 channel[54] and also have pacemaking currents independent of the host myocardium.[55,56] In addition, because of their allogeneic origin, they are at risk for host immune rejection,[53] a potential mechanism for arrhythmogenicity discussed in more detail later. As is possible with introduction of any cell type, the transplanted cells may modify the substrate with ectopic electrical activities, such that an arrhythmogenic focus is generated.

Although the electromechanical coupling of PSC-derived CMs in the heart remains a significant concern, the host environment may play an essential role. Ardehali and colleagues[57] for the first time showed structural and functional integration of hESC-derived cardiovascular progenitors into human fetal hearts. Shiba and colleagues[58] also reported that hESC-derived CMs can electrically couple in guinea pig models and suppress arrhythmias in the injured heart, seemingly by forming a conduction bridge over the scar tissue. Fully understanding the arrhythmogenicity of hPSC cardiac cell transplants requires additional large-animal studies, with precise assessment of electrical activities that are propagated throughout the grafted cells. It is speculated that the proarrhythmic properties of hPSC-derived cardiac cells grafts are caused by their immature electrophysiologic phenotype and may be avoided by the use of in vitro maturation methods before transplantation.[59]

## ELECTROPHYSIOLOGIC STUDIES AND CELL COUPLING

The clinical application of stem cells to replenish new myocytes in the heart relies on electromechanical coupling of the transplanted cells with the host. Also important is the ability of the transplanted cells to generate action potentials and thereby perhaps function as biological pacemakers. This automaticity was studied in in vitro models that revealed that hESCs show spontaneous electrical activity, although with significant rhythmic variation.[60] Automaticity can be studied in vitro using whole-cell voltage clamp and simultaneous patch-clamp/laser scanning confocal calcium imaging.[61] Studies have also shown that the coupling between excitation and contraction is related to calcium-induced calcium release, that is local calcium release from the sarcoplasmic reticulum (calcium clock) and activation of voltage gated ion channels.[60,61] Disruption in either of these mechanisms leads to dysrhythmic beating or, in some cases, suppression of automaticity altogether. Kehat and colleagues[62] also reported electromechanical coupling in vitro. Within 24 hours of coculturing hESC-derived CM (hESC-CMs) with neonatal rat ventricular myocytes, synchronous mechanical activity was detected. High-resolution activation maps that characterize impulse initiation and propagation showed close temporal coupling between graft and host. Electrophysiologic analysis has also shown that hESC-CMs express many of the same ion channels as mature cells.[61,62]

Electromechanical integration of hESC-CMs into injured hearts is essential to improving cardiac function (**Fig. 1**). Several in vivo studies have shown that delivery of hESC-CMs into an injured heart leads to at least partial coupling of the transplanted cells with the host CMs. One group[58] showed that these cells form new force-generating units. The

investigators used genetically modified hESC-CMs that encoded a fluorescent calcium sensor such that after transplantation, epicardial fluorescent transients could be correlated with electrocardiogram to show synchrony with host myocardium. Ardehali and colleagues[57] established that when hESC-derived cardiovascular progenitors are transplanted in human fetal hearts, they are able to migrate and couple with neighboring host CMs, showing synchronous electrical activity. Others have also reported that transplanted hESC-CMs survive and integrate in vivo.[62] Using a pig complete heart block model, Kehat and colleagues showed that the transplanted cells showed automaticity and biological pacing functionality.

For functional integration to occur, the electrical potential generated in 1 cell must be sufficient to propagate through gap junctions and depolarize neighboring cells.[62] It is the disruption of this structure through loss of desmosomes and gap junctions in ischemic disease that leads to arrhythmia in the injured heart.[63] One gap junction of particular importance is Cx43.[20,57,62–64] It has been shown that transplantation of embryonic CMs led to increased electrical stability in the injured heart, particularly improved coupling between graft and host and decreased incidence of ventricular tachycardia, a property that is dependent on Cx43.[20,65] Transplantation of SMs that do not express Cx43 showed significant increase in the rate of arrhythmias. Similar findings were shown in another study in which a hypoxic culture environment served to restore Cx43 in MSCs, thereby curbing the incidence of arrhythmias.[66] Nevertheless, expression of Cx43 is not in itself sufficient to suppress the arrhythmic potential of stem cell transplantation, and various other mechanisms exist.

In addition to electromechanical coupling and formation of gap junctions, another mechanism that may have confounding effects on the induction of arrhythmia is cell fusion. Studies have shown that bone marrow–derived cells selectively fuse with cells in the brain, liver, and heart.[29,67] In sex mismatch studies with transplanted hESC-derived CMs to investigate the degree of cell fusion observed,[57] less than 3.8% of transplanted cells showed evidence of fusion, suggesting that fusion events are rare and perhaps transdifferentiation is the dominant process. The key question of whether these fusions have a role in the formation of new cells or a repair and maintenance function remains unanswered.

## MECHANISMS OF ARRHYTHMOGENICITY

Various mechanisms have been described for the proarrhythmic potential of stem cell

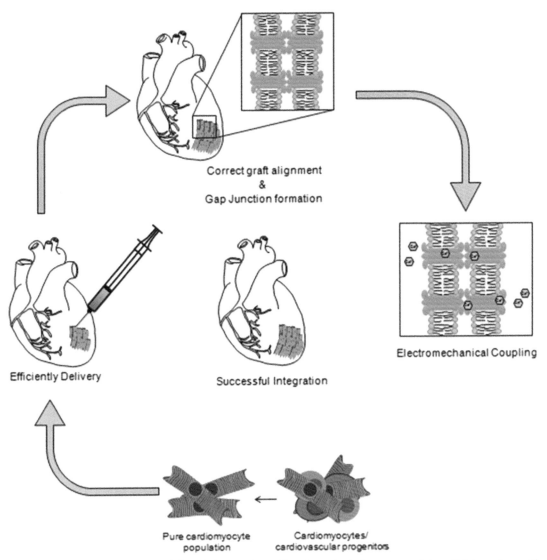

**Fig. 1.** Factors influencing successful graft integration. After transplantation, successful graft integration with host myocardium is dependent on several factors: a cell population with low percentage of noncardiac derivatives, an efficient delivery method that favors cell survival and retention, correct graft alignment and gap junction formation that allows for electromechanical coupling.

transplantation (**Fig. 2**). In part, these mechanisms are largely dependent on the type of cells transplanted, as discussed earlier.

### Reentrant Pathways and Automaticity

In a study by Liao and colleagues,[68] the proarrhythmic risk of hESCs versus hESC-CMs was investigated in a mouse model of MI (CSp-derived cell). Through in vitro and in vivo experimental evidence, the investigators reported increased arrhythmogenesis in the hESC-CM population, particularly prolonged action potential duration,

which led to a higher rate of inducible ventricular tachycardia than the hESC group. One explanation is that the relative difference in action potential duration between transplanted hESC-CMs and intrinsic ventricular CMs facilitates reentrant excitation. Another proposed mechanism is that hESC-CMs can cause abnormal impulse initiations, serving as ectopic arrhythmic foci, early afterdepolarization, or delayed afterdepolarization. The in vivo experiments showed that although CMs integrate with host myocardium, they have immature electrophysiologic properties, which may lead to less organized gap junctions.[65] These

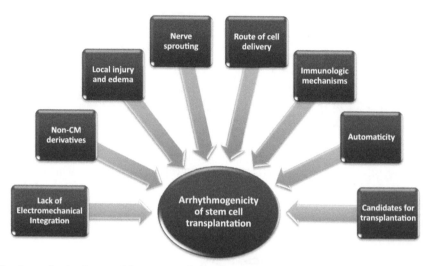

**Fig. 2.** Mechanisms of arrhythmogenicity. Proposed mechanisms for the higher rates of arrhythmia observed with stem cell transplantation include (1) lack of electromechanical integration; (2) transplantation of noncardiomyocyte derivatives; (3) local injury and edema; (4) nerve sprouting resulting in increased sympathetic tone; (5) route of cell delivery, with intramyocardial being more arrhythmogenic than retrograde intracoronary; (6) immunologic mechanisms leading to rejection and inflammation; (7) graft automaticity; and (8) candidates for transplantation, in whom expression of gap junctions such as Cx43 influence the arrhythmogenicity of the graft.

properties predispose the substrate to higher rates of arrhythmia.

However, the reported degree of electrical instability and arrhythmia rate seems to be variable in the literature. One possible explanation for the conflicting data may be differences in heart size and rate of the animal models. Many studies have relied on the murine model for in vivo cell transplantation studies. However, considering that the intrinsic heart rate in mice is approximately 500 to 600 beats per minute, hPSC-CMs fail to couple with the mouse CMs to maintain such an increased contraction rate. Using a macaque model of MI, researchers[3] showed that electrical coupling occurs between graft and host myocardium. All transplanted primates showed electromechanical coupling shown by epicardial fluorescent calcium transients that were synchronous with host electrocardiogram. However, hESC-CM transplanted primates showed arrhythmias, particularly premature ventricular contractions and ventricular tachycardia.[3] This finding was especially evident in the first 2 weeks after transplantation. The coupling rates seen in this large-animal study were higher than seen in experiments by Shiba and colleagues, in which in a guinea pig MI model, only 60% of transplanted hearts showed electrical coupling.[58] When transplanted into uninjured hearts, there was 100% electromechanical coupling, suggesting that graft behavior is more heterogeneous in injured heart models.[58] In addition, hESC-CM transplanted

guinea pigs showed the lowest fraction of premature ventricular contractions and spontaneous ventricular tachycardia as well as overall a higher rate of electrical stability in studies evaluating inducible arrhythmias with programmed electrical stimulation.[20,58] This finding was also seen in similar experiments with mice[69] and rats.[70] Possible mechanisms for observed arrhythmias include the presence of reentrant circuits as well as graft automaticity.[62]

The differences in arrhythmia rate observed in large versus small animals seem to be related, at least in part, to variation in heart size and rate.[3] As mentioned earlier in murine models, graft integration with host myocytes is immature and with slower rates of ventricular action potential conduction.[68] This phenomenon may be accentuated in large hearts in which larger grafts are used, leading to an even slower rate of action potential conduction and predisposing to reentrant loops.[3] This finding may explain why increased arrhythmogenicity is seen in larger animal studies rather than with mice and guinea pigs. An alternative explanation surrounds the species-specific heart rate. Faster heart rates as seen in mice (600 beats/min) and guinea pigs (230 beats/min) favor native conduction pathways over graft automaticity or reentrant loops.[3] Conversely, macaques have rates between 100 and 130 beats/min. This slower rate may have increased susceptibility to graft automaticity and ventricular arrhythmias.

## Impurities in Stem Cell Differentiation

The process of differentiating hSECs from CMs is an imperfect one. The yield of these protocols is never 100%, with isolates often containing noncardiac derivatives, and may be contaminated with residual undifferentiated pluripotent stem cells capable of forming teratomas in vivo. One explanation for arrhythmogenicity with stem cell transplantation may lie in the impurities of the transplanted graft. This hypothesis was tested using a guinea pig chronic infarct model.[71] At 28 days after cardiac cryoinjury, animals were transplanted with hESC-CMs, noncardiac hESC derivatives or vehicle, the latter 2 serving as controls. There was no statistically significant difference in arrhythmia rate between the 3 groups outside the periprocedural period. All animals then underwent electrophysiologic studies to assess the electrical stability. Of the 3 groups, guinea pigs transplanted with noncardiac hESC derivatives showed the highest degree of electrical instability, with a greater incidence of inducible ventricular tachycardia. The hESC-CM and vehicle groups were fairly resistant to arrhythmia. These data suggest that 1 possible mechanism for arrhythmogenicity in stem cell transplantation is impurity in the CM differentiation process. It is suggested that immunologic mechanisms could explain why this situation leads to higher arrhythmia rates.[71] Transplantation of noncardiac derivatives could evoke a stronger and more intense host immune response to the graft, leading to increased rejection and thereby increased arrhythmogenicity. However, this hypothesis was not supported in follow-up immunohistochemical studies.[71] Several investigators[57,72,73] have isolated hESC-derived CMs or cardiovascular progenitors using specific surface markers to circumvent the impurity issue. Identification of markers that allow for prospective isolation of hESC-derived cardiovascular cells at different stages of development is promising and warrants further investigation.

## Confounding Factors

In addition to the mechanisms outlined earlier, perhaps there are confounding factors in the mechanism of arrhythmogenicity in stem cell transplantation that are cell independent.[74] These factors may include local injury or edema induced by myocardial injection[65] as well as variation in transplantation methods. Few head-to-head studies exist comparing delivery methods, but one in particular[75] showed that intramyocardial injection of BMCs was more arrhythmogenic, including higher rates of ventricular tachycardia,

than retrograde intracoronary delivery. One may postulate that injection of cell clusters via the intramyocardial route serves to impede electrical conduction in the host myocardium as well as stimulate cytokine release from inflammatory cells, both of which may lead to higher rates of arrhythmias. It has been also shown that transplantation of MSCs induces nerve sprouting and high sympathetic nerve density.[76] Although increased sympathetic innervations could lead to improved contractility and left ventricular ejection fraction, it could also result in higher rates of arrhythmia in myocardium that is already damaged by ischemia.[77]

## PARACRINE EFFECTS

Several studies have evaluated how paracrine effects influence the graft electrical activity. Some suggest that secretion of soluble factors such as cytokines, chemokines, and growth factors from transplanted cells may lead to beneficial effects. This theory has come to be known as the paracrine hypothesis.[53] Although further work is needed, potential mechanisms for the beneficial effects include the release of cryoprotective molecules that increase native CM survival, neovascularization (including angiogenesis and arteriogenesis), alterations in the extracellular matrix resulting in remodeling that leads to increased scar strength and reduced ventricular dilation, improved cardiac contractility, and recruitment and activation of resident CSCs.[78] Some groups have also studied how the in vitro environment in which cells are cultured affects their arrhythmic potential. Hwang and colleagues[66] investigated the effects of paracrine media (media conditioned by growing cells) under hypoxic or normoxic conditions. Using myocardial infarct models in rats, they injected hypoxic paracrine media, normoxic paracrine media, or MSCs into the infarct border zone. The hypoxic, but not normoxic, paracrine media were found to prevent sudden death in rats by improving conduction in the border zone through recovery of gap junctions, reducing the degree of fibrosis, and better modulating calcium regulatory ion channels, thereby leading to increased electrical stability.

## SUMMARY

Research in cardiac regeneration has come a long way. It has moved from bench to bedside, with promising results in human studies. However, there is still much to learn, particularly how to safely use cell therapy to improve conditions such as congestive heart failure and ischemic heart disease and minimize arrhythmogenicity of cell therapy. Further work is needed to improve methods of cell delivery and transplantation. Newer delivery systems include cell-seeded patches and scaffold-free cell sheets. Cell coupling and engraftment are also of vital importance to reduce risk of reentrant pathways and automaticity, which serve as a nidus for arrhythmia. From cell selection to proper graft alignment, finding ways to curb the proarrhythmic risk of stem cell transplantation is an essential step toward successful clinical application.

# REFERENCES

1. Bolli R, Chugh AR, D'Amario D, et al. Effect of cardiac stem cells in patients with ischemic cardiomyopathy: initial results of the SCIPIO trial. Lancet 2011;378:1847–57.

2. Menasché P, Alfieri O, Janssens S, et al. The Myoblast Autologous Grafting in Ischemic Cardiomyopathy (MAGIC) trial: first randomized placebo-controlled study of myoblast transplantation. Circulation 2008;117:1189–200.

3. Chong JJ, Yang X, Don CW, et al. Human embryonic-stem-cell-derived cardiomyocytes regenerate non-human primate hearts. Nature 2014;510:273–7.

4. Mummery C, Ward-van Oostwaard D, Doevendans P, et al. Differentiation of human embryonic stem cells to cardiomyocytes: role of coculture with visceral endoderm-like cells. Circulation 2003;107:2733–40.

5. Laflamme MA, Murry CE. Heart regeneration. Nature 2011;473:326–35.

6. Snir M, Kehat I, Gepstein A, et al. Assessment of the ultrastructural and proliferative properties of human embryonic stem cell-derived cardiomyocytes. Am J Physiol Heart Circ Physiol 2003;285:H2355–63.

7. Schuldt AJ, Rosen MR, Gaudette GR, et al. Repairing damaged myocardium: evaluating cells used for cardiac regeneration. Curr Treat Options Cardiovasc Med 2008;10:59–72.

8. Lyon AR, Harding SE, Peters NS. Cardiac stem cell therapy and arrhythmogenicity: Prometheus and the arrows of Apollo and Artemis. J Cardiovasc Transl Res 2008;1:207–16.

9. Miyoshi S, Ikegami Y, Itabashi Y, et al. Cardiac cell therapy and arrhythmias. Circ J 2007;71(Suppl A):A45–9.

10. Meng X. Transdifferentiation during heart regeneration. J Stem Cell Res Ther 2014;4:188.

11. Widimsky P, Panicka M, Lang O, et al. Intracoronary transplantation of bone marrow stem cells: background, techniques, and limitations. Eur Heart J 2006;8(Supplement H):H16–22.

12. Oettgen P. Cardiac stem cell therapy need for optimization of efficacy and safety monitoring. Circulation 2006;114:353–8.

13. Siminiak T, Kalmucki P, Kurpisz M. Autologous skeletal myoblasts for myocardial regeneration. J Interv Cardiol 2004;17:357–65.

14. Scharner J, Zammit PS. The muscle satellite cell at 50: the formative years. Skelet Muscle 2011;1:28.

15. Koh GY, Klug MG, Soonpaa MH, et al. Differentiation and long-term survival of C2C12 myoblast grafts in heart. J Clin Invest 1993;92:1548–54.

16. Menasché P, Hagège AA, Vilquin JT, et al. Autologous skeletal myoblast transplantation for severe postinfarction left ventricular dysfunction. J Am Coll Cardiol 2003;41:1078–83.

17. Smits PC, van Geuns RJ, Poldermans D, et al. Catheter-based intramyocardial injection of autologous skeletal myoblasts as a primary treatment of ischemic heart failure: clinical experience with six-month follow-up. J Am Coll Cardiol 2003;42:2063–9.

18. Reinecke H, MacDonald GH, Hauschka SD, et al. Electromechanical coupling between skeletal and cardiac muscle. Implications for infarct repair. J Cell Biol 2000;149:731–40.

19. Gepstein L, Ding C, Rahmutula D, et al. In vivo assessment of the electrophysiological integration and arrhythmogenic risk of myocardial cell transplantation strategies. Stem Cells 2010;28:2151–61.

20. Roell W, Lewalter T, Sasse P, et al. Engraftment of connexin 43-expressing cells prevents post-infarct arrhythmia. Nature 2007;450:819–24.

21. Perumal Srinivasan S, Neef K, Treskes P, et al. Enhanced gap junction expression in myoblast-containing engineered tissue. Biochem Biophys Res Commun 2012;422:462–8.

22. Abraham MR, Henrikson CA, Tung L, et al. Antiarrhythmic engineering of skeletal myoblasts for cardiac transplantation. Circ Res 2005;97:159–67.

23. Kocher AA, Schuster MD, Szabolcs MJ, et al. Neovascularization of ischemic myocardium by human bone-marrow-derived angioblasts prevents cardiomyocyte apoptosis, reduces remodeling and improves cardiac function. Nat Med 2001;7:430–6.

24. Bartunek J, Vanderheyden M, Vandekerckhove B, et al. Intracoronary injection of CD133-positive enriched bone marrow progenitor cells promotes cardiac recovery after recent myocardial infarction: feasibility and safety. Circulation 2005;112:I178–83.

25. Raval AN, Schmuck EG, Tefera G, et al. Bilateral administration of autologous CD133+ cells in ambulatory patients with refractory critical limb ischemia: lessons learned from a pilot randomized, double-blind, placebo-controlled trial. Cytotherapy 2014;16:1720–32.

26. Fuchs S, Baffour R, Zhou YF, et al. Transendocardial delivery of autologous bone marrow enhances collateral perfusion and regional function in pigs with chronic experimental myocardial ischemia. J Am Coll Cardiol 2001;37:1726–32.

27. Handgretinger R, Kuçi S. CD133-positive hemato-poietic stem cells: from biology to medicine. Adv Exp Med Biol 2013;777:99–111.

28. Orlic D, Kajstura J, Chimenti S, et al. Bone marrow stem cells regenerate infarcted myocardium. Pediatr Transplant 2003;7(Suppl 3):86–8.

29. Alvarez-Dolado M, Pardal R, Garcia-Verdugo JM, et al. Fusion of bone-marrow-derived cells with Purkinje neurons, cardiomyocytes and hepatocytes. Nature 2003;425:968–73.

30. Assmus B, Schächinger V, Teupe C, et al. Transplanta-tion of progenitor cells and regeneration enhancement in acute myocardial infarction (TOPCARE-AMI). Circu-lation 2002;106:3009–17.

31. Hare JM, Traverse JH, Henry TD, et al. A randomized, double-blind, placebo-controlled, dose-escalation study of intravenous adult human mesenchymal stem cells (prochymal) after acute myocardial infarc-tion. J Am Coll Cardiol 2009;54:2277–86.

32. Heldman AW, iFede DL, Fishman JE, et al. Transen-docardial mesenchymal stem cells and mononuclear bone marrow cells for ischemic cardiomyopathy: the TAC-HFT randomized trial. JAMA 2014;311:62–73.

33. Hendrikx M, Hensen K, Clijsters C, et al. Reco-very of regional but not global contractile function by the direct intramyocardial autologous bone marrow transplantation: results from a random-ized controlled clinical trial. Circulation 2006; 114:I101–7.

34. Cai B, Wang G, Chen N, et al. Bone marrow mesen-chymal stem cells protected post-infarcted myocar-dium against arrhythmias via reversing potassium channels remodelling. J Cell Mol Med 2014;18: 1407–16.

35. Dai W, Hale SL, Kay GL, et al. Delivering stem cells to the heart in a collagen matrix reduces relocation of cells to other organs as assessed by nanoparticle technology. Regen Med 2009;4:387–95.

36. Hale SL, Dai W, Dow JS, et al. Mesenchymal stem cell administration at coronary artery reperfusion in the rat by two delivery routes: a quantitative assess-ment. Life Sci 2008;83:511–5.

37. Perin E, Dohmann HF, Borojevic R, et al. Transendo-cardial, autologous bone marrow cell transplantation for severe, chronic ischemic heart failure. Circulation 2003;107:2294–302.

38. Strauer BE, Brehm M, Zeus T, et al. Repair of infarcted myocardium by autologous intracoronary mononuclear bone marrow cell transplantation in humans. Circulation 2002;106:1913–8.

39. Bergmann O, Bhardwaj RD, Bernard S, et al. Evidence for cardiomyocyte renewal in humans. Science 2009;324:98–102.

40. Ali SR, Hippenmeyer S, Saadat LV, et al. Existing cardiomyocytes generate cardiomyocytes at a low rate after birth in mice. Proc Natl Acad Sci U S A 2014;111:8850–5.

41. Senyo SE, Steinhauser ML, Pizzimenti CL, et al. Mammalian heart renewal by pre-existing cardio-myocytes. Nature 2013;493:433–6.

42. Nadal-Ginard B, Anversa P, Kajstura J, et al. Cardiac stem cells and myocardial regeneration. Novartis Found Symp 2005;265:142–54 [discussion: 155–7, 204–11].

43. Torella D, Ellison GM, Méndez-Ferrer S, et al. Resi-dent human cardiac stem cells: role in cardiac cellular homeostasis and potential for myocardial regeneration. Nat Clin Pract Cardiovasc Med 2006; 3(Suppl 1):S8–13.

44. Beltrami AP, Barlucchi L, Torella D, et al. Adult cardiac stem cells are multipotent and support myocardial regeneration. Cell 2003;114:763–76.

45. Chugh AR, Beache GM, Loughran JH, et al. Admin-istration of cardiac stem cells in patients with ischemic cardiomyopathy: the SCIPIO trial surgical aspects and interim analysis of myocardial function and viability by magnetic resonance. Circulation 2012;126:S54–64.

46. Hong KU, Bolli R. Cardiac stem cell therapy for cardiac repair. Curr Treat Options Cardiovasc Med 2014;16:324.

47. Messina E, De Angelis L, Frati G, et al. Isolation and expansion of adult cardiac stem cells from human and murine heart. Circ Res 2004;95:911–21.

48. Barile L, Gherghiceanu M, Popescu LM, et al. Human cardiospheres as a source of multipotent stem and progenitor cells. Stem Cells Int 2013; 2013:e916837.

49. Malliaras K, Makkar RR, Smith RR, et al. Intracoro-nary cardiosphere-derived cells after myocardial infarction: evidence of therapeutic regeneration in the final 1-year results of the CADUCEUS trial (CArdiosphere-Derived aUtologous stem CElls to reverse ventricUlar dySfunction). J Am Coll Cardiol 2014;63:110–22.

50. Capricor. Allogeneic heart stem cells to achieve myocardial regeneration (ALLSTAR). Bethesda (MD): National Library of Medicine (US); 2000. NLM Identifier: NCT01458405. Available at: https:// clinicaltrials.gov/ct2/show/NCT01458405. Accessed January 23, 2015.

51. Lian X, Hsiao C, Wilson G, et al. Robust cardiomyo-cyte differentiation from human pluripotent stem cells via temporal modulation of canonical Wnt signaling. Proc Natl Acad Sci U S A 2012;109: E1848–57.

52. Lian X, Zhang J, Azarin SM, et al. Directed cardio-myocyte differentiation from human pluripotent stem cells by modulating Wnt/β-catenin signaling under fully defined conditions. Nat Protoc 2013;8: 162–75.

53. Malliaras K, Marbán E. Cardiac cell therapy: where we've been, where we are, and where we should be headed. Br Med Bull 2011;98:161–85.

54. Lieu DK, Fu JD, Chiamvimonvat N, et al. Mechanism-based facilitated maturation of human pluripotent stem cell-derived cardiomyocytes. Circ Arrhythm Electrophysiol 2013;6:191–201.

55. Laflamme MA, Gold J, Xu C, et al. Formation of human myocardium in the rat heart from human embryonic stem cells. Am J Pathol 2005;167:663–71.

56. Zhu WZ, Santana LF, Laflamme MA. Local control of excitation-contraction coupling in human embryonic stem cell-derived cardiomyocytes. PLoS One 2009;4:e5407.

57. Ardehali R, Ali SR, Inlay MA, et al. Prospective isolation of human embryonic stem cell-derived cardiovascular progenitors that integrate into human fetal heart tissue. Proc Natl Acad Sci U S A 2013;110:3405–10.

58. Shiba Y, Fernandes S, Zhu WZ, et al. Human ES-cell-derived cardiomyocytes electrically couple and suppress arrhythmias in injured hearts. Nature 2012;489:322–5.

59. Yang X, Pabon L, Murry CE. Engineering adolescence: maturation of human pluripotent stem cell-derived cardiomyocytes. Circ Res 2014;114:511–23.

60. Zahanich I, Sirenko SG, Maltseva LA, et al. Rhythmic beating of stem cell-derived cardiac cells requires dynamic coupling of electrophysiology and Ca cycling. J Mol Cell Cardiol 2011;50:66–76.

61. Satin J, Itzhaki I, Rapoport S, et al. Calcium handling in human embryonic stem cell-derived cardiomyocytes. Stem Cells 2008;26:1961–72.

62. Kehat I, Khimovich L, Caspi O, et al. Electromechanical integration of cardiomyocytes derived from human embryonic stem cells. Nat Biotechnol 2004;22:1282–9.

63. Matsushita T, Oyamada M, Kurata H, et al. Formation of cell junctions between grafted and host cardiomyocytes at the border zone of rat myocardial infarction. Circulation 1999;100:II262–268.

64. Reinecke H, Zhang M, Bartosek T, et al. Survival, integration, and differentiation of cardiomyocyte grafts: a study in normal and injured rat hearts. Circulation 1999;100:193–202.

65. Zheng SX, Weng YL, Zhou CQ, et al. Comparison of cardiac stem cells and mesenchymal stem cells transplantation on the cardiac electrophysiology in rats with myocardial infarction. Stem Cell Rev 2013;9:339–49.

66. Hwang HJ, Chang W, Song BW, et al. Antiarrhythmic potential of mesenchymal stem cell is modulated by hypoxic environment. J Am Coll Cardiol 2012;60:1698–706.

67. Nygren JM, Jovinge S, Breitbach M, et al. Bone marrow-derived hematopoietic cells generate cardiomyocytes at a low frequency through cell fusion, but not transdifferentiation. Nat Med 2004;10:494–501.

68. Liao SY, Liu Y, Siu CW, et al. Proarrhythmic risk of embryonic stem cell-derived cardiomyocyte transplantation in infarcted myocardium. Heart Rhythm 2010;7:1852–9.

69. Robey TE, Saiget MK, Reinecke H, et al. Systems approaches to preventing transplanted cell death in cardiac repair. J Mol Cell Cardiol 2008;45:567–81.

70. Fernandes S, Habib M, Caspi O, et al. Human embryonic stem cell-derived cardiomyocytes engraft but do not alter cardiac remodeling after chronic infarction in rats. J Mol Cell Cardiol 2010;49:941–9.

71. Shiba Y, Filice D, Fernandes S, et al. Electrical integration of human embryonic stem cell-derived cardiomyocytes in a guinea pig chronic infarct model. J Cardiovasc Pharmacol Ther 2014;19:368–81.

72. Skelton RJ, Costa M, Anderson DJ, et al. SIRPA, VCAM1 and CD34 identify discrete lineages during early human cardiovascular development. Stem Cell Res 2014;13:172–9.

73. Kattman SJ, Witty AD, Gagliardi M, et al. Stage-specific optimization of activin/nodal and BMP signaling promotes cardiac differentiation of mouse and human pluripotent stem cell lines. Cell Stem Cell 2011;8:228–40.

74. Menasché P. Stem cell therapy for heart failure: are arrhythmias a real safety concern? Circulation 2009;119:2735–40.

75. Fukushima S, Varela-Carver A, Coppen SR, et al. Direct intramyocardial but not intracoronary injection of bone marrow cells induces ventricular arrhythmias in a rat chronic ischemic heart failure model. Circulation 2007;115:2254–61.

76. Pak HN, Qayyum M, Kim DT, et al. Mesenchymal stem cell injection induces cardiac nerve sprouting and increased tenascin expression in a swine model of myocardial infarction. J Cardiovasc Electrophysiol 2003;14:841–8.

77. Makkar RR, Lill M, Chen PS. Stem cell therapy for myocardial repair: is it arrhythmogenic? J Am Coll Cardiol 2003;42:2070–2.

78. Gnecchi M, Zhang Z, Ni A, et al. Paracrine mechanisms in adult stem cell signaling and therapy. Circ Res 2008;103:1204–19.

# Moving?

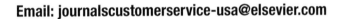

## Make sure your subscription moves with you!

To notify us of your new address, find your **Clinics Account Number** (located on your mailing label above your name), and contact customer service at:

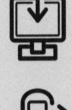

**Email: journalscustomerservice-usa@elsevier.com**

**800-654-2452** (subscribers in the U.S. & Canada)
**314-447-8871** (subscribers outside of the U.S. & Canada)

**Fax number: 314-447-8029**

**Elsevier Health Sciences Division
Subscription Customer Service
3251 Riverport Lane
Maryland Heights, MO 63043**

\*To ensure uninterrupted delivery of your subscription, please notify us at least 4 weeks in advance of move.

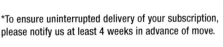

Printed and bound by CPI Group (UK) Ltd, Croydon, CR0 4YY

03/10/2024

01040375-0001